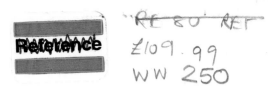

RE 80 REF
£109.99
WW 250

date shown below.

D1615413

Ophthalmic Surgical Procedures

Second Edition

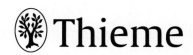

Ophthalmic Surgical Procedures

Second Edition

Peter S. Hersh, MD, FACS
Director, Cornea and Laser Eye Institute
Teaneck, New Jersey
Clinical Professor of Ophthalmology, New Jersey Medical School
Newark, New Jersey
Visiting Research Collaborator, Princeton University
Princeton, New Jersey

Bruce M. Zagelbaum, MD, FACS
Associate Professor of Ophthalmology
New York University School of Medicine
New York, New York
Attending Ophthalmologist, North Shore University Hospital
Cornea Service
Manhasset, New York

Sandra Lora Cremers, MD, FACS
Instructor of Ophthalmology, Massachusetts Eye and Ear Infirmary
Harvard Medical School
Boston, Massachusetts

Laurel Cook Lhowe
Medical Illustrator

Thieme
New York • Stuttgart

Thieme Medical Publishers, Inc.
333 Seventh Avenue
New York, NY 10001

Editorial Director: Michael Wachinger
Managing Editor: J. Owen Zurhellen IV
Editorial Assistants: Dominik Pucek and Cristina Baptista
Vice President, Production and Electronic Publishing: Anne T. Vinnicombe
Production Editor: Martha L. Wetherill
Vice President, International Marketing and Sales: Cornelia Schulze
Chief Financial Officer: Peter van Woerden
President: Brian D. Scanlan
Compositor: Macmillan Publishing Solutions
Printer: The Maple-Vail Book Manufacturing Group
Medical Illustrator: Laurel Cook Lhowe

Library of Congress Cataloging-in-Publication Data

Hersh, Peter S.
    Ophthalmic surgical procedures / Peter S. Hersh, Bruce M. Zagelbaum, Sandra
Lora Cremers ; illustrator, Laurel Cook Lhowe. — 2nd ed.
        p. ; cm.
    Includes bibliographical references and index.
    ISBN 978-0-86577-980-8
    1. Eye—Surgery. I. Zagelbaum, Bruce M. II. Cremers, Sandra Lora. III. Title.
    [DNLM: 1. Ophthalmologic Surgical Procedures—Handbooks. WW 39 H572o 2008]
    RE80.H47 2009
    617.7'1—dc22
                                                                2008040725

Important note: Medical knowledge is ever-changing. As new research and clinical experience broaden our knowledge, changes in treatment and drug therapy may be required. The authors and editors of the material herein have consulted sources believed to be reliable in their efforts to provide information that is complete and in accord with the standards accepted at the time of publication. However, in view of the possibility of human error by the authors, editors, or publisher of the work herein, or changes in medical knowledge, neither the authors, editors, or publisher, nor any other party who has been involved in the preparation of this work, warrants that the information contained herein is in every respect accurate or complete, and they are not responsible for any errors or omissions or for the results obtained from use of such information. Readers are encouraged to confirm the information contained herein with other sources. For example, readers are advised to check the product information sheet included in the package of each drug they plan to administer to be certain that the information contained in this publication is accurate and that changes have not been made in the recommended dose or in the contraindications for administration. This recommendation is of particular importance in connection with new or infrequently used drugs.

Some of the product names, patents, and registered designs referred to in this book are in fact registered trademarks or proprietary names even though specific reference to this fact is not always made in the text. Therefore, the appearance of a name without designation as proprietary is not to be construed as a representation by the publisher that it is in the public domain.

Printed in the United States of America

5 4 3 2 1

ISBN 978-0-86577-980-8

Dedications

To my father, Dr. Donald Hersh, who taught me everything I know; to Beth, James,
and Julia for whom I live; and most of all to my brother, Jimmy.
—PH

I dedicate this book to Alice, Matthew, Jennifer, and Andrew for their love and support;
and to my parents, Pearl and Jack, who have given me the gift of life.
—BZ

I dedicate this work to my parents Nereida and Fernando Lora, whose love has guided me through the years.
To my four sons Lucas, Jacob, John Hendrik, and Joseph, who are true gifts from God, and most
importantly to my wonderful husband Jan-Hein, who is my soul mate in everything. Ik houd van jou!
—SLC

Contents

Contents

Section VIII Oculoplastics

Section IX Vitreoretinal

Foreword

In 1982, my colleagues and I accepted a young residency applicant by the name of Peter S. Hersh to our Harvard University/Massachusetts Eye and Ear Infirmary program. Of course we expected and continue to expect the most of our residents during their three years with us, but Dr. Hersh was exceptional, particularly in surgical skills coupled with mature judgment. Years later his reputation as a surgical teacher has become truly international. It is therefore not surprising, and indeed fortunate, that Dr. Hersh has been willing to share his surgical experience in a most clear and easily comprehensible way. In 1988 his book *Ophthalmic Surgical Procedures* was published, a concise and richly illustrated guide for residents and beginning surgeons. This unusual book was very popular, and it is easy to understand why a fully updated and expanded second edition is needed. Joined now by two co-authors, Bruce M. Zagelbaum and Sandra Lora Cremers, this new second edition has a similar emphasis on illustrations, with many excellent line drawings of the basic procedures,

in a step-by-step format. The addition of several highly experienced section editors has added even more to the book's overall quality. All in all, this surgical text promises to be a national and international bestseller.

Two decades have passed since the first edition was published. It has been out of print for years and, in our library, our copy is kept in a locked cabinet to prevent loss. This new second edition of *Ophthalmic Surgical Procedures* is certainly needed, not the least because of the many new surgical advancements that have been made in the past 20 years. This book is bound to be a very popular guide for surgeons the world over.

Claes H. Dohlman, MD, PhD
Professor of Ophthalmology
Harvard Medical School
Chief Emeritus
Massachusetts Eye and Ear Infirmary
Boston, Massachusetts

Preface to the Second Edition

Both beginning ophthalmic surgeons and experienced practitioners, learning new or relearning old techniques, can travel two avenues. First, and most important, they can watch accomplished surgeons operate, amalgamating key concepts and diverse techniques into a procedure that is clearly understood and can be confidently accomplished. Second, they can research surgical references, subspecialty texts, and journal articles, splicing technical variations and procedural innovations into their personal surgical protocol. Unfortunately, it is often difficult and time consuming to combine information learned while active in the operating room with material culled from reading. *Ophthalmic Surgical Procedures, Second Edition,* has been designed to bridge this gap between surgical observation, active practice, and library study.

Foremost, this book is envisioned as a speedy reference covering a broad range of eye surgical procedures in a clear, easy-to-follow format. Its scope encompasses the commonly performed and basic ophthalmic surgical procedures. Each chapter walks the reader through a procedure via step-by-step instructions, and the most important aspects are illustrated by clear line drawings. Whereas the goal of each chapter remains a succinct, how-to-do-it presentation of a specific procedure, each chapter also includes brief sections on (1) indications; (2) preoperative preparation for surgery; (3) instrumentation required; (4) postoperative care; and (5) complications. Moreover, introductory chapters reviewing surgical instrumentation, sutures, ophthalmic anesthesia, and preoperative and postsurgical care should make the beginning eye surgeon more comfortable in the operating room and in dealing with surgical patients.

In addition to serving as a concise and usable reference, *Ophthalmic Surgical Procedures, Second Edition,* has been specifically designed to be used as a learning and teaching tool. Although the focus of each chapter remains a clear and concise presentation of a surgical procedure, we also envision this text doubling as a surgical workbook. As such, it is meant for frequent reference and active use and, consequently, should be a useful adjunct to the reader's day-to-day learning. The authors hope that students of ophthalmic surgery will continually reshape this book, adding to it to reflect their individual needs, variations in technique, and learning over time. In this way, ophthalmologists-in-training should be able to turn to *Ophthalmic Surgical Procedures, Second Edition,* as a ready reference, quickly read the appropriate chapter, walk into the operating room with a clear overview of the procedure, and make notes in the margins as they learn the nuances of specific techniques or modify individual steps.

Of course, many of the surgical procedures described here can be performed using several variations with equal success. The surgeon must choose from these procedural modifications based on personal preference and individual training. Although each chapter is sufficiently detailed to take the beginning surgeon from preoperative preparation to the final suture, it is not the intention of this book to recommend specific procedures and techniques. Rather, each chapter is intended to form a basic foundation on which to introduce the surgeon to a procedure in general, and with time, study, and practice, to help build a personal portfolio of the many different eye surgical techniques.

Nearly 20 years have passed since the first edition of *Ophthalmic Surgical Procedures* was published. During this time, the procedures covered in the book have evolved dramatically and many have been born anew. And with this passing of time, the breadth of knowledge of a single author diminishes as individual interests continue to focus. Thus, for this new revised edition, we have added section editors and selected contributors who have reviewed, revised, and rewritten the original material, and who also have added new chapters on procedures not included or not developed at the time of the original book. All are respected surgeons who bring specific expertise in their subspecialty fields, as well as teachers who understand the process of explaining and learning new surgical techniques.

Peter S. Hersh, MD
Bruce M. Zagelbaum, MD
Sandra Lora Cremers, MD

Acknowledgments

We gratefully acknowledge artist Laurel Cook Lhowe for her outstanding illustrations, a result of her artistic talents, clear comprehension of eye surgical techniques, and painstaking work during the long hours of writing this book. Our appreciation goes to Esther Gumpert, J. Owen Zurhellen, and Dominik Pucek at Thieme Publishers, for their energetic efforts in bringing this book to fruition. We also would like to thank Paul Guerriero, MD, Barry Pinchoff, MD, Eric Roberts, MD, I. Rand Rodgers, MD, Robert Rothman, MD, and Robert Strome, MD for their help in reviewing the manuscript; and Zandra Ferrufino, MD, Jae Kim, MD, PhD, Neetu Brar, MD, Sarosh Janjua, MD, Stacey Lazar, Helena Wade, Jennifer Horowitz, and Lois Slattery who helped with the behind-the-scenes work to put this book together. We also want to acknowledge our friend and section editor, Mariana Mead, MD, one of the great teachers at the Massachusetts Eye and Ear Infirmary, Harvard Medical School, whose untimely passing was a great loss to all. Finally, our thanks go to our many former teachers, residents, and fellows: your dedication to education and desire to keep learning is a source of inspiration to all of us as teachers and surgeons.

Contributors

Editors

Sandra Lora Cremers, MD, FACS
Instructor of Ophthalmology, Massachusetts Eye and Ear
  Infirmary
Harvard Medical School
Boston, Massachusetts

Peter S. Hersh, MD, FACS
Director, Cornea and Laser Eye Institute
Hersh Vision Group
Teaneck, New Jersey
Clinical Professor of Ophthalmology
Chief, Cornea and Refractive Surgery
Institute of Ophthalmology and Visual Science
New Jersey Medical School
Newark, New Jersey
Visiting Research Collaborator, Princeton University
Princeton, New Jersey

Bruce M. Zagelbaum, MD, FACS
Associate Professor of Ophthalmology
New York University School of Medicine
New York, New York
Attending Ophthalmologist, North Shore University Hospital
Cornea Service
Manhasset, New York

Section Editors

Neelakshi Bhagat, MD, MPH, FACS
Director, Vitreo-Retinal and Macular Surgery
Assistant Professor of Ophthalmology
Institute of Ophthalmology and Visual Science
New Jersey Medical School
Newark, New Jersey

Alan S. Crandall Jr., MD
Clinical Professor and Senior Vice Chair of Ophthalmology
Director of Glaucoma and Cataract
Moran Eye Center
University of Utah
Salt Lake City, Utah

David A. Lee, MD
Professor of Ophthalmology
University of Texas
Houston, Texas
Attending Ophthalmologist
Robert Cizik Eye Clinic
Houston, Texas

Peter S. Levin, MD
Co-Director, Ophthalmic Plastic Surgery
Clinical Adjunct Professor of Ophthalmology
Stanford University School of Medicine
Stanford, California

Mariana D. Mead, MD
[deceased]

John Tong, MD, FACS
Assistant Clinical Professor of Ophthalmology
University of California—Davis Medical Center
Sacramento, California

Marco A. E. Zarbin, MD, PhD, FACS
Professor and Chair
Institute of Ophthalmology and Visual Science
New Jersey Medical School
Newark, New Jersey

Contributors

Nathalie F. Azar, MD
Director, Pediatric Ophthalmology and Adult Strabismus
Associate Professor of Clinical Ophthalmology
Department of Ophthalmology and Visual Sciences
University of Illinois at Chicago
Illinois Eye and Ear Infirmary
Chicago, Illinois

Teresa Chen, MD, FACS
Assistant Professor of Ophthalmology
Harvard Medical School
Director of Clinical Affairs, Glaucoma Service
Massachusetts Eye and Ear Infirmary
Boston, Massachusetts

Bonnie Ann Henderson, MD
Partner, Ophthalmic Consultants of Boston
Assistant Clinical Professor
Harvard Medical School
Boston, Massachusetts

Howard A. Lane, MD, FACS
Clinical Assistant Professor
New York University School of Medicine
Department of Ophthalmology
North Shore University Hospital
Manhasset, New York

Andrea Lora, MD
Ophthalmology Resident Physician
Bascom Palmer Eye Institute
University of Miami, Miller School of Medicine
Miami, Florida

I

Introduction to Ophthalmic Surgery

1

Instrumentation

Several instruments have been designed specifically to facilitate ophthalmic surgical procedures. The following are a few of those most typically used:

Scissors (Fig. 1.1)

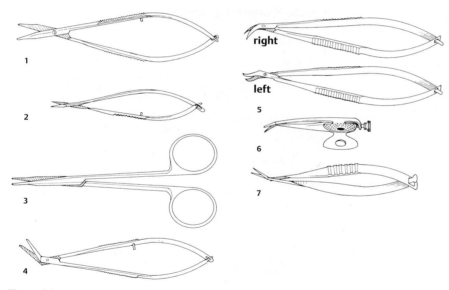

right

left

Figure 1.1

1 Westcott
2 Vannas
3 Stevens
4 Corneoscleral
5 Corneal (right and left)
6 Barraquer iris
7 Long Gills Vannas

Forceps (Fig. 1.2)

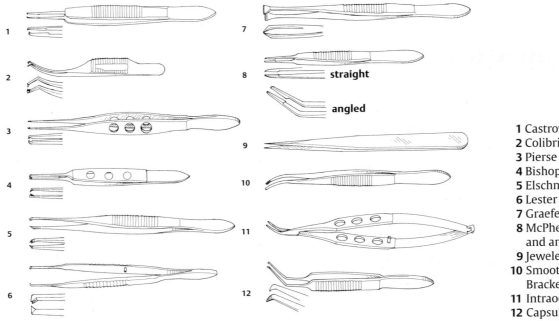

Figure 1.2

1 Castroviejo (0.12 mm)
2 Colibri (0.12 mm)
3 Pierse
4 Bishop-Harmon
5 Elschnig fixation
6 Lester fixation
7 Graefe fixation
8 McPherson tying: straight
   and angled
9 Jeweler's
10 Smooth (e.g., Chandler,
   Bracken)
11 Intraocular lens
12 Capsulorhexis forceps
   (e.g., Utrata)

Blades (Fig. 1.3)

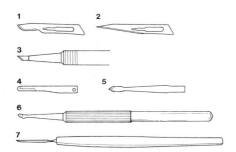

Figure 1.3

1 Bard-Parker #15
2 Bard-Parker #11
3 Sharp microsurgical knife
   (e.g., Beaver #75, Superblade)
4 Beaver #64
5 Keratome (e.g., Beaver #55)
6 Scarifier (e.g., Beaver #57, Grieshaber #681.01)
7 Wheeler knife

Needle Holders (Fig. 1.4)

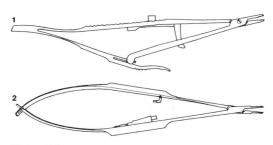

Figure 1.4

1 Kalt
2 Microsurgical needle holder

Spatulas (Fig. 1.5)

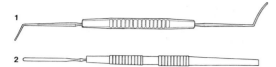

Figure 1.5

1 Cyclodialysis
2 Iris

Muscle Hooks (Fig. 1.6)

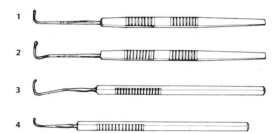

Figure 1.6

1 Graefe
2 Jameson
3 Green
4 Stevens

Hooks and Retractors (Fig. 1.7)

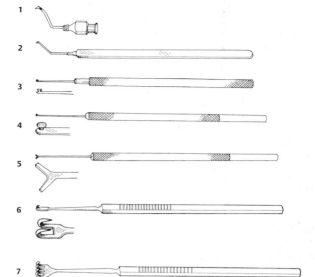

Figure 1.7

1 Cystotome
2 Sinskey hook
3 Kuglen hook
4 Graether collar Button
5 Y hook
6 Double fixation hook
7 Blaire retractor
8 Desmarres retractor

Choppers (Fig. 1.8)

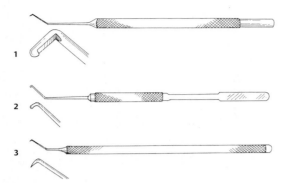

Figure 1.8

1 Nagahara nucleus chopper
2 Mackool phaco chopper
3 Minardi phaco chopper

Lid Speculums (Fig. 1.9)

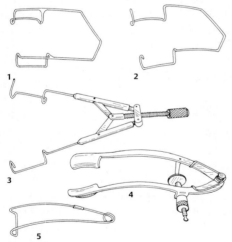

Figure 1.9

1 Barraquer
2 Kratz-Barraquer
3 Lieberman
4 Lancaster
5 Jaffe

Other Instruments (Fig. 1.10)

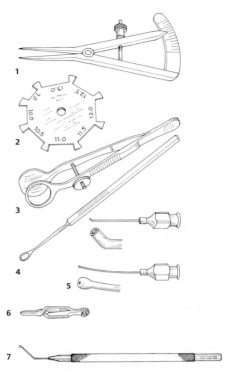

Figure 1.10

1 Castroviejo calipers
2 Stahl caliper
3 Chalazion forceps
4 Lens loop
5 Capsule polishers
6 Serrefine
7 Dreysdale nucleus manipulator

2

Ophthalmic Sutures and Needles

Several sutures have been developed for use in ophthalmic surgery. Many have unique features particularly suited to a specific surgical intervention, while others are essentially interchangeable. Properties such as absorbability, tensile strength, elasticity, handling and tying characteristics, and propensity to incite an inflammatory tissue reaction are all features that determine the surgeon's selection of suture material. Moreover, several surgical needle designs are available, varying in both tip shape and shaft configuration.

This chapter will review the characteristics of the most common types of sutures and needles available to the ophthalmic surgeon.

Suture Material

Note: The tensile strength and duration of a suture depend on the suture material as well as the diameter of the suture and the tissue environment into which it is placed. The absorption characteristics discussed here are approximate and reflect the duration of effective tensile strength, not the length of time residual suture material remains in the tissue.

Nonabsorbable Sutures

1. Nylon (polyamide)
   a. Duration: Losses 10–15% of tensile strength per year.
   b. Tissue reactivity: Minimal
   c. Other characteristics:
      i. Monofilament material.
      ii. High tensile strength.
      iii. Relatively elastic.
      iv. Stiff suture ends.

2. Silk
   a. Materials
      i. Virgin silk: Natural silk filaments (fibrin coated by sericin), twisted together to form a fine diameter suture.
      ii. Braided silk: Degummed silk (sericin removed), braided to form a multifilament suture.
   b. Duration: 3–6 months.
   c. Tissue reactivity: Moderate.
   d. Other characteristics
      i. Easy tying and handling characteristics
      ii. Soft suture ends are well tolerated by patients.
      iii. Inelastic.
      iv. Braided sutures have a tendency to fray when handled.
      v. Braided sutures produce more tissue drag than monofilament materials.
      vi. Multifilament structure may act as a nidus of infection.

3. Polypropylene (e.g., Prolene, Ethicon, Inc.)
   a. Duration: Essentially permanent, retaining tensile strength for over 2 years.
   b. Tissue reactivity: Minimal.
   c. Other characteristics
      i. Monofilament material.
      ii. High tensile strength.
      iii. Most elastic suture.
      iv. Very stiff suture ends.
      v. Since polypropylene is nonabsorbable, it is useful for suturing nonhealing structures (e.g., iris suture, intraocular lenses to iris or sclera).

4. Polyester (Mersilene, Ethicon, Inc.; Dacron, U.S. Surgical/ Davis & Geck)
   a. Duration: Essentially permanent.
   b. Tissue reactivity: Minimal
   c. Other characteristics
      i. Available in braided and monofilament materials.
      ii. Very high tensile strength.
      iii. Less elastic than other monofilament sutures.
      iv. Used in orbital and plastic surgery procedures.

Absorbable Sutures

1. Polyglactin 910 (e.g., Vicryl, Ethicon, Inc.)
   a. Material
      i. Polyglactin 910 is a copolymer of glycolic acid and lactic acid.
      ii. Coated Vicryl: Polyglactin 910 coated with polyglactin 370 and calcium stearate (coating makes suture surface smoother, thus decreasing tissue drag).
   b. Duration: 2–3 weeks (tensile strength decreases before suture mass is absorbed).
   c. Tissue reactivity: Mild
   d. Other characteristics
      i. Available in braided and monofilament materials.
      ii. High tensile strength.
      iii. Undergoes hydrolytic degradation.
      iv. Used in conjunctival closure, small incision cataract wound closure.
2. Polyglycolic acid (e.g., Dexon, U.S. Surgical/Davis & Geck, Inc.)
   a. Material
      i. Dexon S: Braided polyglycolic acid suture without coating.
      ii. Dexon Plus: Polyglycolic acid suture treated with a surface lubricant, Poloxamer 188.
   b. Duration: 2–3 weeks.
   c. Tissue reactivity: Mild.
   d. Other characteristics
      i. Braided material.
      ii. High tensile strength.
      iii. Undergoes hydrolytic degradation.
3. Plain gut
   a. Material prepared from mucosal or submucosal layers of sheep or beef intestines.
   b. Duration: one week.
   c. Tissue reactivity: marked.
   d. Other characteristics
      i. May evoke allergic reaction.
      ii. Undergoes enzymatic degradation.
4. Chromic gut
   a. Material: Plain gut tanned in chromic salts.
   b. Duration: 2–3 weeks.
   c. Tissue reactivity: moderate.
   d. Other characteristics
      i. Mild chromic gut absorbs faster than chromic gut.
      ii. Undergoes enzymatic degeneration.

Suture Needles

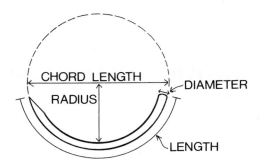

Figure 2.1

1. Needle dimensions (**Fig. 2.1**)
   a. Wire diameter.
   b. Wire length.
   c. Chord length.
   d. Radius of curvature.
   e. Curvature: Segment of total circle that needle encompasses (e.g., half-circle, quarter-circle, 160-degree needle).

Note: Compound-curve needles have a variable curvature allowing for deep suture placement.

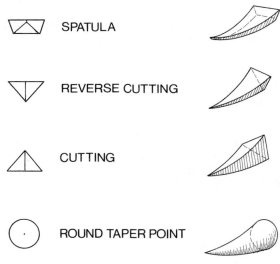

SPATULA

REVERSE CUTTING

CUTTING

ROUND TAPER POINT

Figure 2.2

2. Tip designs (**Fig. 2.2**)
   a. Spatula
      i. Configuration
         I. Four- or six-sided with cutting edges on the sides.
         II. Cuts at tip and sides parallel to tissue plane.
      ii. Characteristics
         I. Displaces tissue above and below needle, avoiding inadvertent penetration of tissue as needle is passed.

II. Maintains needle in tissue plane.

III. Most frequently used microsurgical needle style.

b. Reverse cutting

i. Configuration

I. Triangular with cutting edge at bottom of needle.

II. Cuts at tip and three edges of needle.

ii. Characteristics

I. Suture canal extends deep to path of needle tip.

II. Advantageous for full-thickness suturing of tough tissue (facilitates tissue penetration)

III. May inadvertently perforate tissue during partial-thickness suturing (e.g., sclera during strabismus surgery)

c. Cutting

i. Configuration

I. Triangular with cutting edge at top of needle.

II. Cuts at tip and three edges of needle.

ii. Characteristics

I. Suture canal extends superficial to path of needle tip.

II. May pull out of tissue as needle is passed.

d. Round taper-point needle

i. Configuration

I. Round shaft tapered to a point.

II. Cuts at its tip only.

ii. Characteristics

I. Atraumatic

II. Leaves smallest hole of any needle style

III. Use in easily penetrable tissue where tissue trauma must be minimized (e.g., iris sutures)

3

Preoperative Preparation and Orders

The specific preoperative preparation of the patient who is about to undergo ophthalmic surgery varies widely with the individual surgeon's preferences. The following orders, therefore, are suggestions for ocular surgery in general and should be tailored to the specific procedure planned, the particular needs of the patient, and the specific requirements of the ambulatory surgery center or hospital.

Note: Preoperative administration of topical antibiotics has been shown to decrease lid and conjunctival bacterial colony counts and likely minimizes the risk of postoperative infection. As yet, however, no specific regimen has been rigorously shown to be superior. Following are suggestions of preoperative antibiotics that provide broad prophylactic coverage.

Ambulatory Surgery

Preparation

- Document indications for surgery.
- Explain risks, benefits and alternatives of procedure, carefully addressing the patient's expectations. Document this in the chart.
- Obtain informed consent.
- Discuss suggested method of anesthesia and possible alternatives.
- Give patient the opportunity to ask questions about the surgery.
- Obtain medical clearance from primary care physician.
- Review preparatory and operating room procedures that patient should expect.
- Obtain laboratory evaluation as indicated.

Note: Workup should be tailored to patient's age and medical history. Different surgery centers have different requirements. For example:

- ❏ Complete blood count.
- ❏ Chemistry panel.
- ❏ Electrocardiogram.
- ❏ Chest X-ray (if required for preoperative clearance).
- ❏ Consider pregnancy test for menstruating female.
- Obtain preoperative photos where required (e.g., plastics procedures).

Patient Instructions

- Apply topical antibiotic drops (e.g., moxifloxacin 0.5% [Vigamox, Alcon Laboratories, Inc., Fort Worth, TX, US], gatifloxacin 0.3% [Zymar, Allergan, Inc., Irvine, CA, US]) 4 times per day starting 2 days before surgery.
- Consider a topical nonsteroidal anti-inflammatory agent (e.g., ketorolac tromethamine 0.5%, Acular, Allergan, Inc.) 4 times per day for 4 to 7 days before surgery if history of diabetes, uveitis, or cystoid macular edema.
- Consider lid scrubs or doxycycline, or both, 100 mg orally 2 times per day, 2 weeks before surgery if significant lid disease (e.g., blepharitis, meibomian gland dysfunction).
- Do not eat food after midnight on the night before surgery. You may drink clear liquids up to 8 hours before surgery.

Note: check with surgical facility about specific requirements.

- Take regular systemic medications according to primary care physician's advice on the morning of surgery with small sips of water.

Preoperative Orders

- Antibiotic drops preoperatively (e.g., moxifloxacin 0.5% [Vigamox, Alcon Laboratories, Inc.], gatifloxacin 0.3% [Zymar, Allergan, Inc.]).
- Nothing by mouth.
- Void on call to operating room.

- Additional orders as necessary for planned surgery (see specific surgical procedures).
- Mark the correct eye before giving anesthesia.

In-Hospital Admission for Ocular Surgery

Preparation

- Document indications for surgery.
- Explain risks and benefits of procedure, carefully addressing patient's expectations. Document this in the chart.
- Obtain informed consent.
- Discuss suggested method of anesthesia and possible alternatives.
- Give patient the opportunity to ask questions about the surgery.
- Review the preparatory and operating room procedures patient should expect.
- Obtain medical clearance (history and physical) as indicated.

Hospital Admission Orders

- Diagnosis.
- Diet: Nothing by mouth after midnight on the night before surgery. Patient may drink clear liquids up to 8 hours before surgery.
- Laboratory tests (as indicated).
  - Complete blood count.
  - Chemistry panel.
  - Electrocardiogram.
  - Chest X-ray (if required).
  - Consider pregnancy test for menstruating female.
- Systemic medications: Include patient's usual daily medications.
- Ocular medications.
  - Antibiotic drops every 6 hours (e.g, moxifloxacin 0.5% [Vigamox, Alcon Laboratories, Inc.], gatifloxacin 0.3% [Zymar, Allergan, Inc.]).
  - Additional medications as necessary for planned surgery (see specific surgical procedure).
- Void on call to operating room.

4

Ophthalmic Anesthesia

Many ophthalmic procedures today are safely performed under topical or local anesthesia to avoid the potentially adverse systemic consequences of general anesthetics. Topical anesthesia is rapidly growing in popularity for cataract surgery and minor anterior segment procedures; local anesthesia, including facial nerve blocks, peribulbar, subtenons, and retrobulbar blocks have become the routine for other general ophthalmic surgery. With the revolution of ambulatory surgery, many choices in ophthalmic anesthesia permit surgeons to develop their own versions of the ideal anesthetic techniques.

Local Anesthetic Agents

Note: Several agents may be used for local and regional anesthesia. The following anesthetic agents and additives comprise a mixture that is among the most frequently used in ophthalmic surgery.

- Lidocaine 2%.
  - ❑ Onset of action: Approximately 5–10 minutes.
  - ❑ Duration of action: Approximately 1–2 hours. Approximately 2–4 hours with epinephrine added.
- Bupivacaine 0.75%.
  - ❑ Onset of action: Approximately 15–30 minutes.
  - ❑ Duration of action: Approximately 5–10 hours.
- Epinephrine 1:100,000.
  - ❑ Minimizes systemic absorption of anesthetic agents.
  - ❑ Prolongs duration of action of anesthetic.
  - ❑ Minimizes bleeding (especially important in oculoplastic procedures).
  - ❑ Systemic sympathetic effects may be harmful.
  - ❑ Epinephrine 1:100,000 is available premixed in either the lidocaine or bupivacaine solution.

- Hyaluronidase.
  - ❑ Enhances diffusion of anesthetic mixture through tissues.
  - ❑ Use 75 units per 10 ml of anesthetic solution. To prepare 10 ml of anesthetic solution, mix:
    - Lidocaine 2% with or without epinephrine 1:100,000 (5 ml).
    - Bupivacaine 0.75% (5 ml).
    - Hyaluronidase (75 units).

Therefore, the final concentrations in the anesthetic mixture are lidocaine 1%, bupivacaine 0.375%, epinephrine 1:200,000, and hyaluronidase 7.5 units per ml.

Facial Nerve (Orbicularis/Lid) Block

General Technique

- Use 25G, 1.5 inch disposable needle.
- Raise a small intradermal wheal of anesthesia at the entry site to make subsequent needle manipulations less painful.
- Direction of needle may be changed without removing it from skin.
  - ❑ Withdraw needle until just the tip penetrates the skin.
  - ❑ Rotate needle about its tip.
  - ❑ Advance needle in the new direction.
- Always aspirate syringe before injecting anesthetic to prevent inadvertent intravascular administration.
- Use a total of 3–5 ml of solution.
- Inject anesthesia slowly.
- Apply pressure over the injected area to facilitate effect of anesthetic on the motor nerves and to minimize hemorrhage.

Classic Van Lint Technique (**Fig. 4.1**)

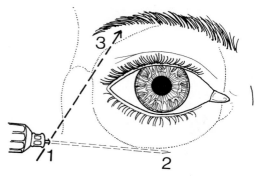

Figure 4.1

- Introduce the needle 1 cm behind the lateral margin of the orbit at the level of the inferior orbital rim.
- Raise a small wheal of anesthetic at the entry site.
- Advance the needle as far as bone and inject ~0.5 ml of anesthetic.
- Advance needle horizontally and inject 1–2 ml subcutaneously along inferotemporal orbital rim while withdrawing needle.
- Similarly, advance needle superonasally and inject along the superotemporal orbital rim.

Modified Van Lint Technique (**Fig. 4.2**)

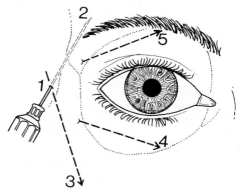

Figure 4.2

- Avoids excessive lid swelling.
- Introduce needle ~1 cm from lateral canthus.
- Raise a small wheal of anesthetic at the entry site.
- Advance needle in the subcutaneous space superiorly and slightly anteriorly and inject 1–2 ml while withdrawing needle. Do not remove needle from skin.
- Similarly, advance needle inferiorly and slightly anteriorly and inject anesthetic.
- Remove needle from skin.

- Optional: Supplement anesthesia with horizontal injections along the orbital rims.
  - ❏ Enter skin ~1 cm inferonasal to original entry site, advance needle along inferior orbital rim, and inject the 1–2 ml subcutaneously while withdrawing needle. (Bending needle to a 30 degree angle may facilitate placement.)
  - ❏ Similarly, enter skin ~1 cm superotemporal to original entry site, advance needle along superior orbital rim, and inject anesthetic.

O'Brien Technique (**Fig. 4.3**)

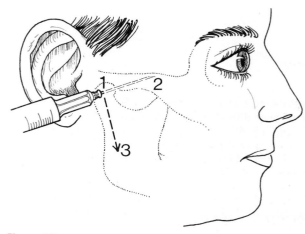

Figure 4.3

- Identify condyloid process of mandible.
  - ❏ Located ~1 cm anterior to the tragus of the ear and inferior to the posterior aspect of the zygomatic process.
  - ❏ May facilitate identification of condyloid process by feeling its movement at the temporomandibular joint as patient opens mouth and moves jaw from side to side.
- Insert needle until the periosteum of the condyloid process is reached.
- Inject ~2 ml of anesthetic solution.
  - ❏ Do not inject into periosteum.
  - ❏ Do not inject into temporomandibular joint space.
- Withdraw needle to its tip and then advance it superiorly and anteriorly over zygomatic arch.
- Inject anesthetic solution as needle is withdrawn.
- Advance needle inferiorly along the posterior edge of ramus of mandible and inject 1–2 ml as needle is withdrawn.

Atkinson Technique (**Fig. 4.4**)

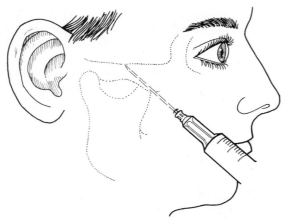

Figure 4.4

- Insert needle subcutaneously at inferior edge of zygomatic bone directly below lateral orbital rim.
- Advance needle across zygomatic arch, aiming ~30 degrees upward toward top of ear.
- Inject ~3–4 ml of anesthetic solution as needle is withdrawn.

Peribulbar Anesthesia

- Advantages
  - Anesthetic agents are deposited outside the muscle cone.
  - Needle is further away from the globe, optic nerve, and dural sheaths.
  - Less pain on injection.
  - Less intraoperative posterior pressure creates a softer eye during surgery.
- Place patient's head flat on a stretcher.
- Apply topical anesthetic (e.g., 0.5% proparacaine).
- Use 27G, 0.5 inch disposable needle. A small skin wheal is raised at the junction of the lateral one third and medial two thirds of the lower lid, just above the orbital rim.
- Direct needle straight back to its full length, avoiding the globe, and inject 1.5 ml of anesthetic agent.
- Remove needle.
- Use 25G, 1.5 inch disposable blunt-tip peribulbar needle (e.g., Atkinson needle).
- Have patient look straight ahead.
  - Stretches periorbital fascial tissues to facilitate needle entry.
  - Decreases the risk of optic nerve penetration.
- Palpate inferior orbital rim.

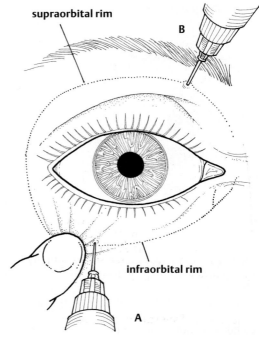

Figure 4.5

- Place needle perpendicularly through skin (**Fig. 4.5A**).
  - Locate needle one third of distance from lateral to medial canthus.
  - Place just superior to inferior orbital rim.
  - Bevel of needle should be directed toward globe.

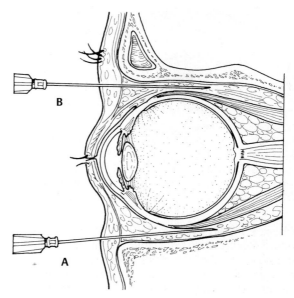

Figure 4.6

- Advance needle straight back (parallel to orbital floor), perforating orbital septum (**Fig. 4.6A**). (Do not redirect needle.)
- Hub of needle should not go beyond the inferior orbital rim.
- Aspirate syringe to ensure that a blood vessel has not been entered.
- Slowly inject 5 ml of anesthetic solution.
- Remove needle.
- Apply pressure to prevent hemorrhage and facilitate diffusion of anesthetic. (Release pressure approximately every 30 seconds to avoid retinal vascular compromise; may use Honan balloon for 10 minutes.)
- Evaluate ocular motility after 10 minutes.
- Optional: Supplement anesthesia with superior injection by the supraorbital notch (**Figs. 4.5B and 4.6B**).
  - Locate needle by the supraorbital notch.
  - Place needle just inferior to the superior orbital rim.
  - Bevel of needle should be directed toward globe.
  - Advance needle straight back.
  - Aspirate syringe to ensure that a blood vessel has not been entered.
  - Slowly inject 5 ml of anesthetic solution.
- Complications.
  - Perforation of eye with peribulbar needle.
  - Intraocular anesthetic injection.
  - Optic nerve impalement with intrathecal injection or optic nerve sheath hematoma.
  - Respiratory and cardiovascular depression.

Subtenons Anesthesia

- Advantages
  - Uses cannula as opposed to needle; therefore less chance of penetrating globe or dural sheath
  - Compression of eye is not required as quantity of anesthetic is small.
  - Effect of anesthesia is very rapid.
  - Reduces patient anxiety, as anesthesia is administered after patient is draped.
  - Gives deeper level of anesthesia compared with topical.
- Apply topical anesthetic (e.g., 0.5% proparacaine).
- Prepare and drape patient in usual sterile manner.
- Use blunt Westcott scissors and 0.12 mm forceps to cut down to bare sclera in inferotemporal quadrant between the inferior and medial rectus muscles (**Fig. 4.7**).
- Dissect down through Tenon capsule to bare sclera.
- Cauterize as necessary to stop bleeding.
- Use 15 mm, 25G blunt tipped cannula; make sure it is through all layers of Tenon capsule.
- Position cannula straight so that it is essentially parallel to the optic nerve (ensures that the anesthetic will encircle the globe).
- Slowly inject 2–3 ml of anesthetic subtenons in the peri-equatorial region.

Note: If chemosis is noted, reposition the cannula under all layers of Tenon capsule.

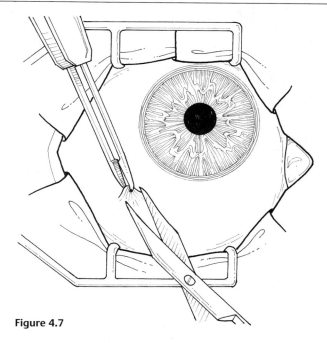

Figure 4.7

- Remove cannula.
- May close conjunctival opening with cautery if needed.
- Complication: subconjunctival hemorrhage may occur at the site of injection.

Retrobulbar Anesthesia

- Place patient's head flat on stretcher.
- Apply topical anesthetic (e.g., 0.5% proparacaine).
- Use 25G, 1.5 inch disposable blunt-tip retrobulbar needle (e.g., Atkinson needle) to minimize possibility of perforating globe.
- Have patient look straight ahead to minimize risk of optic nerve penetration.
- Palpate inferior orbital rim.
- Place needle perpendicularly through skin (**Fig. 4.8**).
  - Locate needle one third of distance from lateral to medial canthus.
  - Place just superior to inferior orbital rim.
  - Bevel of needle should be directed toward globe.
- Inject ~0.5 ml of solution subcutaneously to reduce pain when orbital septum is pierced.
- Advance needle straight back (parallel to orbital floor), perforating orbital septum.
- After septum is perforated and the equator of the globe has been passed (~1 cm of needle penetration), direct needle superonasally at ~30 degree angle (**Fig. 4.9**). Advance needle, piercing intermuscular septum and enter muscle cone.
- Gently move needle from side to side, looking for any movement of eye as a clue that the globe has been penetrated.
- Aspirate syringe to ensure a blood vessel has not been entered.

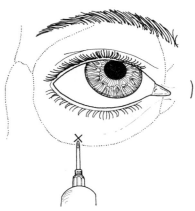

Figure 4.8

- Slowly inject 3–4 ml of anesthetic solution.
- Remove needle.
- Apply pressure to prevent hemorrhage and facilitate diffusion of anesthetic. (Release pressure approximately every 30 seconds to avoid retinal vascular compromise; may use Honan balloon for 10 minutes.)
- Complications.
  - ❏ Retrobulbar hemorrhage.
  - ❏ Central retinal artery occlusion.
  - ❏ Intravascular anesthetic injection.
  - ❏ Perforation of eye with retrobulbar needle.
  - ❏ Intraocular anesthetic injection.
  - ❏ Optic nerve impalement with intrathecal injection or optic nerve sheath hematoma.
  - ❏ Respiratory and cardiovascular depression.

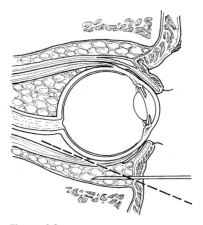

Figure 4.9

Retrobulbar Alcohol Injection

- In a blind, painful eye, retrobulbar alcohol may be injected for long-lasting anesthesia (usually several months). Do not use in an eye with good visual acuity.
- Inject 1–2 ml of routine retrobulbar anesthetic solution as described in *Retrobulbar Anesthesia.*
- Leave retrobulbar needle in place until akinesia is apparent, indicating proper needle placement within the muscle cone.
- Slowly inject 1–2 ml of absolute or 95% alcohol through same needle. A smaller volume of alcohol (e.g., 0.5 ml) may be used to avoid complications, depending on degree of pain relief necessary.
- Complications of retrobulbar alcohol.
  - ❏ Initial discomfort.
  - ❏ Lid swelling.
  - ❏ Conjunctival swelling and proptosis.
  - ❏ Ptosis.
  - ❏ Extraocular muscle paresis.
  - ❏ Periorbital anesthesia.
  - ❏ Decreased visual acuity.

Topical Anesthesia

- Proparacaine hydrochloride 0.5%
  - ❏ Onset of action: Approximately 30 seconds.
  - ❏ Duration of action: Approximately 15–30 minutes.
- Tetracaine hydrochloride 0.5%
  - ❏ Onset of action: Approximately 30 seconds.
  - ❏ Duration of action: Approximately 30+ minutes.
  - ❏ May be deeper penetrating agent than proparacaine.

General Technique

- Advantages:
  - ❏ Least invasive procedure with no chance of penetrating globe or dural sheath.
  - ❏ Compression of eye is not required.
  - ❏ Effect of anesthesia is immediate.
  - ❏ Rapid visual recovery after surgery.
  - ❏ Useful for monocular patients.
- Apply topical anesthetic (e.g., proparacaine); 1 drop in lower fornix, 5 minutes before procedure.
- Optional: Apply 2% Xylocaine gel into inferior fornix.
- Apply anesthetic to the eyelid margins using a soaked surgical spear.
- Prepare and drape patient in usual sterile manner.
- Optional: 1% nonpreserved intracameral lidocaine 0.5 ml may be injected into anterior chamber after paracentesis is made.
- Complications.
  - ❏ Corneal epithelial toxicity (e.g., diffuse punctate keratitis).
  - ❏ Duration of anesthesia is short; supplementation may be required.

5

Ophthalmic Surgical Preparation and Draping Techniques

Preoperative Preparation of Surgical Field

A wide variety of techniques are used by ophthalmic surgeons to prepare the surgical field. In all cases, the surgical eye should be marked before entering the operating room. The following regimen has been shown, along with prophylactic topical antibiotics, to significantly lower the preoperative bacterial colony count.

1. Place 1–2 drops of povidone-iodine 5% solution (e.g., half-strength) directly into the conjunctival fornices.

Note: Omit in patient with known allergy to iodine.

2. Clean skin with cotton balls saturated with povidone-iodine 10% solution.
   a. Start at medial canthus and wipe laterally over lids.
   b. Proceed outward, using progressively wider circular motions to paint skin superiorly over brow and inferiorly down cheek.
   c. Do not return to previously prepared site with the same cotton ball.
   d. Repeat steps 2a, b, and c three times.
   e. With a fresh, povidone-iodine soaked cotton ball, wipe the lids from the medial canthus laterally in one sweep.
3. Do not irrigate the povidone-iodine from the prepared site to avoid releasing meibomian gland secretions.
4. Blot, do not wipe, the prepared area with a sterile towel.

Draping

Note: A wide variety of surgical drapes are available. These include prepackaged, disposable, and one-piece barrier drapes, as well as traditional cloth drapes.

Following is one of many methods of ophthalmic surgical draping.

1. If operating under topical or local anesthesia, place a nasal cannula connected to an oxygen or air source beneath patient's chin to bring fresh air under the drape.
2. Place an instrument stand over patient's chest to lift the drape to minimize claustrophobia and afford easier access to patient; alternatively, use a bridge on the patient's chin to keep the drape lifted.
3. Use a wrist rest for arm support during surgery.
4. Instill lubricating ointment and tape the unoperated eye shut for protection if general anesthesia is used.
5. Cover patient's hair with a surgical cap.

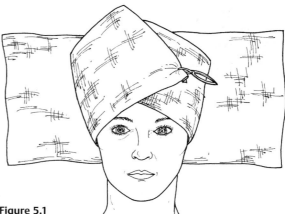

Figure 5.1

6. For oculoplastics procedures: Place a double-layered cloth drape under patient's head, wrap the upper most over the forehead, and secure with a towel clip (**Fig. 5.1**).

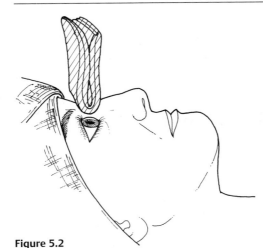

Figure 5.2

7. For intraocular procedures, place a disposable or nondisposable drape over patient's head, leaving eye exposed. Next, place an adhesive plastic drape over the eye, covering the lashes (**Fig. 5.2**).
   a. Field must be dry for drape to stick properly.
   b. May use a drape with a precut hole for the eye.
   c. Over first drape, may use an incise drape.
      i. Place directly over open eye to cover lashes and meibomian glands. May use end of sterile cotton tip applicator or back end of a cellulose sponge on inferior and superior lids to keep eye open as drape is placed.

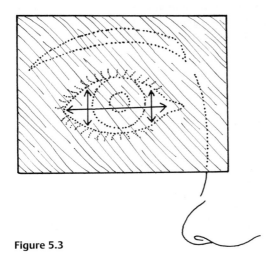

Figure 5.3

ii. Incise the drape from canthus to canthus to expose eye (**Fig. 5.3**).
iii. Optional: Cut relaxing incisions in drape and trim drape over surgical field.

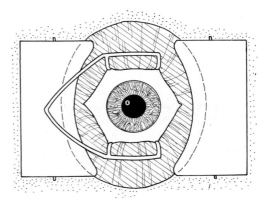

Figure 5.4

iv. Tuck tags around and under lid margin with a lid speculum to completely cover lashes and lid margin (**Fig. 5.4**).

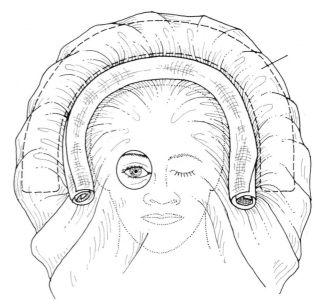

Figure 5.5

v. May tuck the plastic drape into the trough formed by the wrist rest and place a towel in the trough to catch fluids (**Fig. 5.5**).
8. May use "brow tapes" to secure the uppermost drape if necessary.
9. If the lashes are exposed, Steri-Strips may be used to cover and hold them out of the surgical field.

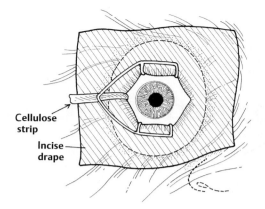

Cellulose
strip

Incise
drape

Figure 5.6

10. May use a cellulose strip (wick) at the lateral canthus to allow excess fluid to drain (**Fig. 5.6**).

6

Patient Instructions for Postoperative Care

Following is an example of a postoperative instruction sheet that may be given to the patient who has undergone intraocular surgery:

Postoperative Instructions

The success of your eye operation depends on a careful postoperative routine. The following suggestions will help to simplify your postoperative course and ensure the most successful result for your eye.

Precautions

1. Always protect your recently operated eye by wearing the glasses or the eye shield provided. You need to wear the shield to bed for at least 1 week after small incision cataract surgery or pterygium surgery; 3 weeks after planned extracapsular cataract surgery, glaucoma, retinal, or corneal transplant surgery; or for 3 days after laser refractive surgery such as laser in-situ keratomileusis (LASIK) or photorefractive keratectomy (PRK).
2. Do not drive for at least 24 hours after surgery. Discuss this with your surgeon.
3. Avoid bending at the waist.
4. Avoid heavy lifting.
5. Avoid vigorous exercise for 2 weeks after intraocular surgery.
6. Do not strain at stool.
7. Keep the operated eye dry. If you need to wash your hair, sit with your head back toward the sink and have someone else shampoo carefully.
8. Do not rub the eye.

Cleaning the Eye

1. Wash your hands before starting.
2. Remove the eye shield.
3. Gently wipe your eyelids and lashes with a cotton ball moistened with warm tap water.
4. Be very gentle, and be careful not to apply pressure to your eyeball and not to get water into the eye.

Applying Medications

1. Gently pull your lower lid down to apply medications. Use drops first, ointments last. Wait a few minutes between drops.
2. Use the following medications:
   a. Topical antibiotic (e.g., moxifloxacin 0.5% [Vigamox, Alcon Laboratories, Inc., Fort Worth, TX, US], gatifloxacin 0.3% [Zymar, Allergan, Inc., Irvine, CA, US]) 4 times each day for one week.
   b. Topical steroid (e.g., prednisolone acetate 1%) 4 times each day until taper is begun.
   c. Optional: Topical nonsteroidal (e.g., ketorolac tromethamine 0.5%, Acular, Allergan, Inc.) drops 4 times per day for a few weeks to months if you are at risk for postoperative cystoid macular edema.
   d. Optional: Short-term pressure-lowering drops as needed.

Signs and Symptoms of Danger

Many patients experience minor discomfort after surgery. However, if you have intense pain in the operated eye, vomiting, or a sudden change in vision, call your surgeon immediately.

II

Cataract

7

Anterior Chamber Paracentesis

Indications

- Diagnostic tap of anterior chamber fluid.
- Central retinal artery occlusion to rapidly decrease intraocular pressure.
- Useful as an adjunct to many intraocular surgical procedures.

Preoperative Procedure

See Chapter 3.

Instrumentation

- Lid speculum
- Fine tissue forceps (e.g., 0. 12 mm Castroviejo or Colibri)
- Wheeler or similar microsurgical knife
- Tuberculin syringe with 30G needle

Operative Procedure

1. Prep and drape eye.
2. Optional: Perform lid block (2% lidocaine plus epinephrine).
3. Place lid speculum.
4. Anesthetize eye.
   a. Apply sterile proparacaine or tetracaine drops.
   b. Apply anesthetic-soaked pledget or cellulose sponge to area of eye that will be grasped with forceps.
5. Grasp eye ~2–3 mm behind limbus near planned entry site with tissue forceps.
6. Perform paracentesis through clear cornea adjacent to limbus (Wheeler knife, #15 blade, or 30G needle) (**Fig. 7.1**)

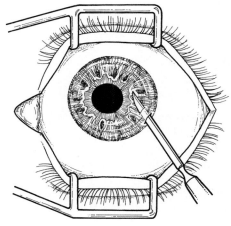

Figure 7.1

   a. Keep blade or needle over iris to avoid lens (aim toward 6 o'clock). Alternatively, aim blade tip toward pupil, perpendicular to entry point, but avoid touching lens (see **Fig. 8.3**, p. 28).
   b. Angle blade or needle slightly toward iris to avoid stripping Descemet membrane (**Fig. 7.2**).

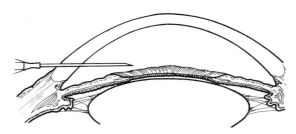

Figure 7.2

c. *Do not touch lens!*
7. Remove blade.
8. Use tuberculin syringe with 30G needle or cannula and follow previously made tract into anterior chamber (**Fig. 7.3**).

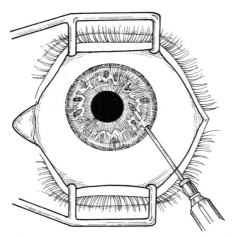

Figure 7.3

9. Slowly withdraw desired amount of aqueous. Alternatively, depress posterior lip of entry site to evacuate fluid.
10. When performed properly, the paracentesis should self-seal. If not, it may be closed with a 10–0 nylon or Vicryl interrupted suture.
11. Apply antibiotic ointment.

Postoperative Procedure

Apply antibiotic drops or ointment 4 times per day for approximately 5 days.

Complications

1. Cataract formation secondary to lens trauma.
2. Bleeding secondary to nicking iris with blade or needle.
3. Detachment of Descemet membrane.
4. Corneal endothelial trauma.
5. Persistent aqueous leak through paracentesis site.

8

Phacoemulsification/Posterior Chamber Intraocular Lens Implantation

Indications

- Small incision phacoemulsification is the standard technique for cataract surgery today.
- Advantages of phacoemulsification over extracapsular cataract extraction:
  - Smaller wound minimizes astigmatism and wound-related postoperative complications.
  - Surgery accomplished within a relatively closed system, allows for greater control over intraocular structures during surgery.
  - May be done under topical anesthesia.
  - Less postoperative discomfort and inflammation.
  - Shorter recovery period.
- Innovations in the methods of phacoemulsification continue (e.g., ultrasound, torsional, laser). Review literature for latest outcomes reports.
- Phacoemulsification generates heat by transforming electrical energy to mechanical energy with the subsequent generation of emulsifying shock waves.

Preoperative Procedure

See Chapter 3.

Before surgery, the surgeon should question the patient about the following:

1. Use of oral medications that are α-1 blockers (e.g., Flomax [tamsulosin]; Cardura [doxazosin]; Hytrin [terazosin]; Uroxatral [alfuzosin]; Minipress [prazosin; Clopixol [zuclopenthixol]) increase the risk of intraoperative floppy iris syndrome (IFIS) (intraoperative miosis, floppy iris, and iris prolapse through wound).
2. Assess dose, duration, and interval since last dose. If patient has used these medications, plan accordingly (see 3d).

3. If patient has an automatic implantable cardiac defibrillator (AICD) or pacemaker, the operating room staff will likely require device information. In general, the AICD should be deactivated as it can inappropriately discharge during surgery. Discussion with patient's cardiologist or anesthesiologist about the generation of AICD (first, second, third, fourth) and the need for deactivation with a "donut" magnet.
4. Note if patient is taking coumadin, aspirin, or plavix (clopidogrel bisulfate [Bristol-Myers Squibb/Sanofi Pharmaceuticals, Inc.]). Patients usually do not have to stop these medications. Most studies show no increased risk of retrobulbar hemorrhage with peribulbar injections. Topical anesthesia is an option if there is a concern; this essentially rules out hemorrhage.
5. On slit lamp examination, carefully assess for the following: size of maximally dilated pupil; pseudoexfoliation; phacodonesis; narrow angle (gonioscopy is recommended); guttae (Fuchs dystrophy), lens subluxation, zonular dialysis.
6. Check eye dominance if planning refractive cataract surgery. Choice of power depends on intraocular lens (IOL) type (i.e., monofocal versus refractive IOL). Some surgeons consider targeting the nondominant eye for reading vision when using monofocal lenses.

Preoperative Surgical Considerations

1. Calculate IOL power:

Numerous formulas for calculating IOL power have been derived based on theoretical optics and empirical data. Check the literature for continued advances in IOL calculations (e.g., IOL master, Holladay II formula). The Sanders-Retzlaff-Kraff (SRK) formula is one of the most basic and widely used.

SRK Formula: Power of IOL = A − 2.5(AL) − 0.9(K), where:

A = constant is determined by the manufacturer of a specific lens. A typical value is A = 118.4 for a posterior chamber IOL. Check with IOL manufacturer for appropriate A-constants for IOL; A-constant may vary if immersion A-scan or IOL Master biometry is used.

K = average keratometry measurement in diopters.

AL = axial length of eye in millimeters measured with A-scan ultrasonography.

Certain formulas are generally recommended for certain axial lengths and IOLs:

   a. For short eyes, AL ≤ 22.0 mm, the Hoffer Q or Holladay II formula is recommended.

   b. For average eyes, AL 22.1–24.4 mm, Hoffer Q, Holladay I or II is recommended.

   c. For medium to long eyes, AL 24.5 to 25.9 mm AL, the Holladay I or II is recommended.

   d. For long eyes, AL ≥ 26.0 mm, SRK/T or Holladay II is recommended.

   e. If using the Crystalens Five-0, the Holladay II is recommended for AL < 22.0; the SRK/T is recommended for AL > 22.0. The Holladay II is recommended for comparison in steep corneas (**Table 8.1**).

2. Determine target postoperative refraction and select proper IOL. Target postoperative refraction may be in part determined by the status of the other eye (e.g., phakic, pseudophakic) and the type of IOL chosen (e.g., refractive lenses). Nomograms for many refractive lenses are available from the IOL manufacturer.

3. Dilate pupil and preoperative drops:

   a. Tropicamide 1%, phenylephrine 2.5%, and Cyclogyl 1%, every 15 minutes starting 1 hour before surgery is a typical regimen. Other regimen examples: Phen/Trop 1 gtt q 5 minutes × 3. Coll 3&38 ¼ 1 gtt q 5 minutes × 3.

   b. Preoperative drop of antibiotic (e.g., moxifloxacin 0.5% [Vigamox, Alcon, Inc., Fort Worth, TX, US], gatifloxacin 0.3% [Zymar, Allergan, Inc., Irvine, CA, US]) 1 drop before surgery.

   c. Optional: Topical nonsteroidal anti-inflammatory agent one drop every 15 minutes × 3 starting 1 hour before surgery (to minimize intraoperative miosis) (e.g., flurbiprofen 0.03% 1 gtt q 5 minutes × 2).

Other topical nonsteroidal anti-inflammatory drugs (NSAIDs) (e.g., nepafenac 0.1% [Nevanac, Alcon, Inc.] 3e times per day, ketorolac tromethamine [Acular, Allergan, Inc.] 4 times daily, or bromfenac ophthalmic solution 0.009% [Xibrom, ISTA, Inc., Alpharetta, GA, US] 2 times per day), can be used for 5–7 days before surgery in patients with a history of diabetes, uveitis, previous cystoid macular edema, epiretinal membrane, or vein occlusion, and then for approximately 3 months after surgery to help prevent cystoid macular edema. Some surgeons use preoperative and postoperative NSAIDs on all patients. Check literature for updated efficacy studies among topical NSAIDs and current practices as indicated.

   d. If pupil dilates poorly or the patient has a history of using α 1A adrenergic antagonists (e.g., tamsulosin hydrochloride [Flomax]), be prepared to use iris hooks (4–0 polypropylene hooks or 6–0 nylon) or alternative method for addressing small pupil for potential IFIS (e.g., Healon 5, intracameral preservative-free epinephrine, preservative-free phenylephrine), Silicone Pupillary Expansion Ring (Graether Pupil Expander [Eagle Vision, Memphis, TN]), Perfect Pupil Injectable (PPI; Milvella, Ltd, Sydney, Australia). Low-flow parameters and lowering the balanced salt solution (BSS) bottle also helps in patients with Flomax. In addition, preoperative atropine 1% drops bid for 4–10 days before surgery may be used, if patient can tolerate potential anticholinergic effects. A preoperative gonioscopy should be considered in potential cases for angle closure (i.e., from anticholinergic effects of atropine).

4. Optional for complicated cases:

For stable uveitis patients with no inflammation for 3 months before surgery, use topical NSAID 4 times daily for 7 days before surgery, then 3 months after surgery to help prevent cystoid macular edema. In case of active uveitis, consider admitting patient the day before surgery for intravenous corticosteroid management.

Many surgeons recommend the use of nonsilicone lenses (e.g., polymethal methacrylate [PMMA] or acrylic) for patients with uveitis to minimize postoperative inflammation and posterior capsular opacification.

If there is a poor red reflex or concern about being able to make a continuous capsulorhexis, consider using a capsular dye to allow easier visualization of the anterior capsule (see Capsular Stains section later in this chapter).

5. Preoperative and intraoperative antibiotic use.

Preoperative and intraoperative antibiotic use (diluted in BSS bottle) is controversial, and there are broad variations in their use. Check the literature for updated information.

Table 8.1 Formulas Recommended for Certain Axial Lengths and Intraocular Lenses

Length	Recommended Formulas
Short eyes (≤ 22.0 mm)	Hoffer Q or Holladay II
Average eyes (22.1–24.4 mm)	Hoffer Q or Holladay I or II
Medium-long eyes (24.5–25.9 mm)	Holladay I or II
Long eyes (≥ 26.0 mm)	SRK/T or Holladay II

Instrumentation

- Honan balloon (optional)
- Lid (phaco) speculum
- Castroviejo calipers
- Fine-toothed forceps (e.g., 0. 12 mm straight Castroviejo and/or Colibri)
- Westcott scissors
- Cellulose sponges
- Cautery (underwater eraser or disposable)
- Scleral incision blade (e.g., Beaver #64, #69)
- Crescent/tunnel incision blade (e.g., Beaver #38, #48)
- Microsurgical knife (e.g., Beaver #75, MVR, MicroSharp, Superblade)
- Viscoelastic substance (e.g., Healon, Amvisc, Viscoat)
- Fine-Thorton 13-mm fixation ring
- Keratome (e.g., Beaver #55, diamond or steel, 2.7 mm to 3.2 mm)
- Cystotome
- Utrata forceps
- Cyclodialysis spatula or vitreous sweep
- Kuglen hook
- Iris hooks (e.g., Grieshaber)
- Drysdale Nucleus Manipulator (to rotate lens)
- Pre-chopper
- Chopper
- Straight and angled McPherson tying forceps
- Needle holder
- Phacoemulsification unit
- Capsule polisher
- Implant blade (e.g., Beaver #47)
- IOL folder or injector system
- IOL forceps
- Sinskey hook
- Vannas scissors
- Sutures: 10–0 nylon, 10–0 Vicryl, 8–0 Vicryl
- Acetylcholine solution (e.g., Miochol)

Operative Procedure

1. Anesthesia: Topical, peribulbar, or retrobulbar plus lid block, or general. (See Chapter 4.)

   Topical: Apply one drop of 0.5% tetracaine 15 minutes before surgery and 1 drop before the start of surgery. Optional: 2% Xylocaine gel in inferior fornix 5 minutes before surgery.

2. Optional: Apply Honan balloon for ~10–15 minutes to decompress eye and orbit, minimizing positive vitreous pressure.

Note: Honan balloons are not used for topical anesthetic cases.

3. Prep and drape. Use Steri-Strips or a brow tape cut in half to fully cover eyelashes.
4. Place lid (phaco) speculum.
5. Ensure adequate pupillary dilation (prefer pupil diameter of 7 mm or more).
6. Optional: Measure "white-to-white" (limbus-to-limbus) with calipers in case an anterior chamber IOL is needed.

Incision Techniques

Scleral Tunnel Technique

1. Prepare a fornix-based conjunctival peritomy at the limbus using Westcott scissors, tissue forceps; ~9 mm for one-piece lens; ~5 mm if a foldable lens is being used. The peritomy is usually centered around 11:00 or 1:00 o'clock on the side of the surgeon's dominant hand.
2. Secure hemostasis with wet-field cautery.
3. Create self-sealing scleral tunnel:
   a. Use a rounded blade (e.g., #64 or #69 Beaver blade) and 0.12 mm forceps to make a partial (50%) thickness, linear incision vertical and perpendicular to sclera, 2 to 3 mm from limbus (**Fig. 8.1**).

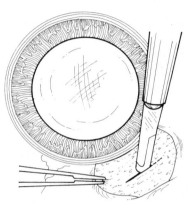

Figure 8.1

   b. Extend partial thickness groove incision 2.7 mm to 3.5 mm if a foldable lens is planned and 6.0 mm if a PMMA lens is planned.
   c. Use crescent or tunnel incision blade (e.g., Beaver #38, #48) to construct a scleral tunnel of same depth into clear cornea. Maintain a surgical plane parallel to the globe by holding the blade flat against the sclera (e.g., keep blade heel down) (**Fig. 8.2**).

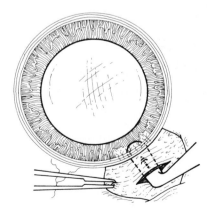

Figure 8.2

d. Continue tunnel construction just past anterior limbal vessels.

4. Perform a paracentesis through clear cornea adjacent to limbus (see **Fig. 7.1**, p. 23). Place at 10 or 2 o'clock on side of nondominant hand, using a microsurgical knife (e.g., Beaver #75, MVR) (**Fig. 8.3**).

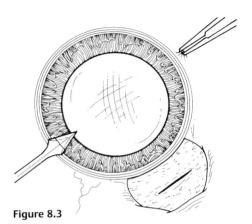

Figure 8.3

5. Optional: Inject 1 ml of 1% nonpreserved intracameral lidocaine (may also use 1:100,000 unpreserved epinephrine to aid in pupil dilation).
6. Inject viscoelastic into anterior chamber through paracentesis port.
7. Use keratome (2.7 mm to 3.2 mm) to slowly enter anterior chamber at the anterior edge of the scleral tunnel, 0.5 mm anterior to the anterior edge of the vascular arcade, on the side of the dominant hand (**Fig. 8.4**).

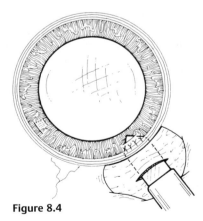

Figure 8.4

Clear Cornea Technique

1. Stabilize and fixate the globe using 0.12 forceps, Fine-Thorton 13-mm fixation ring, or cut end of Wexcel.
2. Perform a paracentesis through clear cornea adjacent to limbus using a microsurgical knife (e.g., Beaver #75, MVR) (see **Fig. 7.1**, p. 23, and **Fig. 8.3**).
   a. Place at 10 or 2 o'clock on side of nondominant hand if a superior wound is used.
   b. **Note:** If working from temporal side, place paracentesis site at 7 or 11 o'clock for right eye, or 1 or 5 o'clock for left eye, on side of nondominant hand.
3. Optional: Inject 1 ml of 1% nonpreserved intracameral lidocaine for topical cases.
4. Inject viscoelastic into anterior chamber through paracentesis port.
5. Using a keratome, create a clear cornea incision at the desired location (superior or temporal). A triplanar or biplanar incision can be made.
6. Techniques may vary depending on the blade manufacturer's specifications.
   a. For a triplanar incision (**Fig. 8.5**):

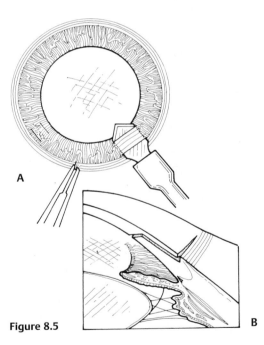

A

Figure 8.5   B

   i. Make first incision in clear cornea and perpendicular to the cornea plane. Place incision in front of the limbal vessels at a depth of ~250 um using a keratome. Optional: An initial 3.0 mm groove may be placed at the anterior edge of the vascular arcade. If an initial groove is made, make the next incision by depressing on the posterior edge of the groove with the diamond or steel blade of choice.
   ii. Flatten the blade against the surface of the eye.

b. For a biplanar incision: Use a straight or angled bi-beveled clear cornea blade.
   i. Place tip of blade just in front of the anterior limbal vessels.
   ii. Gently press down against the globe, along the heel of the blade so as to engage clear cornea to approximately one half depth with the tip.
   iii. Push forward, as the eye is stabilized with a cannula safely placed in the paracentesis (or by holding the conjunctiva/sclera with a 0.12). A wiggle motion is usually not necessary.

7. Construct the second plane of the incision in the corneal stroma parallel to the corneal plane (**Fig. 8.5A**).

   Drive the point of the blade through the stroma until it is 2 mm central to the external incision. Some blades have line marks on the surface to indicate the 2 mm landmark.

8. Point tip of the blade down slightly to nick Descemet's membrane.
9. Reestablish a plane parallel to the stromal plane of the incision and parallel to the iris (**Fig. 8.5B**).
10. Direct the blade toward the anterior apex of the lens and center of the pupil, being careful to avoid the lens and iris.
11. Drive the blade into the anterior chamber to its hub and then come out at the same plane (**Fig. 8.5A**).

Note: Advantages of temporal incision:

   a. No obstruction from brow (especially in deep-set orbits).
   b. Irrigation fluids drain off easier (prevents pooling).
   c. Induces less astigmatism than superior incisions.
   d. Less central endothelial cell loss.

12. Adjust illumination on microscope to improve visualization of the anterior capsule. If there is a poor red reflex, consider using a capsular dye.
13. For small pupils:
   a. Perform synechiae lysis if needed.
   b. Position two Kuglen hooks or Y hook at pupil margin 180 degrees or 90 degrees apart (at different locations) for a few seconds. If small pupil is secondary to an α-1-antagonist, do not stretch pupil with hooks as it can worsen signs of IFIS (see Preoperative Surgical Considerations, 3d).
   c. May use Behler pupil dilator.

d. May use iris hooks.
   i. Create 4 paracentesis sites at 2, 4, 8, and 10 o'clock positions.
   ii. Place paracentesis incisions posteriorly in the limbus and parallel to iris to avoid tenting of the iris when hooks in place.
   iii. Grasp iris hook with fine forceps or needle holder and insert into anterior chamber with hook parallel to the iris plane (**Fig. 8.6**).

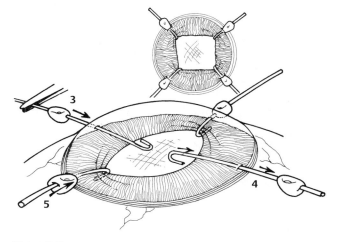

Figure 8.6

   iv. Rotate hook 90 degrees to engage edge of iris.
   v. Slide silicone sleeve down to limbus to secure hook.
   e. Sphincterotomies may be performed in multiple quadrants.

14. Perform a continuous curvilinear capsulorhexis with a cystotome or Utrata capsulorhexis forceps, ~5.0–5.5 mm in diameter. If no red reflex is present (e.g., a white or brunescent cataract), or if visualization of the anterior capsulorhexis is poor, use a capsular dye (see Capsular Stains section later in this chapter).

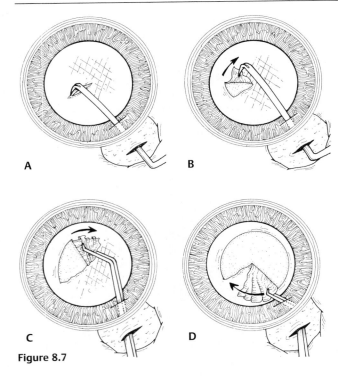

A   B

C   D

Figure 8.7

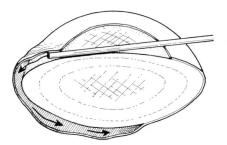

Figure 8.8

a. Place tip of flat or round cannula attached to balanced salt solution filled syringe, under distal anterior edge of capsulorhexis (**Fig. 8.8**).
b. Position cannula toward equator of lens and gently inject balanced salt solution, watching for fluid wave.
c. Optional: Hydrodelineation (**Figs. 8.9A and 8.9B**).

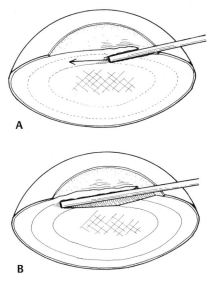

A

B

Figure 8.9

a. Puncture capsule near center of lens with cystotome and direct toward periphery (**Fig. 8.7A**).

Alternatively, use a "pinch-technique." Use Utrata forceps centered over central capsule. Open forceps and then pinch central capsule to create a tear. Gently pull down on initial tear to propagate tear in circular direction or push away for a counterclockwise capsulorhexis.

b. Fold over edge of flap (**Fig. 8.7B**).
c. Irrigate cornea frequently with balanced salt solution to aid visualization.
d. Use Utrata forceps in circular motion to complete rhexis, regrasping capsule flap at intervals (**Figs. 8.7C and 8.7D**).
e. If edge of capsulorhexis becomes difficult to view, or if the chamber shallows, or if rhexis edge starts to head toward equator of lens, inject viscoelastic into anterior chamber to flatten capsule and make rhexis easier.
f. Remove anterior capsule with Utrata forceps.

Note: If the capsule tear extends too far into the periphery, complete the capsulotomy using the "can-opener" technique. (See Chapter 9.)

15. Perform hydrodissection and hydrodelineation with balanced salt solution:

   i. Insert cannula tip in center of lens between endonucleus and epinucleus and between epinucleus and cortex, then minimally retract cannula tip to create a space for fluid to track.
   ii. Gently inject balanced salt solution along track to delineate epinucleus and endonucleus (may see double golden ring).
d. Optional: Gently rotate nucleus or push nucleus toward 6 o'clock to partially separate superior equator of nucleus from cortex (may use cystotome, Kuglen hook, cyclodialysis spatula, or nucleus rotator).

16. Prepare phacoemulsification unit.
    a. Add 0.3–0.5 ml 1:1000 epinephrine to each 500 ml of irrigating solution to help maintain pupil dilation.
    b. Foot pedal functions.
        i. Position 1 = irrigation only.
        ii. Position 2 = irrigation/aspiration
        iii. Position 3 = irrigation/aspiration/phacoemulsification.
    c. Set initial power: Depending on density of nucleus and machine used, may set 50% for moderate densities and up to 90% for hard cataracts.

Note: Power settings will vary depending on machine, nuclear density, phaco tip used, and experience of the surgeon. Surgeon should learn specific settings for particular machine and instrumentation.

    d. Set initial vacuum setting.

Note: Settings will vary depending on machine used and surgeon preference. Vacuum power will be affected by port size and tubing.

    e. Set initial aspiration to 20 (range 10–40).
17. Perform phacoemulsification:

Phacoemulsification Techniques

Standard Divide and Conquer Technique

1. Set phaco power high enough to emulsify nucleus without stressing zonules. If the nucleus moves excessively during phacoemulsification, increase the power setting.
2. Create initial linear groove (**Fig. 8.10**).

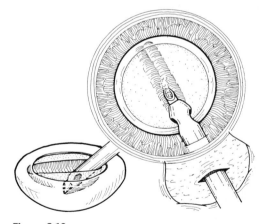

Figure 8.10

a. Sculpt nucleus starting near superior pole from 12 o'clock to 6 o'clock under capsulorhexis.
b. Always be cognizant of capsule edge. A 30 or 45 degree phacoemulsification tip is helpful.
c. Use ultrasound (position 3) while slowly advancing ultrasound tip in superior-to-inferior direction and by skimming off layers.
d. Go back to position 1 or 2 when repositioning for next pass, keeping ultrasound port in view.
e. Use initial groove of 1½ times the width of the phaco tip; use smaller width for softer nucleus to aid in rotating.
f. Continue sculpting until two thirds of the nucleus depth has been reached, watching for red reflex.
3. Position second instrument (e.g., Drysdale nucleus manipulator, cyclodialysis spatula, vitreous sweep, chopper) through the paracentesis to stabilize the nucleus.
4. Rotate nucleus: Use phaco tip and second instrument (e.g., cyclodialysis spatula, Drysdale nucleus manipulator) through the paracentesis to gently rotate nucleus 180 degrees (**Fig. 8.11**).

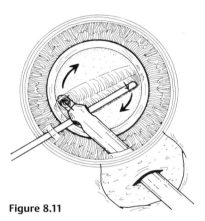

Figure 8.11

5. Continue to sculpt toward 6 o'clock periphery.
6. Rotate lens 90 degrees.

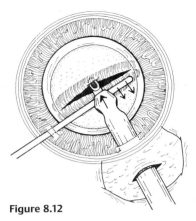

Figure 8.12

7. Fracture nucleus (**Fig. 8.12**):
   a. Place phaco tip and the second instrument deep and against opposite walls of the initial groove or trench.
   b. Using a second instrument (e.g., nucleus rotator, chopper) through the paracentesis port will crack the nucleus in half. A cross-action motion is optional.

Note: Do not push down on the nucleus as this may damage zonules.

Note: Keep foot pedal position 1 (irrigation) at all times to avoid collapse of anterior chamber.

8. Phaco toward inferior periphery (**Fig. 8.13**).

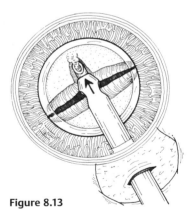

Figure 8.13

9. Rotate lens 180 degrees and phaco toward inferior periphery.
10. Crack both halves in half to make four quadrants (**Fig. 8.14**).

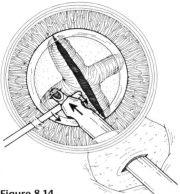

Figure 8.14

Alternatively, all trenches can be grooved before cracking any quadrant. When dividing quadrants, gently push laterally to see red reflex between pieces. Avoid pushing down.

11. Increase vacuum setting on phacoemulsification machine.

Note: Vacuum settings will vary depending on machine used.

12. Complete nucleus removal by emulsifying pie-shaped segments.
    a. Engage one quarter of nucleus with phaco probe using aspiration mode (footswitch position 2) (**Fig. 8.15A**).

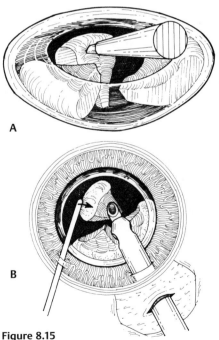

A

B

Figure 8.15

b. Bring nucleus piece to the center of the pupil near the iris plane.

c. Use short bursts of ultrasound to emulsify.

d. Second instrument through paracentesis port will stabilize and help maneuver nucleus pieces (**Fig. 8.15B**).

e. Rotate the nucleus using nucleus rotator or chopper, bringing successive pieces of nucleus to the center of capsulorhexis, and emulsify.

13. Precautions

a. Avoid tumbling of the nucleus, which may cause trauma to the corneal endothelium and posterior capsule.

b. Nucleus rotator or second instrument may be used to manipulate lens material into the port.

c. Viscoelastic may be used to atraumatically push nuclear fragments into proximity of the phaco tip. (This also helps to further protect the corneal endothelium during sonication.)

d. Avoid contact of lens fragments with the cornea.

e. Do not chase fragments through the anterior chamber while the ultrasound is engaged.

f. Decrease power to prevent "chattering" of small nuclear remnants within the anterior chamber.

g. Additional viscoelastic may coat and protect the corneal endothelium.

Chopping Technique

1. Phaco Chop

a. Use 0 or 15 degree phacoemulsification tip to impale the nucleus. Use the least amount of ultrasound needed to fully impale metal phaco tip into nucleus. Then allow vacuum to build (**Fig. 8.16**).

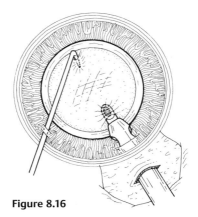

Figure 8.16

b. Use second instrument (Nagahara chopper or variant) through side port.

c. For horizontal chop: place blunt tip chopper into peripheral nucleus at the 6 o'clock periphery under the capsule for a horizontal chop (**Figs. 8.16 and 8.17**).

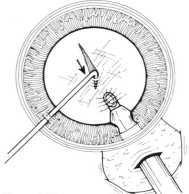

Figure 8.17

d. For a vertical chop: use a sharp-tipped chopper and place it adjacent to the impaled phaco tip (**Fig. 8.17**).

e. Hold nucleus using high vacuum and use chopper to "chop" down and pull toward stab incision for a horizontal chop, and push down, and then out when divided, for a vertical chop (**Fig. 8.17**).

   i. Pull chopper toward phaco tip, then direct chopper to the left and phaco tip to the right to fracture nucleus as the two instruments are separated.

   ii. Rotate nucleus 90 degrees, burying phaco tip into inferior half of nucleus and chop (**Fig. 8.18**).

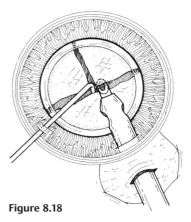

Figure 8.18

f. Rotate nucleus 180 degrees and chop the remaining nucleus in half, resulting in four quarters.

g. Phacoemulsify each quarter separately.

h. Creating multiple pieces by manual chopping decreases overall phaco time.

2. Variants of Phaco Chop

Note: Many variants of phaco chop involve fracturing (chopping) the nucleus into smaller segments before emulsifying.

Bowl and Crack Technique
This technique may be helpful if you cannot divide the nucleus (e.g., poorly constructed trench) or if there is a concern with the integrity of the capsulorhexis and you want to avoid lateral force on the capsule.

1. Set phaco power high enough to emulsify nucleus without pushing the lens and stressing zonules.
2. Sculpt nucleus starting near superior pole from 12 o'clock to 6 o'clock out to the nuclear rim (**Fig. 8.19**).

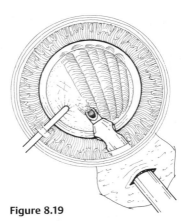

Figure 8.19

   a. Engage ultrasound (foot pedal position 3) while slowly advancing ultrasound tip in superior-to-inferior direction.
   b. In this fashion, continue removing nucleus to form a bowl-shaped nucleus.
   c. May use chopper or Drysdale through paracentesis to stabilize the nucleus.
3. Use phaco tip and second instrument (e.g., Drysdale, chopper) to fracture the peripheral nuclear rim (**Fig. 8.20**).

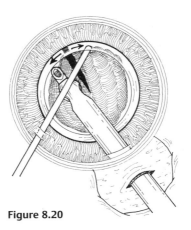

Figure 8.20

4. Rotate nucleus and make a second fracture.
5. Emulsify each section individually (**Fig. 8.21**).

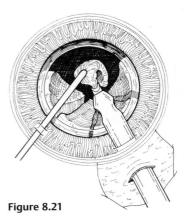

Figure 8.21

6. Remove residual cortical material with the 0.3 mm irrigation/aspiration tip on the phacoemulsification unit.

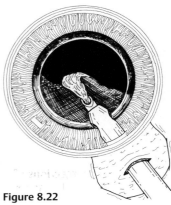

Figure 8.22

   a. Purchase cortex in periphery and strip it toward the center of pupil (**Fig. 8.22**).

Note: If "spider webs" (wrinkling of capsule) appear in posterior capsule, take foot off foot pedal and side kick pedal to reflux. Do not pull on irrigation/aspiration tip, as this will tear capsule.

   b. May use 45 or 90 degree (angled) irrigation/aspiration tip for 12 o'clock cortex.
   c. If subincisional is difficult to remove, consider using split irrigation and aspiration instruments (bimanual "chopsticks"). The paracentesis port may need to be slightly enlarged to fit the irrigation piece. Alternatively, a second paracentesis can be made to avoid anterior chamber shallowing, which can occur if the clear cornea site is used with split irrigation and aspiration (I&A).

7. Optional: Polish posterior capsule centrally using a capsule polisher. Some machines have a capsular polish setting for decreased flow.
8. Inject viscoelastic, such as a cohesive viscoelastic which will be easy to remove, into capsular bag.
9. The wound may need to be enlarged (e.g., Beaver #47) depending on the type of IOL used.
   a. If planning one piece IOL insertion with the scleral tunnel incision, extend the wound at the same depth as the tunnel to 0.5 mm larger than the optic size using the keratome or crescent blade.
   b. Check with IOL manufacturer if using an injector as most wounds do not need to be enlarged.
10. Place posterior chamber intraocular lens into the bag. (See Intraocular Lenses and Lens Insertion Techniques section later in this chapter.)
11. Remove residual viscoelastic with irrigation/aspiration instrument using minimum suction.
12. Optional: Irrigate Miochol into anterior chamber to constrict pupil.
13. Hydrate clear corneal wound site, if constructed, with residual Miochol or BSS.

    Optional: hydrate paracentesis.
14. Check wound for leaks by applying gentle pressure at the wound (cellulose sponges) or behind the wound. Check pressure with palpation using cannula gently pressing against the globe. Inject BSS or release pressure by burping the paracentesis with cannula tip as needed.

    Optional: Close wound if needed with interrupted 10–0 nylon sutures or 10–0 Vicryl sutures.
    a. Interrupted sutures
    b. Mattress / double X suture
15. If needed, reposition conjunctiva and secure with sutures (e.g., 10–0 Vicryl or nylon), or cautery.
16. Administer subconjunctival or subtenons injections of antibiotic (e.g., cephalexin) and steroid (e.g., Decadron or SoluMedrol).
17. Remove lid speculum and lid drape.
18. Optional: Apply topical combination antibiotic/steroid ointment.

Note: Ointments are not generally used for clear cornea. Use topical antibiotic or combination steroid drop antibiotic.

19. Apply patch if not done under topical anesthesia. Place clear Fox shield.

Intraocular Lenses and Lens Insertion Techniques

Polymethalmethacrylate
See Chapter 9.

Foldable Lenses

■ Silicone
■ Acrylic

1. Folding technique: Many lenses can now be loaded into an injector (see IOL manufacturer's specifications). Alternatively, these lenses can be folded manually.

   First-generation acrylic lenses and some first-generation refractive, acrylic lenses may be easier to fold after being slightly warmed (e.g., placed on top of the autoclave or computer monitor, or by irrigating warmed BSS before folding).

   a. Use smooth forceps (e.g., angled McPherson) to remove lens from case by haptic. Be careful not to scratch optic, especially if a refractive IOL.

Note: Irrigate acrylic lens with balanced salt solution. Do not irrigate silicone lenses (they become slippery).

   b. Grasp the lens using holding forceps across the optic with haptics in reverse "S" position (**Fig. 8.23**).

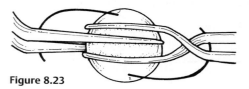

Figure 8.23

   c. Fold lens slowly in a controlled manner with implant forceps; using downward pressure on the optic will allow the lens to fold (**Fig. 8.23**).
   d. Release the holding forceps while closing the implant forceps (**Fig. 8.24**).

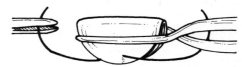

Figure 8.24

2. Alternate folding technique:
   a. Use smooth forceps (e.g., angled McPherson) to remove lens from case by haptic. Be careful not to scratch optic, especially if a refractive IOL.

Note: Irrigate acrylic lens with balanced salt solution. Do not irrigate silicone lens.

   b. Place lens on a flat surface (may use lens case on surgical table).
   c. Place folding forceps paddles on opposite sides of optic, parallel with the reverse "S" haptic direction (**Fig. 8.25**).

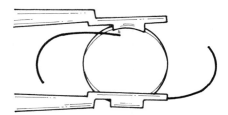

Figure 8.25

   d. Maintain pressure against optic edges and lift lens from surface.

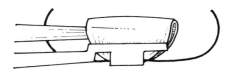

Figure 8.26

   e. Squeeze lens gently, closing folding forceps (**Fig. 8.26**).
   f. Place implant forceps on each side of the folded optic, pushing the superior haptic to the right (**Fig. 8.27**).

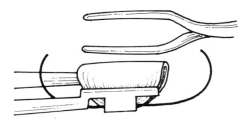

Figure 8.27

   g. Place implant forceps blades on top and parallel to implant forceps.
   h. Remove folding forceps.

   i. Check alignment of folded optic in forceps. A symmetrically folded IOL will fit through a smaller incision than an asymmetric folded one (**Fig. 8.28**).

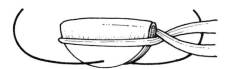

Figure 8.28

3. Optional: Coat leading edge of lens with viscoelastic. The leading haptic may be tucked into the optic's folded gap.
4. Insert inferior haptic and optic through the incision (scleral tunnel or clear cornea), placing the inferior haptic into the capsular bag (**Fig. 8.29**).

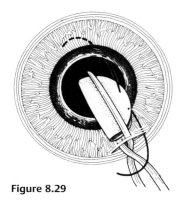

Figure 8.29

5. Rotate the implant forceps 90 degrees so that optic is perpendicular to posterior capsule (**Fig. 8.30**).

Note: Superior haptic remains outside of wound.

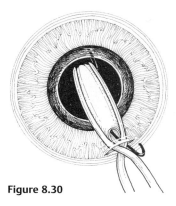

Figure 8.30

6. Open forceps slowly and remove from eye, allowing lens to unfold (**Fig. 8.31**).

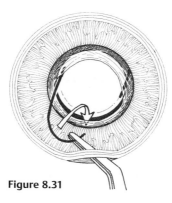

Figure 8.31

7. Grasp superior haptic with angled McPherson forceps.
8. Push haptic into anterior chamber and pronate hand to flex knee of haptic behind iris, releasing haptic into desired position.
9. Center lens using Sinskey hook.

Sulcus Fixed Lens

Note: A sulcus fixed IOL is inserted for cases with unstable posterior capsular support. When placing a sulcus lens, decrease IOL power by 0.5–1.0 D depending on desired target refraction.

1. Open wound to 0.5 mm larger than optic if needed.
2. Ensure that vitreous is not present in anterior chamber.
3. Inject viscoelastic just under inferior iris, over the anterior leaflets of capsule.
4. Grasp superior portion of PMMA IOL with smooth forceps. If using a foldable lens, refer to **Figs. 8.23—8.29**, noting placement will be in sulcus and not in capsular bag.
5. Place inferior haptic into ciliary sulcus, just below the inferior iris.
6. Secure superior haptic with McPherson forceps before releasing IOL to prevent uncontrolled movements.
7. Advance optic into pupil by gently pushing it inferiorly.
8. Place superior haptic.
   a. Grasp with angled McPherson forceps.
   b. Push haptic into anterior chamber.
   c. Pronate hand to flex knee of haptic behind iris.
   d. Release haptic into desired location.
9. Center IOL; spin cautiously if decentered.
10. With the injector system, the trailing haptic can be dialed in with the metal tongue of the injector placed into the anterior chamber during insertion or with a Kuglen or Y hook. Many injector systems do not require the enlargement of the wound.

Anterior Chamber Intraocular Lens

Abbreviated discussion follows. For full discussion, see Chapter 11, Anterior Chamber Intraocular Lens Implantation section.

Note: The insertion of an anterior chamber IOL is used for complicated cases that result in the absence of any posterior chamber support.

1. Ensure that there is no vitreous in anterior chamber, including strands to the paracentesis or cataract incision (see Chapter 12).
2. Irrigate anterior chamber with Miochol to constrict pupil.
3. Reform anterior chamber with viscoelastic.
4. Optional: Place a Sheets glide across the chamber.
   a. The glide guides lens placement and prevents iris tuck by the inferior haptic of IOL. The glide width may need to be cut depending on the incision width.
   b. Bending the glide to give it a slight upward curvature facilitates its accurate placement over the pupil and iris.
5. Place anterior chamber intraocular lens.
   a. Grasp superior haptic with McPherson forceps.
   b. Slide lens across anterior chamber into inferior angle.
   c. Stabilize IOL with forceps in the left hand before releasing IOL forceps to avoid displacement of lens from angle.
   d. Remove Sheets glide. (Stabilize superior haptic with forceps to prevent dislocation of the IOL from the inferior angle while removing glide.)
   e. Ensure that the pupil is round without iris tuck.
   f. Retract posterior lip of wound with tissue forceps and place superior haptic of IOL into superior angle. A Koeppe lens can be used to check haptic position in angle.
   g. Perform iridectomy using Colibri forceps and Vannas scissors (see Chapter 31). If it is too difficult to perform a peripheral iridectomy (PI) at the time of surgery or the PI is not open on post-op day one, a peripheral laser iridotomy may be performed (see Chapter 33, Laser Iridotomy section).
6. Remove residual viscoelastic with I&A instrument using minimum suction.
7. Close wound with interrupted 10–0 nylon sutures (e.g., Alcon CU-5 needle).
   a. Sutures should be ~90% wound depth.
   b. Ensure good wound apposition.
   c. Bury knots on scleral side of wound.
8. Check wound for leaks by applying gentle point pressure at the wound (cellulose sponges).

Sutured in Intraocular Lens

See Chapter 11, Sutured Posterior Chamber Intraocular Lens Implantation section.

Postoperative Procedure

1. Keep patch (if placed) and shield in place until patient is examined on postoperative day 1.
2. Steroid drops (e.g., Pred Forte 1%) 4 times per day, tapered over ~4–6 weeks as inflammation warrants.
3. Topical antibiotics (e.g., moxifloxacin 0.5% [Vigamox, Alcon, Inc.], gatifloxacin 0.3% [Zymar, Allergan, Inc.]) 4 times per day for 1 week.
4. Topical NSAIDs: Check literature for updated efficacy studies of topical NSAIDs agents and current practices as indicated. Current options include nepafenac 0.1% [Nevanac, Alcon, Inc.] 3 times per day; ketorolac tromethamine [Acular, Allergan, Inc.] 4 times per day; bromfenac ophthalmic solution 0.009% [Xibrom, ISTA, Inc.] 2 times per day) to help prevent cystoid macular edema for 1 week to 3 months, depending on surgical time and predisposing factors (diabetes, glaucoma, history of uveitis, etc.).
5. Control intraocular pressure rises as needed with topical drops (brimonidine tartrate 0.1%; timolol maleate 0.25%or 0.5%) or oral medications (i.e., acetazolamide 500 mg by mouth × 1) before burping the wound (where Betadine and a fourth-generation fluoroquinolone antibiotic are given before and after).
6. A patient with active uveitis should continue on oral steroid taper for several months after surgery, depending on inflammation.
7. Explain postoperative management to patient (see Chapter 6).

Follow-up Schedule

1. Postoperative day 1.
2. Postoperative day 4 or 5 (highest incidence of endophthalmitis onset at this time).
3. Two and 4 weeks postoperatively, and then as necessary. Many eye doctors see their patients at 3–6 months, and then at 1 year.
4. Final refraction is usually given after the patient is off steroid drops (around 1 month postoperatively).

Complications

1. Posterior capsule rupture before completion of nucleus removal.
2. In all cases of vitreous loss, consider using Burke's method for vitreous staining:

Vitreous Staining, Kenalog 40 mg/ml (for staining capsular rhexis during surgery)

Materials:
  a. Kenalog 40 mg/ml injection, 0.2 ml
  b. 0.22 μm GV filter (yellow round one)
  c. TB syringes × 2
  d. 3 ml syringe
  e. BSS sterile 15 ml bottle

Methods:
  a. Draw up 0.2 ml Kenalog 40 mg/ml into TB syringe.
  b. Remove needle from TB syringe, replace with 0.22 μm filter, push Kenalog through filter to trap particles.
  c. Open 3 ml syringe, put needle on end of micron filter, and replace TB syringe with 3 ml syringe.
  d. Open BSS bottle; this is a washing process to remove preservatives in the Kenalog. Pull back through the filter BSS to fill up 3 ml syringe. Then push back BSS and discard to recapture crystals of Kenalog in the filter. Repeat 3–4 times, keeping enough BSS for final dilution of 0.8 ml.
  e. On final wash, draw back through the filter BSS q.s. to approx. 0.8 ml
  f. Cap with sterile yellow cap, label, use immediately.
3. If vitreous remains posterior to capsule:
  a. Use viscoelastic to keep vitreous posterior.
  b. Consider using a sheets glide to prevent loss of nuclear fragments.
  c. May carefully continue removal of nuclear material by phacoemulsification. Lower bottle height to avoid further posterior pressure.
  d. Consider enlarging wound and converting to an extracapsular technique if bag is unstable.
4. If vitreous is admixed with nuclear material:
  a. Do not continue phacoemulsification.
  b. Enlarge wound and remove remaining nuclear fragments with lens loop. (If vitreous is adherent, remove some to reduce risk to the retina.)
  c. Remove vitreous in anterior chamber either with an anterior approach or via the pars plana if indicated (see Chapter 12 and Chapter 63).
5. Loss of nuclear fragments into vitreous cavity.
  a. Do not chase after a fragment that has fallen into the vitreous cavity.
  b. Remove vitreous in anterior chamber, either with an anterior approach or via the pars plana if indicated (see Chapter 12 and Chapter 63).
  c. If there is capsular support, a sulcus lens may be placed after vitreous is removed from anterior chamber. Otherwise, place an ACIOL with PI and close the wound (see Chapter 11, Anterior Chamber Intraocular Lens Implantation section).
  d. Enlist the help of a retina colleague at time of incident if possible, before placing IOL and closing wound, or otherwise the following day.
6. Transient increase in intraocular pressure.
7. Hyphema.
8. Corneal endothelial damage and consequent bullous keratopathy.
9. Suprachoroidal effusion or hemorrhage.
10. Posterior capsule opacification.
11. Endophthalmitis: any increased pain or increased light sensitivity after surgery warrants an immediate evaluation.
12. Retinal detachment.
13. Cystoid macular edema.

■ Capsular Stains

Indications

Used in cases where the red reflex on retroillumination is absent (e.g., cases with a dense white cataract, heavily pigmented fundi, or both). Capsular stains allow for better discrimination of the anterior capsule from the underlying lens tissue. Helps decrease risk of incomplete capsulorhexis or radial capsule tears and their associated complications.

Capsular Stain Options

1. Trypan blue 0.1% (Gurr, London, UK, BDH Laboratory Supplies, Poole, UK)
2. Indocyanine green (ICG) 0.5% (Akorn Inc.)
3. Fluorescein sodium 2%
4. Gential violet 0.1% and methylene blue 1% have had reports of corneal endothelial toxicity.
5. Hemocoloration of the capsule with autologous blood

Preoperative Procedure

Dilation of pupil with standard preoperative preparation for cataract extraction.

1. Trypan blue:

   Place 0.1ml of trypan blue 0.1% in phosphate-buffered sodium chloride in sterile 1 ml syringe. Place on surgical table.
2. ICG:

   Prepare ICG: Mix 25 mg ICG vial with 10 ml of aqueous diluent to give a 0.25% solution. Then mix 0.5 ml of this solution with 4.5 ml of BSS. Shake well. Draw into a 5 ml syringe. Pass solution through milipore filter. Place 30 g cannula on syringe.

Instrumentation

- Capsular dye: trypan blue 0.1% in phosphate-buffered sodium chloride or ICG 25 mg vial (Akorn Inc.)
- 1 ml or 5 ml syringe
- Milipore filter
- 15 blade
- 27–30 g cannula
- Viscoelastic (e.g., Healon, Viscoat)
- Cystotome
- Utrata capsular forceps

Operative Procedure

1. Anesthesia: as usual (e.g., retrobulbar with lid block, peribulbar, subtenon's, or topical anesthesia)
2. Prepare and drape eye
3. Place lid speculum
4. Create a small anterior chamber paracentesis through clear cornea at 10 o'clock or 2 o'clock with #15 blade (see Chapter 7). A smaller paracentesis will prevent air from escaping.
5. Via filter, inject a single large air bubble into the anterior chamber. It is not necessary to aspirate aqueous first, as the air bubble will displace aqueous out the paracentesis. The capsule will stain adequately without an air bubble, though many surgeons note a better, more uniform result with an air bubble.
6. Insert syringe and cannula containing the dye. Apply drops of dye uniformly over capsule. (Optional, though not necessary in most cases: use side of cannula to spread dye over capsule.)
7. Wait 1–2 minutes for ICG; wait a few seconds for trypan blue.
8. Inject viscoelastic to displace the air bubble out of the anterior chamber. Inject under and beyond the bubble while burping the paracentesis so the bubble will come out more quickly.
9. Alternatively, make the larger corneal incision to burp out remaining air if needed. With trypan blue, some surgeons first thoroughly irrigate with balanced salt solution to wash out the excess dye before injecting viscoelastic, though this is not necessarily needed.
10. Use cystotome and then capsular forceps as needed to initiate and complete continuous capsulorhexis.
11. Optional: if capsule still poorly defined in certain areas with ICG, inject more ICG under anterior capsular flap once initial flap has been created.
12. Optional: Side illumination can still be of benefit in poorly stained areas.
13. Continue capsulorhexis and rest of procedure as noted in step 10 in beginning section.

Complications

Corneal edema has been reported with gentian violet 0.1% and methylene blue 1% used in combination. This is thought to be due to endothelial toxicity. Endothelial toxicity has not been reported with ICG or trypan blue.

Posterior capsular staining causing a temporary loss of the red reflex with obstruction of the posterior fundus view in post vitrectomized eyes has been reported.

9

Extracapsular Cataract Extraction

Indications

- Visually significant cataract impairing patient's lifestyle.
- Dense cataract obstructing view of fundus.
- Possible advantages of extracapsular over phacoemulsification cataract surgery:
  - Reduced incidence of corneal decompensation in patients with corneal compromise.
  - Ease of removal of hard nucleus.

Preoperative Procedure

See Chapter 3.

1. Calculate intraocular lens (IOL) power.
2. Numerous formulas for the calculation of IOL power have been derived based on theoretical optics and empirical data. The Sanders-Retzlaff-Kraff (SRK) formula is one of the most widely used.
3. *SRK Formula:* Power of IOL = A − (2.5 × AL) − (0.9 × K) where
   a. A = constant is determined by the manufacturer of a specific lens. A typical value is A = 118.4
   b. K = average keratometry measurement in diopters.
   c. AL = axial length of eye in millimeters measured with A-scan ultrasonography.
4. Determine target postoperative refraction:
   a. Target postoperative refraction decisions depend on numerous factors, including patients' desire for good vision for near or distance, eye dominance, refractive and lens status of the other eye, and the type of IOL planned (multifocal, new-generation refractive lenses).
   b. Communication with the patient regarding refractive options assists in choosing appropriate targets.
5. Dilate pupil and preoperative drops:
   a. Tropicamide 1%, phenylephrine 2.5%, and Cyclogyl 1%, every 15 minutes starting 1 hour before surgery is a typical regimen. Other regimen examples: Phen/Trop 1 gtt q 5 minutes × three. Coll 3&38 ¼ 1 gtt q 5 minutes × 3.
   b. Preoperative drop of antibiotic (e.g., moxifloxacin 0.5% [Vigamox, Alcon, Inc., Fort Worth, TX, US], gatifloxacin 0.3% [Zymar, Allergan, Inc., Irvine, CA, US]) 1 drop before surgery.
   c. Optional: Topical nonsteroidal anti-inflammatory drug (NSAID) 1 drop every 15 minutes × 3 starting 1 hour before surgery (to minimize intraoperative miosis) (e.g., flurbiprofen 0.03% 1 gtt q 5 minutes × 2). Other topical NSAID (e.g., nepafenac 0.1% [Nevanac, Alcon, Inc.] 3 times per day, ketorolac tromethamine [Acular, Allergan, Inc.] 4 times per day, or bromfenac ophthalmic solution 0.009% [Xibrom, ISTA, Inc., Alpharetta, GA, US] 2 times per day) can be used for 5–7 days before surgery in patients with a history of diabetes, uveitis, previous cystoid macular edema, epiretinal membrane, or vein occlusion, and then for approximately 3 months after surgery to help prevent cystoid macular edema. Some surgeons use preoperative and postoperative NSAIDS on all patients. Check literature for updated efficacy studies among topical NSAIDs and current practices as indicated.
   d. The use of preoperative (days before surgery) and intraoperative antibiotic use (diluted in balanced salt solution [BSS] bottle: vancomycin 1 mg/0.1ml balanced salt solution; intracameral cefuroxime: 1 mg cefuroxime in 0.1 ml saline 0.9%; intracameral moxifloxacin 100 µg/0.1 ml [1:5 dilution of moxifloxacin with BSS]) is controversial in terms of its proven benefit. Their use varies widely. Check the literature for updated information.
   e. A commonly used regimen is the use of preoperative "pulse" antibiotics: fourth-generation fluoroquinolone used every 10 minutes times 4 doses 1hour before surgery. A fourth-generation fluoroquinolone is then used immediately after surgery and then continued during postoperative week 1 (e.g., moxifloxacin 0.5%

[Vigamox, Alcon, Inc.], gatifloxacin 0.3% [Zymar, Allergan, Inc.]).
6. Recommended:

Use PMMA or acrylic lenses for patients with diabetes, uveitis, or glaucoma.

Instrumentation

- Honan balloon (optional)
- Lid speculum
- Castroviejo calipers
- Fine-toothed tissue forceps (e.g., 0.12 mm straight Castroviejo and/or Colibri)
- Sutures: 4–0 silk, 7–0 Vicryl, 10–0 Vicryl, 10–0 nylon
- Elschnig forceps
- Kalt needle holder
- Fine needle holder
- Westcott scissors
- Cellulose sponges
- Cautery (underwater eraser or disposable)
- Scleral incision blade (e.g., Beaver #64 or #69)
- Microsurgical knife (e.g., Beaver #75M, Superblade)
- Viscoelastic substance (e.g., Healon, Amvisc, Viscoat)
- Cystotome or bent-tipped 1 inch 22 G needle
- Straight and angled McPherson tying forceps
- Left- and right-handed corneoscleral scissors
- Cyclodialysis spatula
- Lens loop
- Muscle hook
- 19 G needle on syringe
- Irrigation/aspiration unit (automated or manual)
- Kuglen or collar button hook
- Sinskey hook
- Jeweler's forceps
- Vannas scissors
- Capsule polisher
- IOL forceps
- Acetylcholine solution (e.g., Miochol)

Operative Procedure

1. Anesthesia: General or retrobulbar plus lid block or peribulbar block. (See Chapter 4.)
2. Optional: Apply Honan balloon for ~10–15 minutes to decompress eye and orbit, minimizing positive vitreous pressure.
3. Prep and drape.
4. Place lid speculum.
5. Place 4–0 silk bridle sutures through insertions of superior and inferior rectus muscle (Elschnig forceps, Kalt needle holder, 4–0 silk, e.g., #734 Ethicon cutting needle, muscle hook) (**Fig. 9.1**).

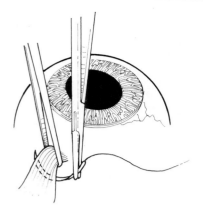

Figure 9.1

a. Facilitate visualization by having assistant rotate eye inferiorly with muscle hook placed in conjunctival fornix.
b. Elevate muscle insertion with Elschnig forceps while slinging the suture beneath the muscle tendon.
6. Prepare a fornix-based conjunctival peritomy at the superior limbus with blunt Westcott scissors and tissue forceps (**Fig. 9.2**).

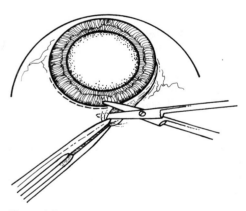

Figure 9.2

7. Secure hemostasis with wet-field cautery.

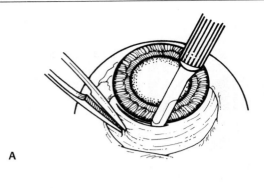

A

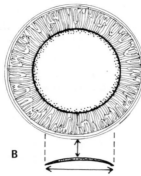

B

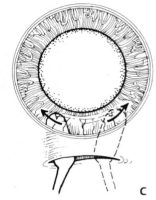

Figure 9.3   C

8. Perform a partial-thickness groove incision at the limbus (e.g., 0.12 mm forceps, #64 or #69 Beaver blade)
(**Fig. 9.3A**).
   a. Place at posterior limbus.
   b. Chord length of groove should be ~11 to 12 mm.
   c. Make incision perpendicular to tissue, approximately
   two thirds scleral thickness deep.
      i. For a small incision, sutureless extracapsular
      cataract extraction (ECCE): use a rounded or
      crescent blade (e.g., #64 or #69 Beaver blade)
      and 0.12 mm forceps to make a partial (50%)
      thickness, 6 mm linear or frowned incision par-
      allel to limbal plane and perpendicular to sclera
      1.5 mm to 2 mm from limbus at desired location
      (e.g., superior). Cauterize as needed (**Fig. 9.3B**).
      ii. Construct a scleral tunnel of same depth onto
      clear cornea. Maintain an even surgical plane
      by holding the blade heel flat against the sclera.
      Advancing with a circular motion to left and to
      right may be helpful (**Fig. 9.3C**).
      iii. Continue tunnel construction just past anterior
      limbal vessels so the internal opening will be
      larger than the external incision. This will help
      with the delivery of the nucleus.
      iv. For a large brunescent cataract, a larger exter-
      nal (e.g., 7 mm) and internal opening may be
      needed. Alternatively, the nucleus can be di-
      vided in half before delivery.
      v. Use a keratome to enter anterior chamber after
      viscoelastic is injected through a paracentesis to
      create a self-sealing corneal valve (see **Fig. 8.4**, p.
      28).
      vi. No further enlargement of the wound with scis-
      sors or keratome is usually needed in small inci-
      sion ECCE.

9. Enter anterior chamber with microsurgical knife; avoid
capsule (**Fig. 9.4**).

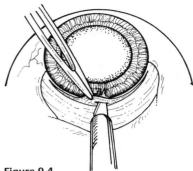

Figure 9.4

10. Instill viscoelastic into anterior chamber.
11. Perform a 360 degree, "can opener" style anterior capsulotomy with a cystotome or bent-tipped 1 inch 22 G
needle, measuring ~5 to 6 mm in diameter (**Fig. 9.5**).

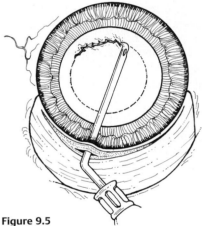

Figure 9.5

Note: A continuous curvilinear capsulorhexis can be used.
However, a relaxing incision should be performed to easily express the nucleus from capsular bag.

12. Remove anterior capsular flap with angled McPherson
forceps (**Fig. 9.6**).

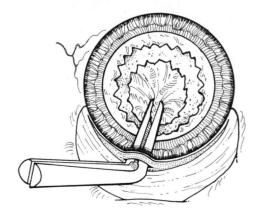

Figure 9.6

18. Irrigate anterior chamber with BSS.
19. Tie preplaced sutures.
20. Place an additional 10–0 nylon suture at 12 o'clock.

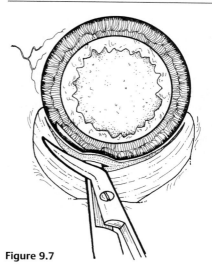

Figure 9.7

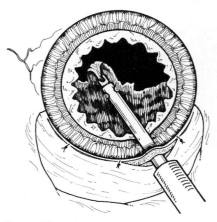

Figure 9.9

13. Extend wound with corneoscleral scissors, angling blades at ~45 degrees to the tissue to create a biplanar incision for traditional ECCE (**Fig. 9.7**).
14. Pre-place 7–0 Vicryl or 10–0 nylon sutures at 10 and 2 o'clock, separated by 7 mm and left untied.
15. Loop sutures out of wound using a cyclodialysis spatula.
16. Optional: Perform hydrodissection with BSS and a 30 G cannula to loosen nucleus
17. Express nucleus (**Figs. 9.8A and 9–8B**).
    a. Apply careful pressure at the limbus at 6 o'clock with a muscle hook and 2 mm posterior to the 12 o'clock with a lens loop.
    b. When the nucleus presents at the wound, the assistant may:
       i. Elevate the cornea.
       ii. Use a 19 G needle or other instrument to spin the nucleus out of eye (**Fig. 9.8B**).

21. Remove residual cortical material with automated irrigation/aspiration (**Fig. 9.9**).
    a. Add 0.3–0.5 ml 1:1000 epinephrine to each 500 ml bottle of irrigating solution to aid in maintaining pupil dilation.
    b. Place irrigation/aspiration tip into capsular fornix.
    c. Engage cortex with suction; aim tip toward underside of anterior capsule edge.
    d. Gently strip cortex from posterior capsule toward the center of the pupil.
    e. May use Kuglen hook or collar button hook to retract iris and better visualize cortex.

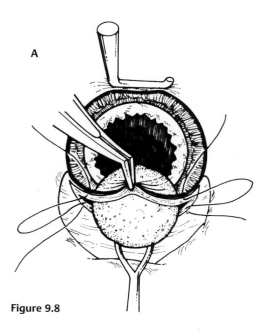

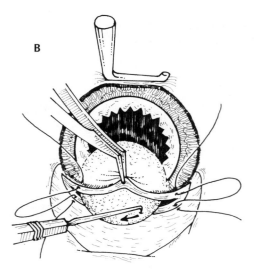

Figure 9.8

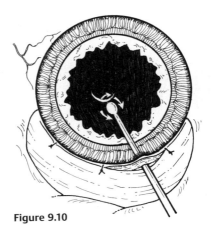

Figure 9.10

22. Optional: Polish posterior capsule centrally with capsule polisher (**Fig. 9.10**).
23. Remove 12 o'clock suture.
24. Irrigate viscoelastic into capsular bag.
25. Place posterior chamber IOL: The standard implant placement of J-loop style haptics is described. Lenses of other styles may require alternative implantation techniques (**Fig. 9.11**).

a. Grasp superior portion of optic with IOL forceps.
b. Place inferior haptic into capsular bag or ciliary sulcus depending upon type of IOL fixation desired. (Secure superior haptic with McPherson forceps before releasing IOL forceps to prevent uncontrolled IOL movements) (**Fig. 9.11A**).
c. Advance optic into pupil by gently pushing it inferiorly (McPherson forceps).
d. Place superior haptic.
   i. Grasp with angled McPherson forceps (**Fig. 9.11B**).
   ii. Push haptic into anterior chamber.
   iii. Pronate hand to flex knee of haptic behind iris. Release haptic into desired location (**Fig. 9.11C**).
26. Center IOL and spin to horizontal position (Sinskey hook). Haptics at 3 and 9 o'clock (**Figs. 9.12A and 9.12B**).

Note: In cases where the posterior capsule is significantly ruptured or with zonular dialysis, lens may be positioned into the ciliary sulcus.

a. Ensure that vitreous is not present in anterior chamber.
b. Inject viscoelastic behind the iris and over the anterior leaflets of capsule.
c. Grasp superior portion of PMMA IOL with smooth forceps.
d. Place inferior haptic into ciliary sulcus, just below the inferior iris.

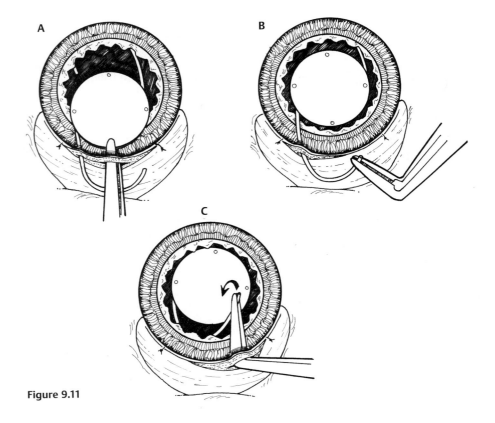

Figure 9.11

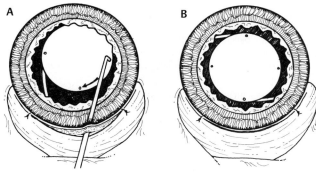

Figure 9.12

e. Secure superior haptic with McPherson forceps before releasing IOL to prevent uncontrolled movements.

f. Advance optic into pupil by gently pushing it inferiorly.

g. Place superior haptic.
   i. Grasp with angled McPherson forceps.
   ii. Push haptic into anterior chamber.
   iii. Pronate hand to flex knee of haptic behind iris.
   iv. Release haptic into desired position.

h. Center IOL; spin cautiously if decentered.

27. Remove viscoelastic with irrigation/aspiration instrument using minimum suction.

28. Irrigate Miochol into anterior chamber to constrict pupil.

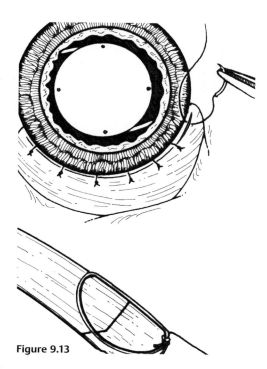

Figure 9.13

29. Close wound with interrupted 10–0 nylon sutures (**Fig. 9.13**).

a. Sutures should be ~90% wound depth.
b. Ensure good wound apposition.
c. Bury knots on scleral side of wound.
d. Remove previously placed 7–0 Vicryl sutures.

30. Check for wound leak by applying gentle point pressure at the wound with cellulose sponges.

31. Remove bridle sutures (if present).

32. Reposition conjunctiva and secure with sutures (e.g., 10–0 Vicryl or nylon), or cautery.

33. Perform subconjunctival or subtenons injections of antibiotic (i.e., cephalexin) and steroid (i.e., Decadron or SoluMedrol).

34. Remove lid speculum.

35. Apply topical combination antibiotic/steroid ointments.

36. Apply patch and place eye shield.

Postoperative Procedure

1. Give patients written instructions for medication use.

2. Keep patch and shield placed until patient is examined on postoperative day 1.

3. Steroid drops (e.g., Pred Forte 1%) 4 times per day, tapered over ~6 weeks as inflammation warrants.

4. Topical antibiotics (e.g., moxifloxacin 0.5% [Vigamox, Alcon, Inc.], gatifloxacin 0.3% [Zymar, Allergan, Inc.]) four times per day for 1 week.

5. Topical NSAIDs: Check literature for updated efficacy studies among topical NSAIDs and current practices as indicated. Current options include nepafenac 0.1% [Nevanac, Alcon, Inc.] 3 times per day; ketorolac tromethamine [Acular, Allergan, Inc.] 4 times per day; bromfenac ophthalmic solution 0.009% [Xibrom, ISTA, Inc.] 2 times per day). Use recommended to help prevent cystoid macular edema for 1 week—3 months, depending on surgical time and predisposing factors (diabetes, glaucoma, history of uveitis, etc.).

6. Control intraocular pressure rises as needed with topical drops (i.e., brimonidine tartrate 0.1%; timolol maleate 0.25% or 0.5%) or oral medications (i.e., acetazolamide 500 mg by mouth × 1) before burping the wound (where Betadine and a fourth-generation fluoroquinolone antibiotic is given before and after).

7. For patient with active uveitis, continue on oral steroid taper for several months after surgery, depending on inflammation.

8. Explain postoperative management to patient (see Chapter 6).

Follow-up Schedule

1. Postoperative day 1.

2. Postoperative day 4 or 5 (highest incidence of endophthalmitis onset at this time).

3. Postoperative week 2, 1 month, 3 months, 6 months, 1 year; then yearly.

Suture Removal

1. May selectively cut sutures for astigmatism control beginning ~6 weeks postoperatively, depending on the stability of the wound, the use of steroid drops, and other risks such as diabetes. Beware of overzealous suture removal, as this may compromise the wound and produce wound gape.
2. Remove loose, exposed, or infiltrated sutures as they appear.
3. Well-buried, quiet sutures may be kept in place indefinitely.
4. Technique
   a. Give drop of sterile tetracaine or proparacaine. Recommended: give one drop of Betadine 10% and/or one drop of antibiotic before suture removal.
   b. Cut suture with scalpel (e.g., #11 Bard-Parker blade or edge of 25 G needle).
   c. Remove suture with jeweler's forceps; may leave in place if ends are buried.
   d. Give drop of antibiotic after suture removal and continue 4 times per day for 3 days.

Complications

1. Posterior capsule rupture.
2. Vitreous loss (see Chapter 12). Also see Chapter 8, Complications section discussing Burke's method for vitreous staining with Kenalog, p. 38.
3. Suprachoroidal effusion or hemorrhage.
4. Hyphema.
5. Transient increase in intraocular pressure.
6. Endophthalmitis.
7. Wound leak.
8. Posterior capsule opacification.
9. Bullous keratopathy.
10. Retinal detachment.
11. Cystoid macular edema.
12. Prolonged corneal edema especially in Fuchs dystrophy.

10

Intracapsular Cataract Extraction/Anterior Chamber Intraocular Lens

Indications

- Selected cases of lens subluxation.
- Selected cases of lens-induced glaucoma.
- Phacoanaphylactic uveitis.
- Selected cases of traumatic cataract with zonular dehiscence.

Preoperative Procedure

See Chapter 3.

1. Examine anterior chamber angle with a gonioscope to inspect for peripheral anterior synechiae (PAS) or other abnormalities that may interfere with or preclude implantation of anterior chamber intraocular lens (IOL).
2. Calculate IOL power.

Numerous formulas for the calculation of IOL power have been derived based on both theoretical optics and empirical data. The Sanders-Retzlaff-Kraff (SRK) formula is one of the most widely used.

SRK Formula: Power of IOL = A − 2.5(AL) − 0.9(K) where

  a. A = constant is determined by the manufacturer of a specific lens. A typical value is A = 116.7.
  b. K = average keratometry measurement in diopters.
  c. AL = axial length of eye in millimeters measured with A-scan ultrasonography.
3. Determine target postoperative refraction.
4. Dilate pupil: Tropicamide 1%, phenylephrine 2.5%, and Cyclogyl 1% every 15 minutes starting 1 hour before surgery.
5. Preoperative drop of antibiotic (e.g., moxifloxacin 0.5% [Vigamox, Alcon, Inc., Fort Worth, TX, US], gatifloxacin 0.3% [Zymar, Allergan, Inc., Irvine, CA, US]) 1 drop before surgery.
6. Optional: Topical nonsteroidal anti-inflammatory agent every 15 minutes starting 1 hour before surgery (to minimize intraoperative miosis).

7. Optional: Topical nonsteroidal anti-inflammatory agent (NSAID) (e.g., nepafenac 0.1% [Nevanac, Alcon, Inc.] 3 times per day, ketorolac tromethamine [Acular, Allergan, Inc.] 4 times per day, or bromfenac ophthalmic solution 0.009% [Xibrom, ISTA, Inc., Alpharetta, GA, US] 2 times per day), for 5–7 days before surgery suggested for diabetics and then for ~3 months after surgery to help prevent cystoid macular edema. This is also suggested for stable uveitic patients who have shown no inflammation for 3 months before surgery. Consider admitting patient 1 day before surgery for intravenous steroid if active uveitis is present. Check literature for updated efficacy studies among topical NSAIDs as indicated.
8. Optional: Treat patient with a hyperosmotic agent to dehydrate vitreous and minimize positive vitreous pressure. The following may be used:
  a. Mannitol 20%, 1–2 g/kg IV given over 1 hour, 90 minutes preoperative.
  b. Mannitol 25%, 50 ml IV push given just before surgery.

Instrumentation

- Honan balloon
- Lid speculum
- Castroviejo calipers
- Fine-toothed forceps (e.g., 0.12 mm straight Castroviejo and/or Colibri)
- Sutures (4–0 silk, 8–0 and 10–0 Vicryl, 10–0 nylon)
- Elschnig forceps
- Kalt needle holder
- Fine needle holder
- Westcott scissors
- Cellulose sponges
- Cautery (underwater eraser or disposable)
- Scleral incision blade (Beaver #64 or #69)
- Microsurgical knife (e.g., Beaver #75M, Superblade)

- Left- and right-handed corneoscleral scissors
- Jeweler's forceps
- Vannas scissors
- Acetylcholine solution (e.g., Miochol)
- Alpha-chymotrypsin 1: 10,000
- Olive-tipped or 30 G cannula
- Iris retractor
- Cryoextractor
- Iris spatula
- Straight and angled McPherson tying forceps
- Viscoelastic substance (e.g., Healon, Amvisc, Viscoat)
- Sheets glide
- IOL forceps

Operative Procedure

1. Anesthesia: Retrobulbar plus lid block, or general. See Chapter 4.
2. Apply Honan balloon for ~20 minutes to decompress eye and orbit, minimizing positive vitreous pressure.
3. Prep and drape.
4. Insert lid speculum.

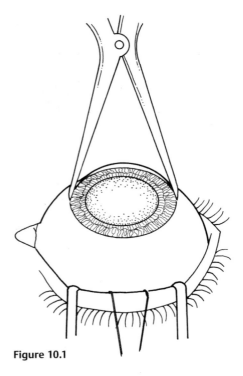

Figure 10.1

5. Measure "white-to-white" (limbus-to-limbus) with calipers. Select size of anterior chamber IOL to approximately equal the white-to-white measurement plus 1 mm (**Fig. 10.1**).

6. Place 4–0 silk bridle sutures through insertions of superior and inferior rectus muscles (see **Fig. 9.1**, p. 41).
7. Prepare a fornix-based conjunctival peritomy at the superior limbus (Westcott scissors, tissue forceps) (see **Fig. 9.2**, p. 41).
8. Secure hemostasis with cautery.

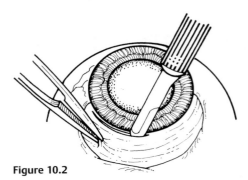

Figure 10.2

9. Perform a partial-thickness groove incision at the limbus (0.12 mm forceps, #64 Beaver blades) (**Fig. 10.2**).
   a. Place at mid-limbus to form an adequate posterior wound lip under which to place anterior chamber IOL.
   b. Chord length of groove should be ~12 mm.
   c. Make incision perpendicular to tissue, approximately two thirds scleral thickness deep.

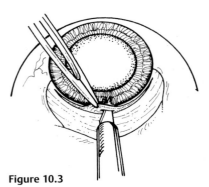

Figure 10.3

10. Enter anterior chamber with microsurgical knife (**Fig. 10.3**).

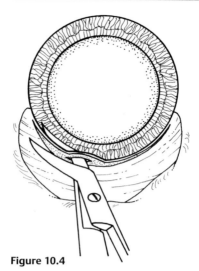

Figure 10.4

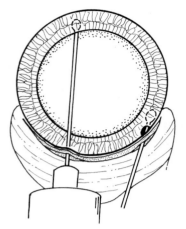

Figure 10.6

11. Extend wound with corneoscleral scissors, angling blades at ~45 degrees to the tissue to create a biplanar incision (**Fig. 10.4**).
12. Pre-place 7–0 Vicryl sutures at 10 and 2 o'clock, separated by 7 mm and left untied.
13. Loop sutures out of wound (cyclodialysis spatula).

15. Irrigate α-chymotrypsin (1:10,000) into posterior chamber (olive-tipped or 30 G cannula) (**Fig. 10.6**).
    a. Use ~0.5 ml of solution.
    b. Irrigate superiorly through iridectomies and inferiorly just under iris.
    c. Allow enzyme to work for 2 minutes.

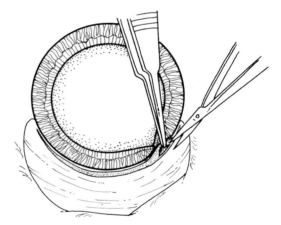

Figure 10.5

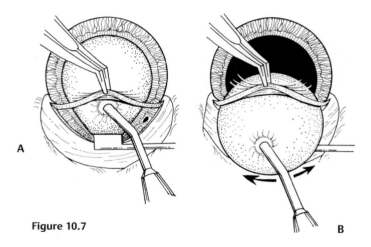

Figure 10.7

14. Perform small peripheral iridectomy (jeweler's forceps, Vannas scissors) (**Fig. 10.5**).

    Place iridectomy so as not to interfere with IOL haptics.

16. Irrigate anterior and posterior chambers with balanced salt solution to remove α-chymotrypsin and zonular fragments.
17. Cryoextract lens (**Figs. 10.7A and 10.7B**).
    a. If pupil is not sufficiently large, perform sphincterotomy or sector/keyhole iridectomy.
    b. Have assistant retract cornea.
    c. Dry lens with cellulose sponge.

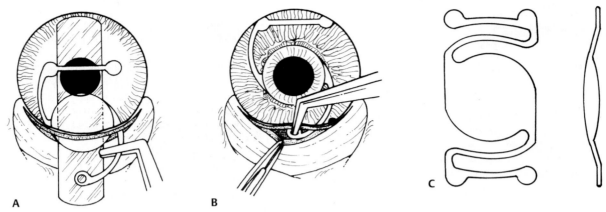

Figure 10.8

d. Retract superior iris (iris retractor or cellulose sponge).
e. Place cryoprobe midway between center of lens and superior equator.
f. Activate cryoprobe and allow ice ball to form.
g. Gently rock lens while slowly elevating superior pole from eye.
h. If cryoprobe inadvertently freezes to iris or cornea, irrigate with balanced salt solution (BSS) to thaw adhesions.
18. Reposition iris with BSS.
19. Tie preplaced Vicryl sutures.
20. Irrigate anterior chamber with Miochol to constrict pupil.
21. Reform anterior chamber with viscoelastic.
22. Optional: Place Sheets glide over iris into inferior angle.
    a. The glide guides lens placement and prevents iris tuck by the inferior haptic of IOL.
    b. Bending the glide to give it a slight upward curvature facilitates its accurate placement over the pupil and iris.
23. Place anterior chamber IOL (**Figs. 10.8A–10.8C**).
    a. Grasp superior haptic with smooth (e.g., McPherson) forceps.
    b. Slide lens across anterior chamber into inferior angle.
    c. Stabilize IOL with forceps in left hand before releasing IOL forceps to avoid displacing lens from angle.
    d. Remove Sheets glide. (Stabilize superior haptic with forceps to prevent dislocation of the IOL from the inferior angle while removing glide.)
    e. Ensure the pupil is round without iris tuck.
    f. Retract posterior lip of wound with tissue forceps and place superior haptic of IOL into superior angle. (Avoid iridectomy sites.)
    g. A 3-point or 4-point fixation anterior chamber intraocular lens (ACIOL) may be used (**Fig. 10.8C**).
24. Irrigate/aspirate residual viscoelastic from anterior chamber.

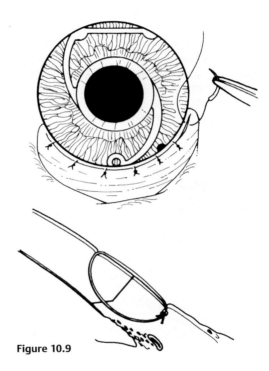

Figure 10.9

25. Close wound with interrupted 10–0 nylon sutures (e.g., Alcon CU-5) (**Fig. 10.9**).
    a. Sutures should be ~90% wound depth.
    b. Ensure good wound apposition.
    c. Bury knots on scleral side of wound.
    d. Remove previously placed 7–0 Vicryl sutures.
26. Check for wound leak by applying gentle point pressure at the wound (cellulose sponges).
27. Remove bridle sutures.
28. Reposition conjunctiva and secure with sutures (e.g., 10–0 Vicryl or nylon), or cautery.
29. Perform subconjunctival injections of antibiotic (e.g., cephalexin) and steroid (e.g., Decadron or SoluMedrol).
30. Remove lid speculum.
31. Apply topical combination antibiotic/steroid ointment.
32. Apply patch and place Fox shield.

Postoperative Procedure

1. Keep patch and shield placed until patient is examined on postoperative day 1.
2. Steroid drops (e.g., Pred Forte 1%) 4 times per day, tapered over 6 weeks as inflammation warrants.
3. Topical antibiotics (e.g., moxifloxacin 0.5% [Alcon, Inc.], gatifloxacin 0.3% [Allergan, Inc.]) 4 times per day for 1 week.
4. Topical nonsteroidal anti-inflammatory agent (e.g., nepafenac 0.1% [Nevanac, Alcon, Inc.], ketorolac tromethamine [Acular, Allergan, Inc.]) recommended 4 times daily to help prevent cystoid macular edema (CME) for 1 week to 3 months, depending on surgical time and predisposing factors (e.g., diabetes, glaucoma, history of uveitis, CME, prior intraocular surgery).
5. Control intraocular pressure rises as needed: recommend maximal medical treatment (brimonidine tartrate 0.1%; timolol maleate 0.25% or 0.5%; acetazolamide 500 mg by mouth × 1) before burping the wound (where Betadine and a fourth-generation fluoroquinolone antibiotic is given before and after).
6. Explain postoperative management to patient (see Chapter 6).

Follow-up Schedule

1. Postoperative day 1.
2. Postoperative day 4 or 5 (highest incidence of endophthalmitis onset at this time).
3. 2 to 4 weeks, 3 months, 6 months, 1 year, and then yearly.

Suture Removal

1. May selectively cut sutures for astigmatism control beginning ~6 weeks postoperatively. (Do this judiciously because overzealous suture removal may compromise wound and produce overcorrection.)
2. Remove loose, exposed, or infiltrated sutures as they appear.
3. Well-buried, quiet sutures may be kept in place indefinitely.
4. Technique
   a. Give drop of sterile tetracaine or proparacaine; then give drop of Betadine 10%.
   b. Cut suture with scalpel (e.g., #11 Bard-Parker blade or edge of 25 G needle).
   c. Remove suture with jeweler's forceps or leave in place if ends are buried.
   d. Give drop of sterile antibiotic (e.g., moxifloxacin 0.5% [Alcon, Inc.], gatifloxacin 0.3% [Allergan, Inc.]) and continue 4 times per day for 3–7 days.

Complications

1. Capsule rupture during lens extraction.
2. Vitreous loss (see Chapter 12).
3. Suprachoroidal effusion or hemorrhage.
4. Hyphema.
5. Transient increase in intraocular pressure (secondary to α-chymotrypsin and/or viscoelastic substance.
6. Iris tuck by the lens.
7. Pupillary block.
8. Wound leak.
9. Endophthalmitis.
10. Bullous keratopathy.
11. Retinal detachment.
12. Cystoid macular edema.

11

Secondary Intraocular Lens Placement

■ Anterior Chamber Intraocular Lens Implantation

Indications

- Monocular aphakia in contact lens intolerant patient in absence of posterior capsule support.
- Selected cases of binocular aphakia in which patient is unable to wear either contact lenses or aphakic spectacles.
- Patients with macular degeneration may, in particular, benefit from the optical consequences of intraocular lenses (no ring scotoma, less magnification of central scotoma) compared with aphakic spectacle correction.

Contraindications

- Low corneal endothelial cell count
- Cystoid macular edema
- Uveitis
- Peripheral anterior synechiae
- Rubeosis
- Need for anterior vitrectomy when placing implant
- Narrow angle glaucoma

Preoperative Procedure

See Chapter 3.

1. Examine anterior chamber angle with gonioscope to inspect for peripheral anterior synechiae, angle depth, and location of any peripheral iridectomies.
2. Assess corneal endothelial integrity with careful slit lamp examination, pachymetry, and/or specular microscopy.
3. Examine macula under the slit lamp with a fundus contact lens and/or fluorescein angiography for signs of cystoid macular edema.

4. Determine the need for anterior vitrectomy before lens is implanted. For instance, an eye with an intact hyaloid face and vitreous behind the iris plane may not require vitrectomy. In contrast, an eye with a disrupted hyaloid face and vitreous in the anterior chamber will require an anterior vitrectomy. This will prevent uncontrolled vitreous loss as well as vitreous incarceration by the implant or in the surgical wound. In select cases, a small amount of loose vitreous may be held back by a viscoelastic substance irrigated into the anterior chamber or by a lens glide, obviating vitrectomy.
5. Calculate intraocular lens (IOL) power: Numerous formulas for calculating IOL power have been derived based on theoretical optics and empirical data. The Sanders-Retzlaff-Kraff (SRK) formula is one of the most widely used.

   SRK Formula: Power of IOL = $A - 2.5(AL) - 0.9(K)$

   where
   a. A = constant is determined by the manufacturer of a specific lens. A typical value is A = 115.1.
   b. K = average keratometry measurement in diopters.
   c. AL = axial length of eye in millimeters measured with A-scan ultrasonography.

Note: Set ultrasound unit for aphakic, not cataractous, eye.

6. Optional: Topical nonsteroidal anti-inflammatory agent (NSAID) every 15 minutes × 3 starting 1 hour before surgery (to minimize intraoperative miosis).
7. Optional: If a vitrectomy is not planned, a hyperosmotic agent may be administered to dehydrate vitreous in an effort to keep it posterior to the iris plane during surgery. The following may be used:
   a. Mannitol 20%, 1–2 g/kg IV given over 1 hour, 90 minutes preoperative.
   b. Mannitol 25%, 50 ml IV push given just before surgery.

Instrumentation

- Honan balloon
- Lid speculum
- Castroviejo calipers
- Sutures (10–0 nylon, 10–0 Vicryl)
- Elschnig forceps
- Kalt needle holder
- Fine needle holder
- Fine toothed tissue forceps (e.g., 0.12 mm straight Castroviejo and/or Colibri)
- Westcott scissors
- Cellulose sponges
- Cautery (underwater eraser or disposable)
- Scarifier (e.g., Beaver #64, #69)
- Microsurgical knife (e.g., Beaver #75M, MVR, Micro-Sharp, Superblade)
- Microvitrectomy suction/cutting instrumentation
- Acetylcholine solution (e.g., Miochol)
- Viscoelastic substance (e.g., Healon, Amvisc, Viscoat)
- Left- and right-handed corneoscleral scissors
- Straight and angled McPherson tying forceps
- Lens (e.g., Sheets) glide
- IOL forceps

Operative Procedure

1. Anesthesia: Topical, peribulbar, or retrobulbar plus lid block; or general if indicated.

    (See Chapter 4.)

2. Apply Honan balloon for ~10–15 minutes to decompress eye and orbit. This minimizes positive vitreous pressure.

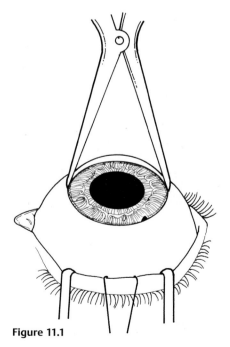

Figure 11.1

3. Optional: Perform surgery using a temporal incision to avoid the original incision, peripheral anterior synechiae, and peripheral iridectomies.
4. Prep and drape.
5. Place lid speculum.
6. Measure horizontal "white-to-white" (limbus-to-limbus) with calipers. Select size of anterior chamber IOL to approximately equal the white-to-white measurement plus 1 mm (**Fig. 11.1**).

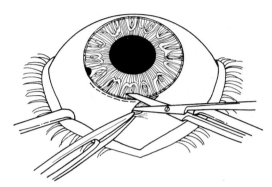

Figure 11.2

7. Prepare a fornix-based conjunctival peritomy at the limbus (Westcott scissors, tissue forceps) (**Fig. 11.2**).
8. Secure hemostasis with cautery.

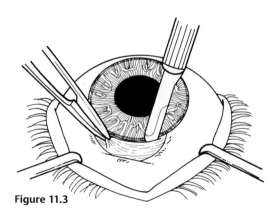

Figure 11.3

9. Perform a partial-thickness groove incision at the limbus (0.12 mm forceps, #64 or #69 Beaver blade) (**Fig. 11.3**).
    a. Chord length of groove should be ~7 mm.
    b. Place at mid-limbus to form an adequate posterior wound lip under which to place the anterior chamber IOL.

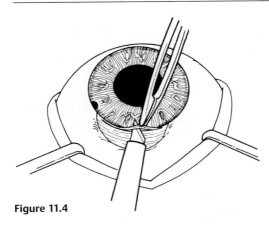

Figure 11.4

10. Enter anterior chamber with microsurgical knife (**Fig. 11.4**).

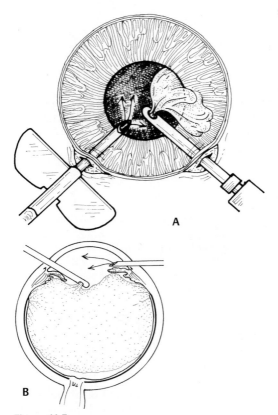

Figure 11.5

11. If necessary, perform anterior vitrectomy (see Chapter 12) (**Figs. 11.5A and 11.5B**).
    a. May use microvitrectomy suction/cutting instrument and separated infusion sleeve through paracentesis.
    b. Vitrectomy instrument parameters:
       i. Cutting rate: ~800 cps.
       ii. Suction: start at ~50–75 mm Hg and increase as necessary.

c. Vitrectomy is complete when:
   i. the wound is free of vitreous
   ii. the anterior chamber is free of vitreous
   iii. the pupil is not peaked
   iv. positive vitreous pressure is relieved with the iris fallen back posteriorly.
d. Alternatively, vitrectomy may be performed using an open-sky technique after wound is extended in step 14.
12. Irrigate Miochol into the anterior chamber to constrict pupil.
13. Irrigate viscoelastic into the anterior chamber to maintain chamber depth and, in some cases, to keep vitreous back.

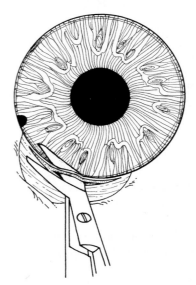

Figure 11.6

14. Extend wound with corneoscleral scissors (**Fig. 11.6**).
15. Optional: Place Sheets glide over iris into opposite angle (**Fig. 11.7**).
    a. The glide guides lens placement and prevents iris tuck by the leading haptic of IOL.
    b. In select cases, the glide may help keep anterior vitreous from interfering with lens placement.
    c. Bending the glide to give it a slight upward curvature facilitates its accurate placement over the pupil and iris.

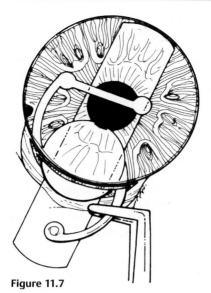

Figure 11.7

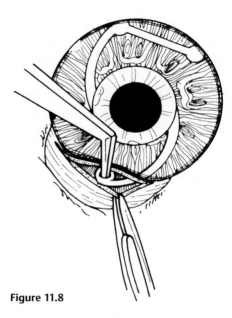

Figure 11.8

16. Place anterior chamber IOL (**Fig. 11.8;** see also **Figs. 10.8C**, p. 50).
    a. Grasp haptic with IOL or McPherson forceps.
    b. Slide lens across anterior chamber into opposite angle.
    c. Stabilize IOL with forceps in left hand before releasing IOL forceps to avoid displacement of lens from angle.
    d. Remove lens glide. (Stabilize superior haptic with forceps to prevent dislocation of the IOL from the inferior angle while removing glide.)
    e. Ensure that the pupil is round without iris tuck.
    f. Retract posterior lip of wound with tissue forceps and place trailing haptic of IOL onto angle.
17. Remove residual viscoelastic with irrigation/aspiration using minimum suction.

18. Perform a peripheral iridectomy if one is not already present (jeweler's forceps, Vannas scissors) (see Chapter 31).
19. Close wound with interrupted 10–0 nylon sutures (e.g., Alcon CU-5 needle).
    a. Sutures should be ~90% wound depth.
    b. Ensure good wound apposition.
    c. Bury knots on scleral side of wound.
20. Check for wound leak by applying gentle point pressure at the wound (cellulose sponges).
21. Reposition conjunctiva and secure with sutures (e.g., 10–0 Vicryl or nylon), or cautery.
22. Perform subconjunctival injections of gentamicin and SoluMedrol.
23. Remove lid speculum.
24. Apply topical combination antibiotic/steroid ointment.
25. Apply patch if not done under topical anesthesia.
26. Place eye shield.

Postoperative Procedure

1. Keep patch (if placed) and shield placed until patient is examined on postoperative day 1.
2. Steroid drops (e.g., Pred Forte 1%) 4 times per day, tapered over ~4 weeks as inflammation warrants.
3. Topical antibiotic 4 times per day for 1 week.
4. Control intraocular pressure rises as needed.
5. Explain postoperative management to patient (see Chapter 6).

Follow-up Schedule

1. Postoperative day 1.
2. Postoperative day 4 or 5 (highest incidence of endophthalmitis onset at this time).
3. Two and 4 weeks postoperatively and then as necessary.

Suture Removal

1. May selectively cut sutures for astigmatism control beginning ~6 weeks postoperatively. (Do this judiciously, as overzealous suture removal may compromise wound and produce overcorrection.)
2. Remove loose, exposed, or infiltrated sutures as they appear.
3. Well-buried, quiet sutures may be kept in place indefinitely.
4. Technique
    a. Give drop of sterile tetracaine or proparacaine and 5% betadine.
    b. Cut suture with scalpel (e.g., #11 Bard-Parker blade or edge of 25 gauge needle).
    c. Remove suture with jeweler's forceps or leave in place if ends are buried.
    d. Give drop of antibiotic and continue 4 times per day for 5 days.

Complications

1. Vitreous incarceration in the wound.
2. Iris tuck by the intraocular lens.
3. Pupillary block by lens or vitreous.
4. Suprachoroidal effusion or hemorrhage.
5. Hyphema.
6. Transient increase in intraocular pressure.
7. Wound leak.
8. Endophthalmitis.
9. Corneal endothelial damage and consequent bullous keratopathy.
10. Retinal detachment.
11. Cystoid macular edema.

■ Posterior Chamber Intraocular Lens Implantation

Indications

■ Monocular aphakia in contact lens intolerant patient in the presence of posterior capsule support or intact anterior capsulorhexis.

■ Selected cases of binocular aphakia in which patient is unable to wear either contact lenses or aphakic spectacles.

■ Patients with macular degeneration may, in particular, benefit from the optical consequences of intraocular lenses (no ring scotoma, less magnification of central scotoma) compared with aphakic spectacle correction.

■ Secondary posterior chamber IOL implantation can be performed via a scleral tunnel or clear cornea approach. Additionally it may be placed in the capsular bag if enough capsular support is available or in the sulcus if the capsule is compromised. For a full discussion of each technique, please see Chapter 8.

Contraindications

■ If inadequate capsular support present, a scleral or iris sutured IOL is indicated (see Sutured Posterior Chamber Intraocular Lens Implantation section later in this chapter).

■ Cystoid macular edema.

■ Active uveitis.

Preoperative Procedure

See Chapter 3.

1. Carefully assess capsular integrity, presence of vitreous in anterior chamber, and zonular dialysis through a well-dilated pupil.
2. Make a preliminary determination of possible in-the-bag or sulcus implantation and choose the IOL powers accordingly. For sulcus implantation, the following general rule is used:
   a. If the planned in-the-bag IOL power is +28.5 D through +30.0 D, subtract 1.50 D power for sulcus implantation.
   b. If the planned in-the-bag IOL power is +17.5 D through +28.0 D, subtract 1.00 D power for sulcus implantation.
   c. If the planned in-the-bag IOL power is +9.5 D through +17.0 D, subtract 0.50 D power for sulcus implantation.
   d. If the planned in-the-bag IOL power is +5.0 D through +9.0 D, no change in IOL power for sulcus implantation is needed.
3. Examine anterior chamber angle with gonioscope to inspect for peripheral anterior synechiae, angle depth, and location of any peripheral iridectomies if an anterior chamber IOL will be needed instead of a posterior chamber IOL (PCIOL).
4. Assess corneal endothelial integrity with careful slit lamp examination, pachymetry, and/or specular microscopy.
5. Examine macula under the slit lamp with a fundus contact lens and/or fluorescein angiography for signs of cystoid macular edema.
6. Determine the need for anterior vitrectomy before lens is implemented. For instance, an eye with an intact hyaloid face and vitreous behind the iris plane may not require vitrectomy. In contrast, an eye with a disrupted hyaloid face and vitreous in the anterior chamber will require an anterior vitrectomy. This will prevent uncontrolled vitreous loss as well as vitreous incarceration by the implant or in the surgical wound. In select cases, a small amount of loose vitreous may be held back by a viscoelastic substance irrigated into the anterior chamber or by a lens glide, obviating vitrectomy.
7. Calculate IOL power: Numerous formulas for calculating IOL power have been derived based on theoretical optics and empirical data. The SRK formula is one of the most widely used.

   SRK Formula: Power of IOL = $A - 2.5(AL) - 0.9(K)$

   where:
   a. A = constant is determined by the manufacturer of a specific lens. A typical value is A = 118.4.
   b. K = average keratometry measurement in diopters.
   c. AL = axial length of eye in millimeters measured with A-scan ultrasonography.

   Note: Set ultrasound unit for aphakic, not cataractous, eye.

8. Optional: Topical NSAID every 15 minutes × three starting 1 hour before surgery to minimize intraoperative miosis.

Instrumentation

■ Honan balloon (optional)
■ Lid (phaco) speculum
■ Castroviejo calipers if using a scleral tunnel incision
■ Fine toothed forceps (e.g., 0. 12 mm straight Castroviejo and/or Colibri)
■ Westcott scissors if using a scleral tunnel incision
■ Cellulose sponges
■ Cautery if using a scleral tunnel incision (underwater eraser or disposable)
■ Scleral incision blade (e.g., Beaver #64, #69) if using a scleral tunnel incision
■ Crescent/tunnel incision blade (e.g., Beaver #38, #48) if using a scleral tunnel incision

- Viscoelastic substance (e.g., Healon, Amvisc, Viscoat, Provisc)
- Fine-Thorton 13-mm fixation ring (optional)
- Keratome (e.g., Beaver #55, diamond or steel, 2.7 mm to 3.2 mm)
- Cystotome
- Utrata forceps
- Cyclodialysis spatula or vitreous sweep
- Kuglen hook
- Straight and angled McPherson tying forceps
- Needle holder
- IOL folder or injector system
- IOL forceps
- Sinskey hook
- Vannas scissors
- Sutures: 10–0 nylon, 10–0 Vicryl, 8–0 Vicryl
- Acetylcholine solution (e.g., Miochol)

Operative Procedure

1. Anesthesia: Topical, peribulbar, or retrobulbar plus lid block, or general. (See Chapter 4.)
   a. Topical: Apply 1 drop of 0.5% tetracaine 15 minutes before surgery and 1 drop before surgery starts.
   b. Optional: 2% Xylocaine gel in inferior fornix 5 minutes before surgery.
2. Optional: Apply Honan balloon for ~10–15 minutes to decompress eye and orbit, minimizing positive vitreous pressure

Note: Honan Balloon are not used for topical anesthetic cases.

3. Prep and drape. A brow tape cut in half to fully cover eyelashes and glands may be preferable to Steri-Strips in certain cases.
4. Place lid (phaco) speculum.
5. Ensure adequate pupillary dilation (prefer pupil diameter of 7 mm or more).
6. Incision techniques
   a. Scleral tunnel technique
      i. Prepare a fornix-based conjunctival peritomy at the limbus using Westcott scissors, tissue forceps; ~9 mm for a one-piece lens; 5 mm for a foldable lens. The peritomy is usually centered around 11 or 1 o'clock on the side of the surgeon's dominant hand.
      ii. Secure hemostasis with wet-field cautery.
      iii. Create self-sealing scleral tunnel:
         A. Use a rounded blade (e.g., #64 or #69 Beaver blade) and 0.12 mm forceps to make a partial (50%) thickness, linear incision vertical and perpendicular to sclera, 2 to 3 mm from limbus (see **Fig. 8.1**, p. 27).
         B. Extend partial thickness groove incision 3.5 mm if a foldable lens is planned and 6.0 mm if a polymethyl methacrylate (PMMA) lens is planned.
         C. Use crescent or tunnel incision blade (e.g., Beaver #38, #48) to construct a scleral tunnel of same depth on to clear cornea. Maintain a surgical plane parallel to the globe by

holding the blade flat against the sclera (e.g., keep blade heel down) (see **Fig. 8.2**, p. 27).
         D. Continue tunnel construction just past anterior limbal vessels.
      iv. Perform a paracentesis through clear cornea adjacent to limbus (see Chapter 7). Place at 10 or 2 o'clock on side of nondominant hand, using a microsurgical knife (e.g., Beaver #75, MVR) (see **Fig. 8.3**, p. 28).
      v. Optional: Inject 1 ml of 1% nonpreserved intracameral lidocaine
      vi. Inject viscoelastic into anterior chamber through paracentesis port.
      vii. Use keratome (2.65 mm to 3.20 mm) to slowly enter anterior chamber at the anterior edge of the scleral tunnel, 0.5 mm anterior to the anterior edge of the vascular arcade, on the side of the dominant hand (see **Fig. 8.4**, p. 28).
   b. Clear cornea technique
      i. Stabilize and fixate the globe using 0.12 forceps or Fine-Thorton 13 mm fixation ring.
      ii. Perform a paracentesis through clear cornea adjacent to limbus using a microsurgical knife (e.g., Beaver #75, MVR) (see **Fig. 7.1**, p. 23, and **Fig. 8.3**, p. 28).
         A. Place at 10 or 2 o'clock on side of nondominant hand if a superior wound is used.
         B. Note: If working from temporal side, place paracentesis site at 7 or 11 o'clock for right eye, or 1 or 5 o'clock for left eye, on side of nondominant hand.
      iii. Optional: Inject 1 ml of 1% nonpreserved intracameral lidocaine for topical cases.
      iv. Inject viscoelastic into anterior chamber through paracentesis port.
      v. Using a keratome, create a clear cornea incision at the desired location (superior or temporal). A triplanar or biplanar incision can be made.
      vi. Techniques may vary depending on the blade manufacturer's specifications.
         A. For a triplanar incision (see **Fig. 8.5**, p. 28):
            I. Make first incision in clear cornea and perpendicular to the cornea plane. Place incision in front of the limbal vessels at a depth of ~250 μm using a keratome. Optional: An initial 3.0 mm groove may be placed at the anterior edge of the vascular arcade. If an initial groove is made, make the next incision by depressing on the posterior edge of the groove with the diamond or steel blade of choice.
            II. Flatten the blade against the surface of the eye.
         B. For a biplanar incision: Use a straight or angled bi-beveled clear cornea blade.
            I. Place tip of blade just in front of the anterior limbal vessels.
            II. Gently press down against the globe, along the heel of the blade so as to engage clear cornea to approximately one half depth with the tip.

III. Push forward, as the eye is stabilized with a cannula safely placed in the paracentesis (or by holding the conjunctiva/sclera with a 0.12). A wiggle motion is usually not necessary.

vii. Construct the second plane of the incision in the corneal stroma parallel to the corneal plane. Drive the point of the blade through the stroma until it is 2 mm central to the external incision. Some blades have line marks on the blade's surface to indicate the 2 mm landmark (see **Fig. 8.5A**, p. 28).

viii. Point tip of the blade down slightly to nick Descemet's membrane.

ix. Reestablish a plane parallel to the stromal plane of the incision and parallel to the iris (see **Fig. 8.5B**, p. 28).

x. Direct the blade toward the anterior apex of the lens and center of the pupil being careful to avoid the lens and iris.

xi. Drive the blade into the anterior chamber to its hub and then come out at the same plane (see **Fig. 8.5A**, p. 28).

xii. Inject more viscoelastic into the bag or sulcus depending where the PCIOL placement is planned. Do not overinflate: use enough viscoelastic to inflate the bag or to separate the posterior iris from the anterior capsular surface for sulcus implantation.

7. Intraocular Lens Implantation: See Chapter 8.

Polymethylmethacrylate (PMMA)

See Chapters 8 and 9 for implantation technique.

Foldable Lenses

- Silicone
- Acrylic
  1. Folding Technique: Many lenses can now be loaded into an injector (see IOL manufacturer's specifications). Alternatively, these lenses can be folded manually.

First-generation acrylic lenses and some first-generation refractive, acrylic lenses may be easier to fold after being slightly warmed (e.g., placed on top of the autoclave or computer monitor, or by irrigating warmed balanced salt solution [BSS] prior to folding).

  a. Use smooth forceps (e.g., angled McPherson) to remove lens from case by haptic. Be careful not to scratch optic, especially if a refractive IOL.

Note: Irrigate acrylic lens with BSS. Do not irrigate silicone lens.

  b. Grasp the lens using holding forceps across the optic with haptics in reverse "S" position (see **Fig. 8.23**, p. 35).
  c. Fold lens slowly in a controlled manner with implant forceps; using downward pressure on the optic will allow the lens to fold (see **Fig. 8.23**, p. 35).
  d. Release the holding forceps while closing the implant forceps (see **Fig. 8.24**, p. 35).

2. Alternate Folding Technique:
  a. Use smooth forceps (e.g., angled McPherson) to remove lens from case by haptic. Be careful not to scratch optic, especially if a refractive IOL.

Note: Irrigate acrylic lens with BSS. Do not irrigate silicone lens.

  b. Place lens on a flat surface (may use lens case on surgical table).
  c. Place folding forceps paddles on opposite sides of optic, parallel with the reverse "S" haptic direction (see **Fig. 8.25**, p. 36).
  d. Maintain pressure against optic edges and lift lens from surface.
  e. Squeeze lens gently, closing folding forceps (see **Fig. 8.26**, p. 36).
  f. Place implant forceps on each side of the folded optic, pushing the superior haptic to the right (see **Fig. 8.27**, p. 36).
  g. Place implant forceps blades on top and parallel to implant forceps.
  h. Remove folding forceps.
  i. Check alignment of folded optic in forceps. A symmetrically folded IOL will fit through a smaller incision than an asymmetric folded one (see **Fig. 8.28**, p. 36).

3. Optional: coat leading edge of lens with viscoelastic. The leading haptic may be tucked into the optic's folded gap.

4. Insert inferior haptic and optic through the incision (scleral tunnel or clear cornea), placing the inferior haptic into the capsular bag (see **Fig. 8.29**, p. 36).

5. Rotate the implant forceps 90 degrees so that optic is perpendicular to posterior capsule (see **Fig. 8.30**, p. 36).

Note: Superior haptic remains outside of wound.

6. Open forceps slowly and remove from eye, allowing lens to unfold (see **Fig. 8.31**, p. 37).
7. Grasp superior haptic with angled McPherson forceps.
8. Push haptic into anterior chamber and pronate hand to flex knee of haptic behind iris, releasing haptic into desired position.
9. Center lens using Sinskey hook.

Sulcus Fixed Lens

Note: A sulcus fixed IOL is inserted for cases with unstable posterior capsular support.

1. Open wound to 0.5 mm larger than optic.
2. Ensure that vitreous is not present in anterior chamber.
3. Inject viscoelastic just under inferior iris, over the anterior leaflets of capsule.
4. Grasp superior portion of PMMA IOL with smooth forceps. If using a foldable lens, refer to **Figs. 8.23–8.29**, pp. 35–36, noting placement will be in sulcus and not in capsular bag.
5. Place inferior haptic into ciliary sulcus, just below the inferior iris.

6. Secure superior haptic with McPherson forceps before releasing IOL to prevent uncontrolled movements.
7. Advance optic into pupil by gently pushing it inferiorly.
8. Place superior haptic.
   a. Grasp with angled McPherson forceps.
   b. Push haptic into anterior chamber.
   c. Pronate hand to flex knee of haptic behind iris.
   d. Release haptic into desired location.
9. Center IOL; spin cautiously if decentered.
10. With the injector system, the trailing haptic can be dialed in with the metal tongue of the injector placed into the anterior chamber during insertion or with a Kuglen or Y hook. Many injector systems do not require the enlargement of the wound.
11. Remove residual viscoelastic with irrigation/aspiration using minimum suction.
12. Close wound with interrupted 10–0 nylon sutures (e.g., Alcon CU-5 needle).
    a. Sutures should be ~90% wound depth.
    b. Ensure good wound apposition.
    c. Bury knots on scleral side of wound.
13. Check for wound leak by applying gentle point pressure at the wound (cellulose sponges).
14. Reposition conjunctiva and secure with sutures (e.g., 10–0 Vicryl or nylon), or cautery if a scleral tunnel incision performed.
15. Perform subconjunctival injections of gentamicin and SoluMedrol.
16. Remove lid speculum.
17. Apply topical combination antibiotic/steroid ointment.
18. Apply patch if not done under topical anesthesia.
19. Place eye shield. Apply clear shield if done under topical anesthesia.

Postoperative Procedure

1. Keep patch (if placed) and shield placed until patient is examined on postoperative day 1.
2. Steroid drops (e.g., Pred Forte 1%) 4 times per day, tapered over ~4 weeks as inflammation warrants.
3. Topical antibiotic 4 times per day for 1 week.
4. Control intraocular pressure rises as needed.
5. Explain postoperative management to patient (see Chapter 6).

Follow-up Schedule

1. Postoperative day 1.
2. Postoperative day 4 or 5 (highest incidence of endophthalmitis onset at this time).
3. Two and 4 weeks postoperatively and then as necessary.

Suture Removal

1. May selectively cut sutures for astigmatism control beginning ~6 weeks postoperatively. (Do this judiciously, as overzealous suture removal may compromise wound and produce overcorrection.)

2. Remove loose, exposed, or infiltrated sutures as they appear.
3. Well-buried, quiet sutures may be kept in place indefinitely.
4. Technique
   a. Give drop of sterile tetracaine or proparacaine and 5% betadine.
   b. Cut suture with scalpel (e.g., #11 Bard-Parker blade or edge of 25 gauge needle).
   c. Remove suture with jeweler's forceps or leave in place if ends are buried.
   d. Give drop of antibiotic and continue 4 times per day for 5 days.

Complications

1. Vitreous incarceration in the wound.
2. Iris tuck by the intraocular lens.
3. Pupillary block by lens or vitreous.
4. Suprachoroidal effusion or hemorrhage.
5. Hyphema.
6. Transient increase in intraocular pressure.
7. Wound leak.
8. Endophthalmitis.
9. Corneal endothelial damage and consequent bullous keratopathy.
10. Retinal detachment.
11. Cystoid macular edema.

■ Sutured Posterior Chamber Intraocular Lens Implantation

Indications

1. Selected cases as part of the primary or secondary cataract surgery if not enough capsular support for a posterior chamber IOL (within capsular bag or sulcus fixated).
2. Select cases of intraocular lens exchange for a dislocated or subluxed IOL.
3. Select cases of eyes with extensive peripheral anterior synechiae or insufficient iris tissue to support an ACIOL.
4. Sutured PCIOLs may be preferable to ACIOLs in certain situations. In either procedure, exercise caution for patients with a history of glaucoma, low corneal endothelial cell counts, chronic uveitis, or chronic cystoid macular edema.

Preoperative Procedure

See Chapter 3.

1. Before surgery, carefully examine patient's sclera for previous or current filtering bleb, scleral ectasia, or conjunctival scarring.

See also Chapter 8 for full discussion on preoperative issues and IOL calculations and power recommendations.

2. Calculate IOL power.
   a. Advances in IOL power calculations continue. Numerous formulas for the calculation of IOL power have been derived based on both theoretical optics and empirical data. The SRK formula is one of the most widely used.
   b. *SRK Formula:* Power of IOL = A − 2.5(AL) − 0.9(K) where
      i. A = constant is determined by the manufacturer of a specific lens. A typical value is A = 118.4.
      ii. K = average keratometry measurement in diopters.
      iii. AL = axial length of eye in millimeters measured with A-scan ultrasonography.
3. Dilate pupil: Tropicamide 1%, phenylephrine 2.5%, and cyclopentolate 1%, every 15 minutes starting 1 hour before surgery.
4. Optional: Topical NSAID (e.g., nepafenac 0.1% [Nevanac, Alcon, Inc., Fort Worth, TX, US], ketorolac tromethamine [Acular, Allergan, Inc., Irvine, CA, US]) 1 drop every 15 minutes × 3 starting 1 hour before surgery (to minimize intraoperative miosis).

Instrumentation

- Honan balloon (optional)
- Eyelid speculum
- Castroviejo calipers
- 8-line or 12-line radial keratotomy marker
- Fine-toothed forceps (e.g., 0. 12 mm straight Castroviejo or Colibri)
- Elschnig forceps (or other nonlocking forceps)
- Westcott scissors
- Cellulose sponges
- Cautery (underwater eraser or disposable)
- Scarifier (Beaver #64, #69)
- Corneoscleral scissors (right and left)
- Microsurgical knife (e.g., Beaver #75, MVR, MicroSharp, Superblade)
- Viscoelastic substance (e.g., Healon, Amvisc, Viscoat)
- Keratome (e.g., Beaver #55, diamond or steel, 2.9 mm to 3.2 mm)
- Vitrectomy set
- Straight and angled McPherson tying forceps
- IOL forceps
- Vannas scissors
- Fine needle holder
- Hook (Sinsky, Kuglen)
- Sutures: 10–0 nylon, 8–0 and 10–0 Vicryl, 8–0 chromic
- 10–0 polypropylene suture on Ethicon CIF-4, Ethicon STC-6, Ethicon TG 160–8. or Ethicon TG-160–6 needle. Ethicon BV-100–4 can be used for iris-sutured PC IOLs
- Alcon pair pack fixation suture
- Acetylcholine solution (e.g., Miochol)
- Choose appropriate PCIOL with eyelets on haptics to aid in suture fixation and large (7 mm) optic to prevent decentration (Pharmacia U152S, Alcon CZ70BD,

or C540MC). Some surgeons use a 6.5 mm optic (e.g., P366UV, Bausch & Lomb Inc.).

Techniques

Numerous techniques are available to suture an IOL into a stable position. The following techniques are classic. Multiple variations or combinations of techniques are described here. Check the literature for long-term studies. Techniques include:

1. Ab Interno Technique
   a. Classic ab interno (two-point fixation)
   b. Classic ab interno (one-point fixation)
   c. Lane technique (to avoid scleral flaps)

2. Ab Externo Technique
   a. Classic ab externo (one-point fixation)
   b. Small incision ab externo
   c. Modified ab externo technique for sutured IOLs

3. Iris-sutured Intraocular Lens Technique

General Considerations

1. The two key issues with any technique are:
   a. Proper positioning and the stability of the lens to avoid lens rotation and therefore induced refractive error.
   b. Suture placement and durability to avoid long-term suture breakage, which can lead to a dislocated IOL, and to avoid postoperative pain from too tight an iris sutured knot.
2. Technique for suturing PCIOL
   a. Lens used is a Bausch & Lomb Model 6190B one-piece, PMMA with optic size 6.50 mm, biconvex, length 12.75 mm, displaying haptics with two midloop eyelets.
   b. Either 50% thickness limbal-based triangular scleral flaps or circumferential 60% thickness scleral incisions are created, centered at the 3 and 9 o'clock positions.
   c. For small pupil: Flexible iris retractors are placed at 2, 4, 8, and 10 o'clock via limbal incisions created with a sharp blade, and the pupil is dilated widely (**Fig. 11.18A**).
   d. If the eye has not previously undergone vitrectomy, a conventional 3-port vitrectomy is done. Peripheral vitreous is dissected meticulously.

Operative Procedure

1. Anesthesia: Peribulbar or retrobulbar plus lid block, or general (see Chapter 4).
2. Optional: Apply Honan balloon for ~10–15 minutes to decompress eye and orbit, minimizing positive vitreous pressure.

3. Prep and drape.
4. Place eyelid speculum.
5. Ensure adequate pupillary dilation (prefer pupil diameter of 7 mm or more).
6. Optional: Use a 8- or 12-line radial keratotomy marker painted with permanent marker or methylene blue to mark the cornea, as this will ensure the transscleral sutures are 180 degrees apart.
7. Prepare fornix-based conjunctival peritomies using Westcott scissors and tissue forceps:
   a. Create a 4 clock hour peritomy from 11 to 3 o'clock.
   b. Create a small peritomy at 8 o'clock.
   c. Optional: may create 3 separate peritomies: one for the 12 o'clock lens incision site, and one each for the 2 and 8 o'clock scleral flap sites.
8. Secure hemostasis with cautery.
9. Create scleral flaps:

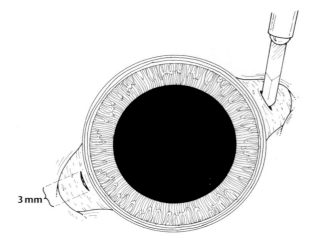

Figure 11.10

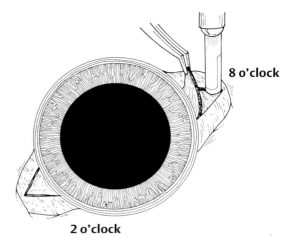

Figure 11.9

a. Perform partial-thickness scleral (triangular or rectangular) flaps at the 8 o'clock and 2 o'clock position (0.12 forceps, #64 or #69 Beaver blade) (**Fig. 11.9**).
   i. Scleral flaps should be ~2 mm by 2 mm in size if rectangular or have a 2 mm base at limbus if triangular.
   ii. **Note:** Avoid the ciliary vessels at 3 and 9 o'clock positions.
b. Alternative: Create scleral grooves instead of flaps:

Make a single vertical groove 3 mm wide and 1 mm posterior to the limbus of 50% thickness at the 8 o'clock and 2 o'clock positions (**Fig. 11.10**).

10. Create incision:
   a. Perform a partial-thickness groove incision at the 12 o'clock limbus (0.12 forceps, #64 or #69 Beaver blade) (see **Fig. 10.2**, p. 48).
      i. Place at posterior limbus
      ii. Chord length of groove should be ~7.0–7.5 mm.
      iii. Make incision perpendicular to tissue, approximately two thirds scleral thickness deep.
   b. Enter anterior chamber with a microsurgical knife; avoid capsule (see **Fig. 10.3**, p. 48).
   c. Extend wound with corneoscleral scissors, angling blades at ~45 degrees to the tissue to create a biplanar incision (see **Fig. 10.4**, p. 49).
11. If necessary, perform bimanual anterior vitrectomy (see Chapter 12).
12. Instill viscoelastic into the anterior chamber.
13. Place intraocular lens.

I. Ab Interno Technique

A. Classic ab interno (two point fixation)
   1. Prepare suture and IOL:
      a. Using a double-armed polypropylene suture with the appropriate needle for the ab interno pass (Ethicon CIF-4, Ethicon STC-6, Ethicon TG-160–6), pass each end through each haptic eyelet.
      b. Tie the suture around the haptic or

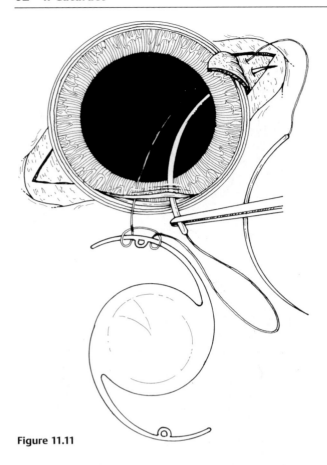

Figure 11.11

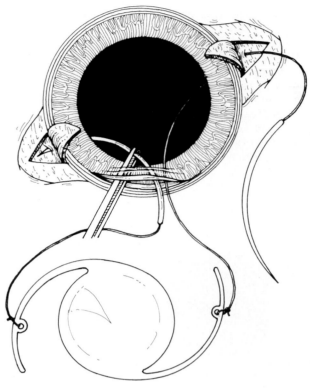

Figure 11.12

pass (Ethicon TG-160–6, Ethicon CIF-4, Ethicon STC-6).

b. Cut a 6-inch double-armed 10–0 polypropylene suture into two equal segments (half).

c. Use a girth hitch to attach the polypropylene suture to the haptic (**Fig. 11.11**).

2. Pass the needle tied to the inferior haptic through the surgical incision, under the iris and aim for the inferior ciliary sulcus at the 8 o'clock position, providing counter pressure on the sclera with 0.12 forceps and exiting 0.75 mm posterior to the limbus (**Fig. 11.11**).

3. Pass the fellow needle of the double-armed suture on a similar path exiting the eye 0.75 mm posterior to the limbus and lateral to the first suture so that the sutures are ~1.0–1.5 mm apart (**Fig. 11.11**).

4. Pass the second set of sutures with short needles (e.g., Ethicon TG 160–8) under the superior iris at 2 o'clock position using counter pressure; each suture should exit ~0.75 mm posterior to the limbus and ~1.0–1.5 mm apart.

5. Carefully secure the IOL into position in the ciliary sulcus with the appropriate amount of suture tension to avoid lens decentration.

6. Tighten and tie the inferior and then the superior sutures with a small 2–1-1 surgeon's knot (see **Fig. 11.18H**).

7. Carefully cut the ends short.

8. Rotate the knots internally if possible.

B. Classic ab interno (one-point fixation)

1. Prepare suture and IOL:

a. Choose the appropriate needle for the ab interno

c. Tie each free end to the eyelet of each haptic using several square knots (**Fig. 11.12**).

2. Pass the needle tied to the inferior haptic through the surgical incision, under the iris and aim for the inferior ciliary sulcus at the 8 o'clock position, providing counter pressure on the sclera with 0.12 forceps, and exit ~0.75 mm posterior to the limbus (**Fig. 11.12**).

3. Pass the second needle for the superior haptic under the superior iris at 2 o'clock position using counter pressure and exit ~0.75 mm posterior to the limbus (**Fig. 11.12**).

4. Use the lens forceps to introduce the IOL into the anterior chamber; the inferior haptic is introduced first.

5. Position the inferior haptic in the inferior ciliary sulcus at the 8 o'clock position while the assistant adjusts the tension of the sutures externally.

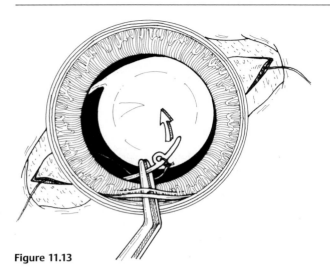

Figure 11.13

6. Place superior haptic:
   a. Grasp with angled McPherson forceps and push haptic into anterior chamber (**Fig. 11.13**).
   b. Pronate hand to flex knee of haptic behind iris (**Fig. 11.13**).
   c. Release haptic into desired position at 2 o'clock periphery (**Fig. 11.13**).

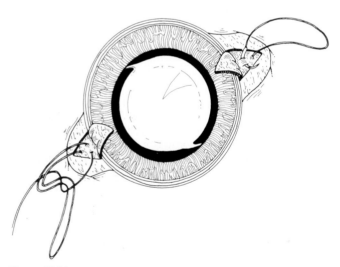

Figure 11.14

7. Tie the suture to itself by passing each needle in the scleral bed to create a loop to be tied to itself (**Fig. 11.14**).
8. Optional: Use a second 10–0 polypropylene suture with a half-circle needle to take a short bite in the 8

o'clock scleral bed just anterior to the exit of the first suture.
   a. Tie the short end of the second suture to the first suture to form the hybrid suture.
   b. Tie the long end of the second suture to the hybrid suture in a 2–1–1 square knot.
9. Remove viscoelastic with irrigation/aspiration instrument using minimum suction.
10. Irrigate Miochol into anterior chamber to constrict pupil.
11. Close superior wound with interrupted 10–0 nylon sutures.
    a. Sutures should be ~90% wound depth
    b. Ensure good wound apposition
    c. Bury knots on scleral side of wound.
12. Check for wound leak by applying gentle point pressure at the wound with cellulose sponges.
13. Close the scleral flaps at their corners using 10–0 nylon or 8–0 Vicryl suture on a spatula needle.
14. Reposition conjunctiva at all sites and secure with sutures (e.g., 10–0 Vicryl or nylon).
15. Perform subconjunctival injections of antibiotic and steroid.
16. Remove eyelid speculum.
17. Apply topical combination antibiotic/steroid ointment.
18. Apply patch and place Fox shield.
C. Lane technique to avoid scleral flaps
   1. Create a 1–2 o'clock hour peritomy at the 2 o'clock and 8 o'clock positions.
   2. Secure hemostasis with cautery.
   3. Create incision:
      a. Perform a partial-thickness groove incision at the 12 o'clock limbus (0.12 forceps, #64 or #69 Beaver blade) (see **Fig. 10.2**, p. 48).
         i. Place at posterior limbus
         ii. Chord length of groove should be ~7 mm– 7.5 mm.
         iii. Make incision perpendicular to tissue, approximately two thirds scleral thickness deep.
      b. Enter anterior chamber with a microsurgical knife; avoid capsule (see **Fig. 10.3**, p. 48).
      c. Extend wound with corneoscleral scissors, angling blades at ~45 degrees to the tissue to create a biplanar incision (see **Fig. 10.4**, p. 49).
   4. If necessary, perform bimanual anterior vitrectomy (see Chapter 12).
   5. Instill viscoelastic into the anterior chamber.
   6. Prepare suture and IOL:
      a. Use a double-armed polypropylene suture with a short needle for the ab interno pass (e.g., Ethicon CIF-4, Ethicon TG-160–6).
      b. Pass a double-armed polypropylene suture through each haptic eyelet.
      c. Optional: Tie the suture around the haptic.
   7. Pass one end of the double-armed polypropylene suture under the iris aiming for the inferior ciliary

sulcus at the 8 o'clock position, providing counter pressure on the sclera with 0.12 forceps and exit ~0.75 mm posterior to the limbus (see **Fig. 11.11**).

8. Pass the other needle of the double-armed suture on a similar path so that it exits 0.75 mm posterior to the limbus at the 8 o'clock position, and 1.0–1.5 mm apart from the other suture (see **Fig. 11.11**).

9. Repeat this for the fixation of the superior haptic. Pass these under the iris, through the superior ciliary sulcus and out through the sclera 0.7 mm posterior to the limbus and 1.0–1.5 mm away from each other.

10. Pass the inferior haptic behind the iris into the ciliary sulcus, while carefully drawing the suture ends through the sclera with tying forceps.

11. Repeat this for the superior haptic, ensuring that the IOL is centered.

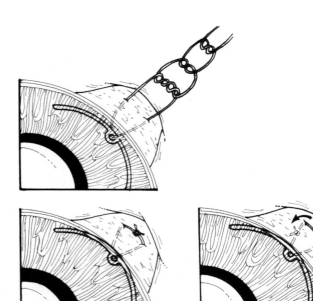

Figure 11.15

12. Tighten and tie the inferior and then the superior sutures with a small 2-1-1 surgeon's knot. Trim the suture ends short (**Fig. 11.15**).

13. Rotate the knots internally (**Fig. 11.15**).

14. Remove viscoelastic with irrigation/aspiration instrument using minimum suction.

15. Irrigate Miochol into anterior chamber to constrict pupil.

16. Close superior wound with interrupted 10–0 nylon sutures.
    a. Sutures should be ~90% wound depth.
    b. Ensure good wound apposition.
    c. Bury knots on scleral side of wound.

17. Check for wound leak by applying gentle point pressure at the wound with cellulose sponges.

18. Reposition conjunctiva at peritomy sites and secure with sutures (e.g., 10–0 Vicryl or nylon).

19. Perform subconjunctival injections of antibiotic and steroid.

20. Remove eyelid speculum.

21. Apply topical combination antibiotic/steroid ointment.

22. Apply patch and place Fox shield.

II. Ab Externo Technique

A. Classic ab externo (one point fixation) (see **Figs. 11.18A–11.18I**)

1. Create scleral flaps (or grooves) and posterior limbal incision (or scleral tunnel) as discussed above (Steps 1–12). (See **Fig. 11.9 and Figs. 10.2–10.4**, pp. 48–49.)

2. Use an appropriate needle with 10–0 polypropylene suture for the ab externo pass (Ethicon STC-6 long straight needle, Alcon Pair Pack Fixation Suture).

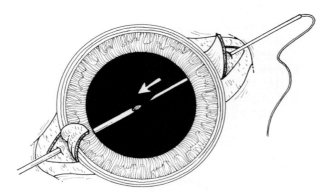

Figure 11.16

3. Pass the long straight needle through the sclera, under the partial thickness scleral flap at the 2 o'clock position ~0.75 mm posterior to the limbus, entering the eye in the superior ciliary sulcus (**Fig. 11.16**).

Note: The needle should be visualized behind the pupil.

4. Pass a 26, 27, or 28 gauge hollow needle, under the partial thickness scleral flap at the 8 o'clock position ~0.75 mm posterior to the limbus, entering the eye in the inferior ciliary sulcus (**Fig. 11.16**).

Note: The tip of the hollow needle should be visualized behind the pupil.

5. Dock the long straight solid needle inside the tip of the hollow needle, and withdraw the hollow needle with the solid needle inside of it, from its entry beneath the 8 o'clock scleral flap (**Fig. 11.16**).

Note: The suture should be visualized crossing eye beneath the pupil.

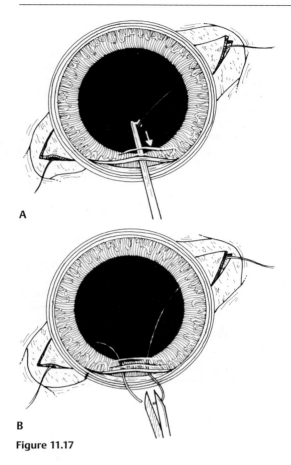

A

B

Figure 11.17

6. Use a Sinskey or Kuglen hook to pull the suture out through the superior surgical wound (**Fig. 11.17A**).
7. Cut the loop of the suture in half (**Fig. 11.17B**).
8. Tie one end to the eyelet of the superior haptic and one end the eyelet of the inferior haptic (see **Fig. 11.12**).
9. Use the lens forceps to introduce the IOL into the anterior chamber; the inferior haptic is introduced first.
10. Position the inferior haptic in the inferior ciliary sulcus at the 8 o'clock position while the assistant adjusts the tension of the sutures externally.
11. Place superior haptic (see **Fig. 11.13**):
    a. Grasp with angled McPherson forceps and push haptic into anterior chamber.
    b. Pronate hand to flex knee of haptic behind iris.
    c. Release haptic into desired position by 2 o'clock periphery.
12. Adjust the tension of the inferior and superior sutures symmetrically.
13. Tie the suture to itself by passing each needle within the scleral bed to create a loop to be tied to itself (see **Fig. 11.14**).
14. Optional: Use a second 10–0 polypropylene suture with a half-circle needle to take a short bite in the 8 o'clock scleral bed just anterior to the exit of the first suture.

a. Tie the short end of the second suture to the first suture to form the hybrid suture.
b. Tie the long end of the second suture to the hybrid suture in a 2–1–1 square knot.
15. Close the scleral tunnel with 10–0 nylon.
16. Close the scleral flaps at their corners using 10–0 nylon or 8–0 Vicryl suture on a spatula needle.
17. Suture the conjunctiva with 10–0 Vicryl or nylon suture.

B. Small incision ab externo
1. Create scleral flaps or grooves as discussed above (Steps 1–9). (See **Fig. 11.9 and Figs. 10.2—10.4**, pp. 48–49.)
2. If necessary, perform bimanual anterior vitrectomy (see Chapter 12).
3. Create a clear corneal incision superiorly using a keratome.
   a. Make first incision in clear cornea and perpendicular to the corneal plane; place incision in front of the limbal vessels at a depth of ~250 μm (e.g., 3 mm keratome).
   b. Flatten the blade against the surface of the eye.
   c. Construct the second plane of the incision in the corneal stroma parallel to the corneal plane.
   d. Drive the point of the blade through the stroma until it is 2 mm central to the external incision.
   e. Point tip of blade down slightly to nick Descemet membrane.
   f. Reestablish a plane parallel to the stromal plane of the incision and parallel to the iris.
   g. Direct the blade toward the center of the pupil, being careful to avoid the iris.
   h. Drive the blade slowly into the anterior chamber to its hub and then come out in the same plane.
4. Instill viscoelastic into the anterior chamber.
5. Use an appropriate needle with 10–0 polypropylene suture for the ab externo pass (Ethicon STC-6 long straight needle, Alcon Pair Pack Fixation Suture) (see **Fig. 11.16**).
6. Pass the long straight needle through the sclera, under the partial thickness scleral flap at the 8 o'clock position ~0.75 mm posterior to the limbus, entering the eye in the superior ciliary sulcus (see **Fig. 11.16**).

Note: The needle should be visualized behind the pupil.

7. Pass a 26, 27, or 28 gauge hollow needle under the partial thickness scleral flap at the 2 o'clock position ~0.75 mm posterior to the limbus, entering the eye in the inferior ciliary sulcus (see **Fig. 11.16**).

Note: The tip of the hollow needle should be visualized behind the pupil.

8. Dock the long straight solid needle inside the tip of the hollow needle, and withdraw the hollow needle with the solid needle inside of it, from its entry beneath the 8 o'clock scleral flap.

Note: The suture should be visualized crossing eye beneath the pupil.

9. Use a Sinskey or Kuglen hook to pull the suture out through the superior surgical wound (see **Fig. 11.17A**).
10. Cut the loop of the suture in half (see **Fig. 11.17B**).
11. Tie one end to the superior haptic and the other end to the inferior haptic of the foldable IOL (see **Fig. 11.12**).
12. Enlarge wound if needed to 4 mm. Otherwise, if using a foldable lens, fold the lens in a standard IOL holder and folder as recommended by the IOL manufacturer (see **Figs. 8.23—8.28**, pp. 35–36, with appropriate text).
13. Place superior haptic (see **Fig. 11.13**):
    a. Grasp with angled McPherson forceps and push haptic into anterior chamber.
    b. Pronate hand to flex knee of haptic behind iris.
    c. Release haptic into desired position at 2 o'clock periphery.
14. Gently pull on the two sutures until the IOL is properly centered with the superior and inferior haptics in the ciliary sulcus at the 2 o'clock and 8 o'clock positions (see **Fig. 11.14**).
15. Tie the suture to itself by passing each needle in the scleral bed to create a loop to be tied to itself (see **Fig. 11.14**).

Optional: Use a second 10–0 polypropylene suture with a half-circle needle to take a short bite in the scleral bed just anterior to the exit of the first suture. Tie the short end of the second suture to the first suture to form the hybrid suture. Tie the long end of the second suture to the hybrid suture in a 2–1–1 square knot.

16. Close the clear corneal wound with 10–0 nylon or 10–0 Vicryl suture.
17. Suture the conjunctiva with 10–0 Vicryl or nylon suture.

C. Modified ab externo technique for sutured IOLs
1. A long 27 gauge bent needle is inserted ab externo 1 mm posterior to the limbus at 3 o'clock and exited at 9:15 o'clock in a ciliary sulcus location (**Fig. 11.18A**).
2. A straight, 16 mm long needle, carrying Ethicon 10–0 polypropylene (Prolene) suture, is swaged blunt end first into the barrel of the 27 gauge needle and maximally advanced (**Fig. 11.18B**).
3. The entire assembly is withdrawn into the vitreous cavity.
4. The entire assembly is directed out of the eye through the ciliary sulcus at 8:45 o'clock (**Fig. 11.18C**).
5. The 27 gauge needle is withdrawn from the eye. This maneuver creates an intraocular loop of 10–0 Prolene suture centered at the 9 o'clock position with two externalized sutures under the scleral flap (**Fig. 11.18D**).

6. A scleral tunnel or partial thickness beveled limbal incision for PCIOL implantation is fashioned at 12 o'clock. If a limbal incision is made, the anterior chamber is entered with a sharp blade at 12 o'clock only (**Fig. 11.18E**).
7. The loop of 10-0 Prolene is externalized through the scleral tunnel using a hook (**Fig. 11.18F**).
8. A long 27 gauge bent needle is inserted ab externo 1 mm posterior to the limbus at 9 o'clock (between the Prolene sutures) and exited at 3:15 o'clock in a ciliary sulcus location. The same steps are followed in the 3 o'clock scleral bed to create the second externalized loop of 10-0 Prolene.
9. The loop is twisted and passed through the eyelet attached to the haptic. The Prolene suture is looped around the haptic without a knot. (**Fig. 11.18G**).
10. The scleral tunnel is widened as needed or the limbal incision is opened fully with a sharp blade to accommodate the IOL.
11. The PCIOL is introduced into the eye; the haptics are seated in the ciliary sulcus, and the lens is centered in the sulcus by pulling up on the externalized sutures (**Fig. 11.18H**).

One can avoid intraocular suture tangles by pulling gently on the externalized sutures under the flaps so the sutures are under mild tension. As the PCIOL is guided into the ciliary sulcus with one hand, the surgeon can use the other hand to pull up further on the free suture ends associated with the haptic that is entering the eye.

12. The externalized sutures are tied and trimmed slightly long so that they lie flat against the sclera. The knots are buried under the scleral flaps, which are sewn shut with 10-0 nylon suture (**Fig. 11.18I**).
13. The scleral tunnel is closed with 10-0 nylon suture; the sclerotomies are closed with 7-0 Vicryl, and the conjunctival incisions are closed with 6-0 plain gut.

III. Iris-Sutured Intraocular Lens Technique

1. The iris-sutured technique generally takes less time than scleral flap techniques. The IOL can be sutured to the iris under local anesthesia with intracameral lidocaine and, for patients on coumadin, usually without significant intraocular bleeding.
2. A three-piece IOL must be used. If placed in the sulcus, one-piece acrylic IOL is known to cause iris chafing at the junction of the IOL haptic and optic and intraocular inflammation, and is thus not used for iris-sutured IOLs. Check with the IOL manufacturer before planned iris suturing of IOL as needed.
3. A foldable or nonfoldable three-piece IOL can be sutured to the iris as part of a routine cataract surgery where there is no longer capsular support, in case of a dislocated IOL, or as a secondary IOL procedure.

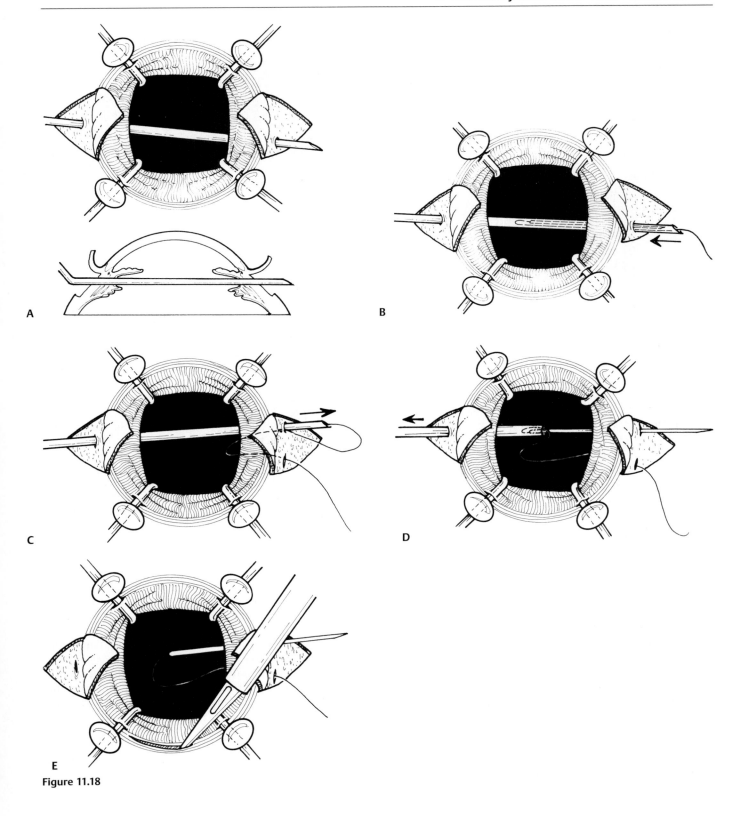

E
Figure 11.18

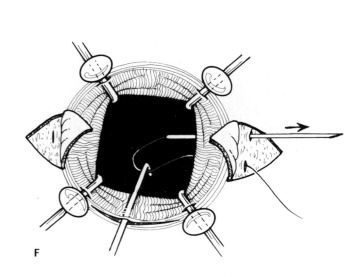

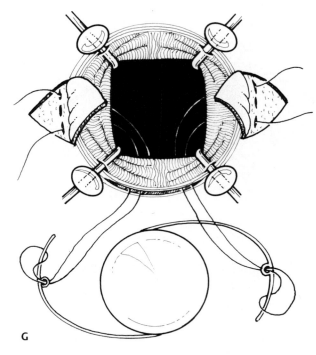

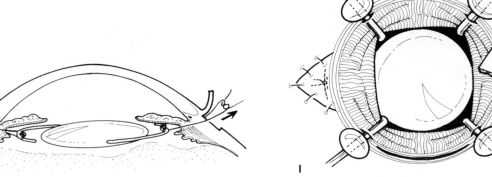

Figure 11.18 *(Continued)*

4. In an atrophic iris, a CIF-4 needle may be preferable to an STC-6 needle as the diameter of the needle is slightly smaller and less likely to cause damage.
5. Procedure:
    a. Anesthesia: Peribulbar is recommended. Topical anesthesia with intracameral lidocaine can be used.
    b. If vitreous is present, perform an anterior vitrectomy (see Chapter 12) before placing the IOL i or suturing the iris.
    c. Prepare suture and IOL: Use an Ethicon CIF-4 or Ethicon STC-6, 10–0 double-armed polypropylene suture. The CIF-4 may be easier to use because of its curvature in most cases.
    d. Place two limbal paracenteses 2 to 3 clock hours from the planned iris suture placement in a convenient position to tie suture ends easily. Place paracentesis on dominant hand side to allow a second instrument (e.g., Y hook or Kuglen hook) to prolapse IOL optic up through pupil (**Fig. 11.19**).
    e. Instill viscoelastic into the anterior chamber through paracentesis port.
    f. Inject Miochol into anterior chamber to constrict pupil before placing the suture.
    g. Place IOL haptics into sulcus, being careful to keep IOL optic above pupillary plane if there is no posterior capsular support.
    h. Use second instrument through paracentesis to lift IOL optic up at its haptic junction to allow the haptic to tent up the iris. This allows visualization of where the iris suture is to be passed.

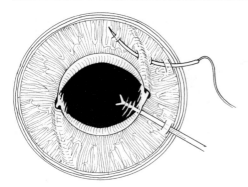

Figure 11.19

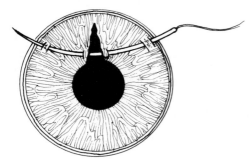

Figure 11.20

i. Pass 10–0 polypropylene suture through the paracentesis, into iris on proximal side of haptic, under haptic, and then up through distal side of iris and out through the opposite peripheral clear cornea (**Figs. 11.19 and 11.20**).
j. Cut the needle off.
k. Introduce Kuglen hook through paracentesis and engage a loop of suture.

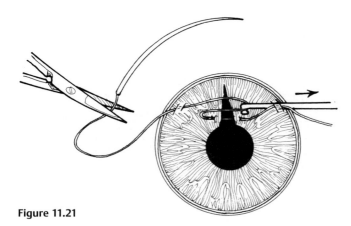

Figure 11.21

l. Retract Kuglen hook through paracentesis, while holding opposite suture end with tying forceps (**Fig. 11.21**).

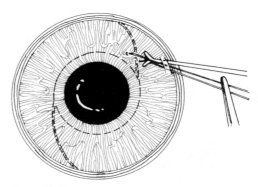

Figure 11.22

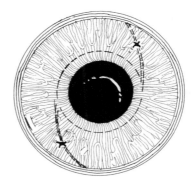

Figure 11.23

m. Pull iris to wound and tie the suture securely with four throws (3–1–1–1) or (1–1–1–1). Avoid making ties too tight as it can cause sutures to break or potential postoperative pain (**Figs. 11.22 and 11.23**).
n. **Note:** If the iris is not flaccid enough to allow the knot to tie outside the paracentesis, may make suture loops inside the anterior chamber and slide knot down to iris plane with a Y hook (**Fig. 11.22**).
o. After knot is tightened, cut suture ends short by drawing knot through wound (**Fig. 11.23**).
    (Also see **Figs. 11.24 and 11.25**.)
p. Alternatively, the surgeon may introduce a sharp knife (e.g., Wheeler blade) through paracentesis to cut suture ends without putting traction on iris.
q. Hydrate the paracentesis with balanced salt solution and check integrity; place interrupted 10–0 nylon suture if necessary.
r. Remove viscoelastic with irrigation/aspiration instrument using minimum suction.
s. Close superior wound if created and needed with interrupted 10–0 nylon sutures.
    i. Sutures should be ~90% wound depth.
    ii. Ensure good wound apposition.
    iii. Bury knots on scleral side of wound.
t. Perform subconjunctival injections of antibiotic and steroid.
u. Remove eyelid speculum.
v. Apply topical combination antibiotic/steroid ointment.
w. Apply patch and place Fox shield.

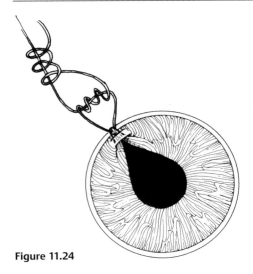

Figure 11.24

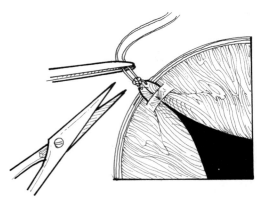

Figure 11.25

Postoperative Procedure

Also see Chapter 8 for postoperative procedure.

1. Keep patch (if placed) and shield in place until patient is examined on postoperative day 1.
2. Steroid drops (e.g., Pred Forte 1%) 4 times per day, tapered over ~4–6 weeks as inflammation warrants.

3. Topical antibiotics (e.g., moxifloxacin 0.5% [Alcon, Inc.], gatifloxacin 0.3% [Allergan, Inc.]) 4 times per day for 1 week.
4. Control intraocular pressure rises with β blockers (e.g., Timoptic) or carbonic anhydrase inhibitors.
5. Avoid using prostaglandin analogs in the immediate postoperative period to avoid medication-induced iritis or cystoid macular edema.
6. Explain postoperative management to patient (see Chapter 6).
7. Follow-up schedule:
   a. Postoperative day 1.
   b. Postoperative day 4 or 5 (highest incidence of endophthalmitis onset at this time).
   c. Two, 4, and 6 weeks postoperatively and then as necessary.

Complications

1. Hyphema
2. Vitreous hemorrhage
3. Corneal endothelial damage and consequent bullous keratopathy
4. Suprachoroidal effusion or hemorrhage
5. Suture exposure and endophthalmitis
6. Increased risk of retinal detachment, choroidal hemorrhage
7. Cystoid macular edema
8. Glaucoma
9. Lens dislocation
10. Uveitis
11. Induced astigmatism from lens tilt
12. Postoperative pain

12

Anterior Segment Vitrectomy Procedures

Indications

This chapter will review several anterior segment vitrectomy procedures that use anterior and posterior segment instrumentation, including management of (1) vitreous loss at cataract surgery, (2) late complications of vitreous in the anterior chamber, (3) inadequate pupillary space, (4) lens surgery, (5) hyphema, and (6) epithelium in the anterior chamber.

General Principles

- Incision site: Limbus versus pars plana.
  - Choose limbal approach if mechanical objectives or problems are anterior to the pars plana; this approach has less risk of retinal damage (because of vitreous incarceration in the pars plana sclerotomy site, with secondary vitreoretinal traction and retinal tear formation).
  - A pars plana approach offers better access to retroiridal space (e.g., for lysis of iridovitreal adhesions), use of intraocular illumination, and access to the posterior two thirds of the vitreous cavity.
- Tissue engagement in the vitrectomy probe. Stiff tissue is best incarcerated and cut with the vitrectomy machine set to low cutting rate (e.g., 100–300 cpm) and high vacuum (e.g., 200–300 mm Hg), as these settings enable greater molding of the tissue to the cutting port (**Table 12.1**). If vacuum is high, infusion pressure must be increased to prevent globe collapse.

Table 12.1 Tissue Engagement in the Vitrectomy Probe

Tissue Engagement	Stiff	Soft
Port Size	Large	Small
Cutting Rate	Slow	Fast
Infusion Pressure	High	Low
Vacuum	High	Low

- Cutting mechanism: Guillotine versus rotary cutting. New rotary cutters offer highly efficient vitreous removal. Guillotine cutters may provide more effective cutting of stiff tissue without inducing traction on the tissue.
- Techniques for cutting stiff tissue:

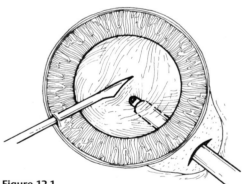

Figure 12.1

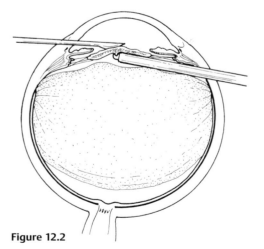

Figure 12.2

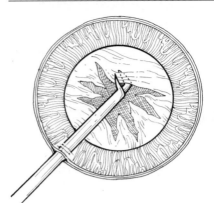

Figure 12.3

- ❏ Chopping block (**Figs. 12.1 and 12.2**).
- ❏ Intraocular scissors (**Fig. 12.3**).
- ❏ Diathermy.
- ■ Management of bleeding
  - ❏ Increase intraocular pressure by increasing the infusion pressure, as vitrectomy incisions are watertight (a hydraulically closed system).
  - ❏ Diathermy.
- ■ Vitrectomy via limbal incisions (e.g., management of vitreous loss at cataract surgery).
  - ❏ Excise enough vitreous to prevent vitreous prolapse into the anterior chamber (anterior to the plane of the iris diaphragm).
  - ❏ Excise vitreous along pupillary-axis: direct probe into center of pupillary space.
  - ❏ Work in anterior one third vitreous cavity: place probe just posterior to iris diaphragm with cutting port in clear view at all times. (Operating microscope does not permit focus on probe tip if it is advanced deeper than anterior ~1/3 of vitreous cavity unless special lenses are used.)
  - ❏ Infusion: Sleeve versus second instrument.
    - ■ Infusion sleeve offers simultaneous fluid infusion and vitreous removal through a single incision. However, the incision is somewhat large (to accommodate the sleeve), and the infusion is directed at the probe tip, which may impair efficient incarceration of vitreous into the probe.
    - ■ Second instrument offers bimanual capabilities (e.g., displacement of iris peripherally to visualize residual peripheral lens cortex) but requires a second entry site. Usually this limbal site has already been created during the cataract surgery.
  - ❏ Illumination: fiber optic probe versus coaxial illumination of the operating microscope.
    - ■ Fiber optic probe can be used externally (probe placement at limbus with visualization by scleral scatter) or internally (through a separate incision). Fiber optic probe probably offers better visualization of vitreous strands in the anterior chamber and better visualization of the anterior vitreous cavity than coaxial illumination of the scope.

- ■ Coaxial illumination of the operating microscope avoids need for second instrument in the eye but offers more limited view of vitreous cavity and vitreous prolapse into the anterior chamber.
- ■ Instrument removal: Steps to avoid vitreous prolapse into anterior chamber and limbal incision.
  - ❏ Lower intraocular pressure.

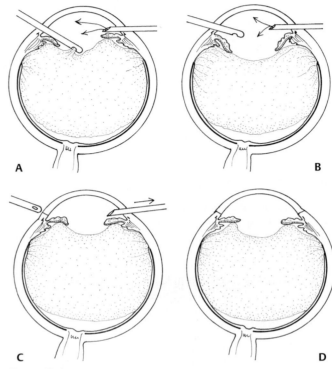

Figure 12.4

- ❏ Some surgeons infuse air to prevent vitreous incarceration in wounds (**Figs. 12.4A,B**).
- ❏ Withdraw instruments (**Figs. 12.4C,D**).
- ❏ If air has been infused, replace air with balanced salt solution.

Preoperative Procedure

See Chapter 3.

Pupil management: For procedures requiring good visualization behind the iris (e.g., excision of retained peripheral lens cortex) dilate the pupil preoperatively (e.g., Cyclogyl 1% plus phenylephrine 2.5% every 15 minutes × 3, starting 1 hour before surgery) or use flexible iris retractors intraoperatively. In other cases (e.g., anterior vitrectomy preceding placement of a secondary intraocular lens [IOL]), dilation may be unnecessary.

Instrumentation

- Lid speculum
- Vitrectomy suction/cutting instrumentation. In this chapter, the Alcon Accurus vitrectomy machine (Alcon, Inc., Fort Worth, TX, US) is used for illustrative purposes. The authors recognize that other excellent machines are available and have no financial interest in the Accurus system.
- Sutures (10–0 nylon, 7–0, 8–0 Vicryl, 6–0 plain gut)
- Fine-toothed tissue forceps (e.g., 0.12 mm straight Castroviejo or Colibri)
- Needle holder
- Lens loop
- 23 gauge butterfly infusion needle or cannula
- Acetylcholine solution (e.g., Miochol)
- Cyclodialysis spatula or vitreous sweep
- Tuberculin syringe with 30 gauge cannula
- Cellulose sponges
- Jeweler's forceps
- Vannas scissors
- Westcott scissors
- Cautery (underwater eraser or disposable)
- Microsurgical knife (e.g., Beaver #75M blade)
- 20-gauge microvitreoretinal (MVR) blade
- Gills-Vannas or 20 gauge vitreous scissors
- 20 gauge intraocular forceps

Operative Procedure

Managing Vitreous Loss at Cataract Surgery

At the time of posterior capsule or zonular rupture, the extent of capsular damage and the presence or absence of vitreous loss must be assessed. In select cases demonstrating adequate capsular support, a posterior chamber intraocular lens (PCIOL) can be fixated in the ciliary sulcus. Removal of prolapsed vitreous with automated instruments permits complete vitreous excision from the anterior chamber while minimizing vitreoretinal traction, compared with vitreous removal from the anterior chamber using cellulose sponges and scissors to directly cut the vitreous strands. Following is a description of the management of an eye with significant operative capsular disruption and vitreous loss.

1. Take measures to limit extent of loss of vitreous.
   a. If a posterior rent is noted and it is unclear if vitreous has moved forward, gently inject viscoelastic into capsular bag through paracentesis site before removing phaco tip or allowing anterior chamber to shallow.
   b. Loosen the bridle sutures and inspect for any other external source of positive vitreous pressure (e.g., lid speculum).
   c. Examine for any ocular source of positive vitreous pressure (e.g., choroidal effusion or hemorrhage, retrobulbar hemorrhage).
2. If the lens nucleus remains in situ, use viscoelastic to "trap" nuclear remnants in anterior chamber. Use a lens loop to remove it (avoid posterior vitreous pressure and further vitreous loss). Low-flow phacoemulsification

may be used to remove the remaining nucleus if there is no vitreous and depending on the size of the nuclear remnant and the size of the capsular tear. A Sheets glide placed under "trapped" fragments may be useful.

3. If the wound is not a self-sealing corneal incision, close with interrupted sutures (e.g., 10–0 nylon) leaving spaces (~2 to 3 mm) to place vitrectomy instruments.
   a. A securely closed anterior chamber will minimize infusion rate necessary to maintain anterior chamber and facilitate control of anterior chamber depth.
   b. Alternatively, anterior vitrectomy may be performed using an open-sky technique through the unsutured limbal incision without infusion.

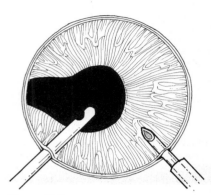

Figure 12.5

4. Keep anterior chamber formed during vitrectomy with infusion needle. Use 23 gauge butterfly on cannula for infusion when using a bimanual technique. **Figure 12.5** shows cannula placement to limit AC entry of needle) (**Fig. 12.5**).

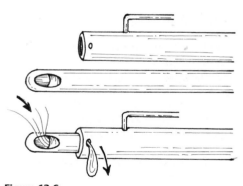

Figure 12.6

Alternatively, an infusion sleeve may be placed directly over the vitrectomy probe. This approach has the disadvantage of greater wound distortion (sleeve adds bulk) and the tendency of fluid currents directed at probe tip to hinder efficient incarceration of vitreous at the cutting port. Many surgeons prefer a separate irrigation port for this reason (**Fig. 12.6**).

5. Place vitrectomy probe into anterior chamber.
   a. Start irrigation before placement to prevent loss of anterior chamber volume.

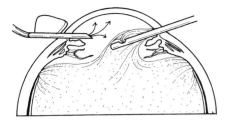

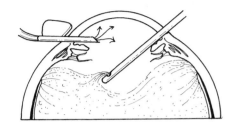

Figure 12.8

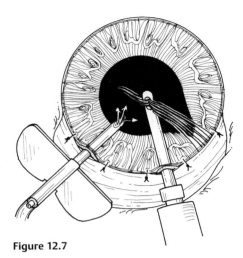

Figure 12.7

b. Always observe position of the infusion cannula and vitrectomy probe to avoid trauma to the corneal endothelium (**Fig. 12.7**).
c. Keep instrument tip near center of pupil. (Do not make abrupt movements with probe.)
d. Cutting rate, vacuum, and infusion pressure settings: Alcon provides different vitrectomy probes that have different cutting rates and different mechanisms of action. For example, the Accurus 800 and 2500 probes have guillotine action, and the InnoVit probe has rotary action. The settings outlined below are just suggestions. Different surgeons prefer different settings.
   i. Accurus 800 probe: cutting rate 800 cpm, vacuum 150 mm Hg, infusion pressure 25–35 mm Hg.
   ii. InnoVit probe: cutting rate 1200 cpm, vacuum 75–125 mm Hg, infusion pressure 35 mm Hg.
   iii. Accurus 2500 probe: cutting rate 2500 cpm, vacuum 75–150, infusion pressure 35 mm Hg.
e. To avoid iris damage, turn the cutting port so that it faces posteriorly and try to avoid high vacuum, as it may inadvertently incarcerate iris in vitrectomy probe.
f. The iris should fall back posteriorly when adequate vitrectomy is complete.
6. Remove any residual cortical and unneeded capsular material.
   a. Aspirate cortex and cut as necessary. Most cortex can be removed with aspiration alone. The cutting mechanism should be activated only with the cutting port in clear view to reduce the risk of creating a tear in the posterior capsule.
   b. Cutting rate (if necessary): Approximately 150–300 cpm.
   c. Vacuum: 100–180 mm Hg and adjust as necessary.

d. May feed capsular flaps into vitrectomy probe using infusion needle (**Fig. 12.8**).
7. Remove instruments from eye.
   a. Use the tips of the two instruments to sweep any adherent vitreous from each other before removal.
   b. Remove vitrectomy probe before irrigation needle.
8. Irrigate anterior chamber with acetylcholine solution to constrict pupil.

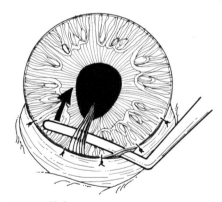

Figure 12.9

9. Examine anterior chamber for any vitreous as evidenced by peaking of the pupil (**Fig. 12.9**).
10. Sweep wound with a vitreous sweep in all areas of suspected vitreous incarceration.
    a. Enter anterior chamber ~90 degrees from suspected vitreous strand.
    b. Place tip into angle and rotate centrally toward pupil.
    c. Observe pupil for any movement during sweep, indicating overriding vitreous strands in this area.
    d. Any pupil peaking should be remedied by this maneuver as vitreous strands are swept from the wound.

e. Sometimes illumination of the anterior chamber with a fiber optic endoilluminator and scleral scatter will reveal vitreous strands in the anterior chamber.

11. Perform additional vitrectomy if anterior chamber is not free of all vitreous or positive vitreous pressure remains present.

12. Consider performing peripheral iridectomy (jeweler's forceps and Vannas scissors or just use the vitrectomy probe).

13. Check wound with dry cellulose sponge for any further evidence of vitreous at wound.

14. When the anterior vitrectomy is complete, the anterior chamber should be clear of vitreous and pupil should be round (**Fig. 12.10A**).

If vitreous prolapses through the limbal wound (**Figs. 12.10B and 12.10C**), a scleral flap may be used to tamponade site (**Figs. 12.10D–12.10F**).

a. Elevate half-thickness of scleral flap after prolapsed vitreous is cut (**Fig. 12.10D**).

b. Close flap anteriorly to cover fistula (**Figs. 12.10E and 12.10F**).

15. Close wound completely with interrupted 10–0 nylon sutures. Optional: Remove 7–0 Vicryl sutures placed earlier in procedure.

16. Complete the procedure as described in Chapter 9.

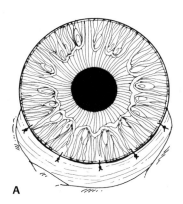

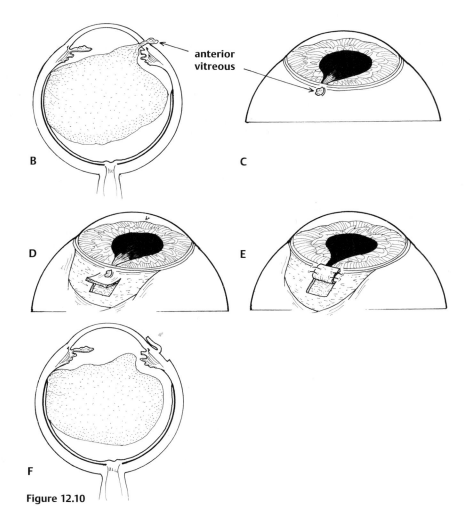

anterior vitreous

Figure 12.10

Secondary Vitrectomy for Treatment of Late Anterior Segment Vitreous Complications

Vitreous in the anterior segment, whether postsurgical or posttraumatic, may cause complications such as corneal endothelial decompensation involving the visual axis, aphakic pupillary block glaucoma (unresponsive to laser iridotomy), a persistent filtering cicatrix (vitreous wick syndrome), and chronic cystoid macular edema (secondary to vitreous incarceration in the wound or iridovitreal adhesions). The following will focus on anterior vitrectomy through a limbal approach. For select cases, a pars plana approach may be preferable.

1. Anesthesia: General or retrobulbar plus lid block.
2. Prep and drape. Adhesive-backed plastic efficiently keeps lashes out of surgical field. If there is a concern about patient head movement under local anesthesia, consider taping the patient's head to the stretcher.
3. Place lid speculum.
4. Prepare fornix-based peritomies at 2 and 10 o'clock, each measuring ~4 mm (Westcott scissors, 0.12 mm forceps).
5. Secure hemostasis with cautery.
6. Enter anterior chamber at each of the two sites (MVR blade).
   a. Entry can be at the limbus or 3 mm posterior to the limbus through the pars plana.

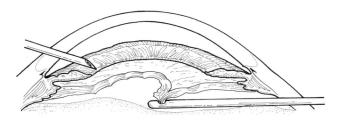

Figure 12.11

   b. A pars plana approach probably permits more effective access to the retroiridal space and more efficient lysis of iridovitreal adhesions, as adhesions are often present peripheral to the pupillary margin (**Fig. 12.11**).

A pars plana approach requires placement of an infusion cannula inferotemporally, 3 mm posterior to the limbus or the use of an infusing light pipe. (See Chapter 63.)

7. Place a 23 gauge butterfly infusion needle through one entry site and start irrigation to maintain the anterior chamber. Alternatively, an infusion sleeve may be placed on the vitrectomy instrument.

For pars plana approach, place pars plana infusion cannula or use an infusing light pipe as described in Chapter 63.

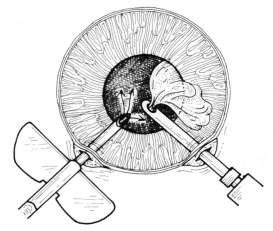

Figure 12.12

8. Place vitrectomy probe into anterior chamber (**Fig. 12.12**).
9. Perform anterior vitrectomy.
   a. Cutting rate and vacuum:
      i. Accurus 800 probe: Cutting rate 800 cpm, vacuum 75–100 mm Hg, infusion pressure 25–35 mm Hg.
      ii. InnoVit probe: Cutting rate 1000 cpm, vacuum 75–100 mm Hg, infusion pressure 35 mm Hg.
      iii. Accurus 2500 probe: Cutting rate 2500 cpm, vacuum 75–100, infusion pressure 35 mm Hg.
   b. If a pars plana approach is used, hold the probe 2–3 mm posterior to the iris diaphragm, activate vacuum and cutting, and slowly sweep the probe behind the iris with the port rotated away from the iris diaphragm toward the pupillary space (to avoid inadvertent iridectomy). If the iris leaflets move during this maneuver, peripheral iridovitreal adhesions probably are present. When the anterior vitrectomy is complete, this sweeping motion will not disturb the iris. The maneuver should be completed with the probe introduced through both the temporal and nasal incisions.
   c. If membranous tissue is to be removed with vitrectomy probe, increase vacuum (~180–300 mm Hg) and decrease cutting rate (~100–300 cpm) to incarcerate firm material into vitrector port. Keep vitrectomy port in view at all times when working at these settings to avoid creating peripheral vitreoretinal traction.
   d. Remove equipment from eye.
      i. Use the tips of the two instruments to sweep any adherent vitreous from each other.
      ii. Remove vitrectomy probe first, then remove irrigation cannula.
   e. Irrigate anterior chamber with Miochol to constrict pupil
   f. Examine anterior chamber for any vitreous as suggested by peaking of pupil or scleral scatter with fiber optic probe.
   g. Sweep the anterior chamber with a vitreous sweep to free any vitreous incarcerated in the wound.
   h. Perform additional vitrectomy if necessary until vitreous is neither in the anterior chamber nor incarcerated in the wound, and the iris has fallen back posteriorly.

i. Close limbal wound with interrupted 10–0 nylon sutures (use 7–0 Vicryl for sclerotomies).
j. Inject subconjunctival cefazolin (100 mg) and Decadron (4–8 mg). If patient is allergic to penicillin, consider using vancomycin (50 mg).
k. Remove lid speculum.
l. Apply topical antibiotic and steroid ointments.
m. Apply patch and place Fox shield.

Inadequate Pupillary Space

Membranous cataract, occluded or updrawn pupil, and retained lens material obstructing the pupillary space can be treated with anterior segment vitrectomy techniques. The objective is to clear the visual axis. A limbal approach is preferred.

1. Prepare the eye and entry sites and place the vitrectomy and irrigation probes as described above (Steps 1–8, Managing Vitreous Loss at Cataract Surgery, earlier in this chapter).
2. Set the initial vitrectomy parameters for membrane and lens removal and adjust as necessary.
   a. Cutting rate: Approximately 100–300 cpm.
   b. Vacuum: Approximately 150–230 mm Hg.
3. Several maneuvers may facilitate removal of the abnormal material.
   a. The irrigating needle may be used to present tissue to the vitrectomy probe.
   b. A dense membrane may first be sectioned to form edges, which can be incarcerated in the vitrectomy port and cut (irrigation needle, Gills or Vannas scissors, 20 gauge intraocular scissors, or MVR blade).
4. After the membrane and/or lens material has been excised adequately, perform an anterior vitrectomy as described above in steps 1–17 above (see Managing Vitreous Loss at Cataract Surgery section earlier in this chapter).

Lens Surgery with Use of Vitrectomy Instruments in the Anterior Chamber

Clinical settings in which surgeons may prefer to excise lens material using vitrectomy instrumentation include congenital or juvenile cataract, subluxed, disrupted lens, complicated cataract (e.g., traumatic cataract with lens and vitreous admixed), and microcornea or compromised corneal endothelium. Types of congenital or juvenile cataract that can be removed readily via vitrectomy instrumentation include anterior polar, lamellar, or nuclear cataract; posterior lentiglobus; persistent hyperplastic primary vitreous (PHPV); and total cataract (rubella, trauma, metabolic, etc.). The indications for surgery include prevention of amblyopia, improvement of vision, and prevention of glaucoma or phthisis. A limbal approach is probably safer for most cases (particularly if the surgeon is not highly skilled at examining the peripheral retina), because the pars plana is small in most of these eyes, and the instruments are likely to pass close to or through the vitreous base. Visual results depend on timing of cataract onset and intervention, postoperative optical correction or occlusion, and associated pathology (e.g., foveal hypoplasia in PHPV).

1. Congenital, juvenile cataract.
   a. Surgical technique (limbal approach).
   b. Prepare the eye and entry sites and place the vitrectomy and irrigation probes as described above (see Steps 1–8, Managing Vitreous Loss at Cataract Surgery, earlier in this chapter).
   c. Set the initial vitrectomy parameters for membrane and lens removal and adjust as necessary.
      i. Cutting rate: Approximately 100–300 cpm. In patients of this age, much of the lens material can be removed with aspiration alone. Activation of the cutting mechanism should be done only with the cutting port in clear view to reduce the risk of creating an unplanned tear in the posterior capsule.
      ii. Vacuum: Approximately 150–300 mm Hg.
   d. Remove cortex and nucleus. To facilitate removal of lens material, the irrigating needle may be used to present lens material to the vitrectomy probe.
   e. Excise central anterior and posterior capsule. If the patient is able to sit at a slit lamp cooperatively, the surgeon can defer the capsulotomy and anterior vitrectomy (see below) and plan to perform Nd:YAG capsulotomy after surgery at an appropriate time.
   f. Limited anterior vitrectomy (no vitreous to wound!).
   g. No peripheral iridectomy.
   h. Consider placement of IOL, depending on patient's age.
   i. Complications:
      i. Early: infection, corneal decompensation, intraocular hemorrhage.
      ii. Late: amblyopia, glaucoma, secondary membrane, macular edema, retinal detachment.
2. Persistent hyperplastic primary vitreous.
   a. Surgical technique: Limbal approach, as pars plana may be quite small (or not exist), and the retina may be drawn anteriorly over the ciliary processes.
   b. Follow steps 1a–1e.
   c. Incise retrolenticular membrane and anterior vitreous.
   d. Apply diathermy to persistent hyaloid vessels.
   e. Follow steps 1f–1g.
   f. At the time of instrument removal, some surgeons prefer to infuse air into the anterior chamber to reduce the chance of vitreous incarceration in the wounds.
3. Traumatic cataract surgery
   a. Approach
      i. Limbal: If posterior capsule intact and lens material is soft.
      ii. Pars plana: If posterior capsule ruptured or lens material is hard (e.g., older patient).
   b. Indications
      i. Lens extraction as a primary procedure: lens is opaque; lens fibers are flocculent.
      ii. Lens extraction as a secondary procedure: small rupture in anterior or posterior capsule is present; exam is inconclusive.
   c. Surgical objectives
      i. Close wound.
      ii. Clear visual axis.

iii. Prevent adherent leukoma, synechiae and secondary glaucoma, updrawn pupil, membranous cataract, vitreoretinal traction, macular edema.

d. Surgical technique: Limbal approach.

   i. Anesthesia: General. (Retrobulbar anesthesia not
advisable with open globe but can be done if cir-
cumstances mandate.)

   ii. Prep and drape. Adhesive-backed plastic efficiently
keeps lashes out of surgical field. Care must be ex-
ercised so as not to apply pressure to open globe.

   iii. Place lid speculum. Self-retaining speculum (e.g.,
Maumenee-Park) may transmit less pressure to
open globe.

   iv. Close corneal wound with 10–0 nylon suture. Close
scleral wound with 8–0 black silk posterior to the
limbus. Posterior to the muscle insertion, consider
using 6–0 black silk suture.

   v. Enter anterior chamber at 2 and 10 o'clock (20
gauge MVR blade).

   vi. Place a 23 gauge butterfly infusion needle through
one entry site and start irrigation to maintain
formed anterior chamber.

   vii. Introduce vitrectomy probe into anterior chamber.

   viii. Clear posterior corneal surface (remove adherent
vitreous, blood, necrotic tissue).

   ix. Necrotic tissue can be manipulated off cornea and
into vitrectomy probe with infusion needle.

   x. Vitrectomy settings:

     A. Accurus 800 probe: cutting rate 800 cpm, vac-
uum 75–100 mm Hg, infusion pressure 25–35
mm Hg.

     B. InnoVit probe: cutting rate 1000 cpm, vacuum
75–100 mm Hg, infusion pressure 35 mm Hg.

     C. Accurus 2500 probe: cutting rate 2500 cpm,
vacuum 75–100, infusion pressure 35 mm Hg.

   xi. Excise lens material.

     A. First remove vitreous from anterior chamber
and, if posterior capsule is ruptured, anterior
vitreous cavity with vitrectomy probe.

     B. Sometimes lens material can be removed with
the vitrectomy probe. If nucleus is hard, use
phacoemulsification.

     C. Aspirate peripheral cortex centrally.

     D. Leave posterior capsule if intact. If capsule
ruptured, excise vitreous with limited anterior
vitrectomy. In some cases, anterior capsular
rupture is small enough to permit anterior capsular support of a sulcus-fixated PCIOL, even if
the posterior capsule is ruptured.

   xii. Infuse air bubble (optional).

   xiii. Place IOL, if appropriate.

   xiv. Perform peripheral iridectomy with vitrectomy
probe (vacuum 50–150 mm Hg, cutting 800–2500
cpm).

4. Membranous cataract: Surgical technique.

a. Limbal approach: see Steps 3.d.i–vi.

b. Lyse posterior synechiae (with MVR blade or with intraocular vertical and horizontal scissors).

c. Lyse corneal attachments using Sinskey hook, retinal
pick, MVR blade, or intraocular forceps and scissors.

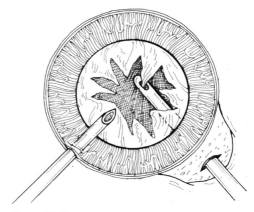

Figure 12.13

d. Incise membrane with an MVR blade or intraocular
scissors. It may be necessary to divide the fibrous tissue into wedge-shaped pieces to facilitate incarceration into the vitrectomy probe for proper cutting with
the guillotine mechanism (**Fig. 12.13**).

e. Extract incised tissue with vitrectomy probe (using
relatively slow cutting rate [e.g., 300 cpm] and relatively high vacuum [e.g., 300 mm Hg]).

f. Perform anterior vitrectomy, removing anterior ~1/4–
1/3 of vitreous gel.

Postoperative Procedure

1. Keep patch and shield placed until patient is examined
on postoperative day 1.

2. Steroid drops (e.g., prednisolone acetate 1%) as degree of
inflammation warrants.

3. Topical antibiotics (e.g., moxifloxacin 0.5% [Alcon, Inc.],
gatifloxacin 0.3% [Allergan, Inc., Irvine, CA, US]) 4 times
per day.

4. Scopolamine 0.25% or atropine 1% drops twice per day.

5. Control intraocular pressure with a topical β-adrenergic
antagonist (e.g., timolol), α-adrenergic agonist (e.g., brimonidine tartrate 0.2%), and carbonic anhydrase inhibitors (e.g., dorzolamide) as necessary.

6. Discharge patient when stable.

Complications

1. Transient increase in intraocular pressure.

2. Hyphema.

3. Persistent inflammation with synechia formation and
fibrotic changes in the anterior segment.

4. Vitreous strands remaining incarcerated in wound.

5. Cystoid macular edema.

6. Retinal tear or detachment.

7. Endophthalmitis.

8. Choroidal hemorrhage.

9. Vitreous hemorrhage.

10. Epithelial downgrowth.

13

Traumatic Cataract Surgery with Capsular Tension Ring

Indications

- Zonular weakness, zonular dialysis, or zonule loss following trauma
- Lens subluxation
- Support of capsular bag *during* phacoemulsification
- Prevention of capsular bag aspiration during irrigation/aspiration of cortex
- Support of capsular bag *after* phacoemulsification
- Improvement of intraocular lens (IOL) centration
- Reduced risk of capsular fibrosis and posterior capsule striae.

Preoperative Procedure

1. Perform a careful slit lamp examination of the cornea, anterior chamber, iris, and lens.
2. Measure the intraocular pressure.
3. Observe closely for phacodonesis, zonular dehiscence, and vitreous in the anterior chamber.
   a. Quantitate the number of clock hours of zonular dehiscence.
   b. Document the exact areas of zonular compromise (helpful in guiding which direction the capsular tension ring [CTR] is placed).
4. Perform dilated ophthalmoscopy to rule out an intraocular foreign body (avoid scleral depression if ruptured globe suspected).
5. B-scan ultrasonography, computed tomography (CT), magnetic resonance imaging (MRI) (if no metallic foreign body suspected), or ultrasound biomicroscopy (UBM) may be indicated to rule out an occult foreign body.
6. Perform A-scan and keratometry measurements of both eyes. (Fellow eye measurements may be necessary in cases of severe corneal trauma.) See Chapter 8.

Timing of Procedure

At the Time of Initial Corneoscleral and Iris Repair

If surgical visualization is adequate, consider removal of a traumatic cataract, preferably with IOL implantation.

Delayed Procedure

Severely traumatized eyes (e.g., with significant fibrinous reactions and corneal or iris injuries) may be delayed for cataract extraction until the eye is less inflamed after ruptured globe repair.

Elective Procedure

Dislocated or subluxated lenses with intact anterior capsules may be removed electively, unless intraocular pressure is elevated.

Preoperative Procedure

See the section on Conjunctival Lacerations in Chapter 28 for complete preoperative supportive measures.

Pupil Dilation

1. Tropicamide 1%, phenylephrine 2.5%, and cyclopentolate 1% every 15 minutes (for 3 total doses) beginning 1 hour before surgery.
2. Optional: Topical nonsteroidal anti-inflammatory agent (e.g., flurbiprofen 0.3% [Ocufen, Allergan, Inc., Irvine, CA, US]) every 30 minutes beginning 2 hours before surgery to minimize intraoperative miosis.

Preoperative Antibiotic Drops

Antibiotic drops (e.g., moxifloxacin 0.5% [Vigamox, Alcon, Inc., Fort Worth, TX, US], gatifloxacin 0.3% [Zymar, Allergan, Inc.]) are administered before surgery.

Instrumentation

- CTRs
  - ❏ Morcher; distributed by FCI Ophthalmics Inc.
  - ❏ Three sizes available: 14 (12.3 mm): for axial lengths < 24 mm (all compress 2–3 mm); 14A (14.5 mm): for axial lengths > 28 mm; 14c (13 mm): for axial lengths 24–28 mm
- Morcher CTRs
- Type 14, MR-1400
  - ❏ For normal eyes
  - ❏ Expanded 12.3 mm
  - ❏ Compressibility 10 mm
  - ❏ Bulbus length < 24 mm
- Type 14A, MR-1410
  - ❏ For highly myopic eyes
  - ❏ Expanded 14.5 mm
  - ❏ Compressibility 12 mm
  - ❏ Bulbus Length > 28 mm
- Type 14c, MR-1420
  - ❏ For normal or myopic eyes
  - ❏ Expanded 13 mm
  - ❏ Compressibility 11 mm
  - ❏ Bulbus length 24–28 mm
- Smooth forceps
  - ❏ (Recommended) Capsular ring injector (Geuder)
  - ❏ Iris retractors (disposable nylon or titanium)
  - ❏ Y-hook (e.g., Osher Y-hook)
  - ❏ 24 gauge cannula
  - ❏ 0.12 mm straight Castroviejo forceps
  - ❏ Cellulose sponges
  - ❏ Barraquer or Lieberman lid speculum
  - ❏ Kalt needle holder
  - ❏ Phacoemulsification instrumentation
  - ❏ Microvitrectomy suction/cutting instrumentation
  - ❏ 10–0 nylon sutures
  - ❏ Keratome (e.g., 3 mm)
  - ❏ Hemostats
  - ❏ Wetfield cautery
  - ❏ Microsurgical knife (e.g., Superblade, 15 degree)
  - ❏ Viscoelastic substance (e.g., Healon, Amvisc, Viscoat)
  - ❏ Cystotome
  - ❏ Capsulorhexis forceps (e.g., Utrata)
  - ❏ Cyclodialysis spatula
  - ❏ Lens loop
  - ❏ Kuglen hook
  - ❏ Intraocular lens forceps
  - ❏ Sinskey hook
  - ❏ Acetylcholine solution (e.g., Miochol)
  - ❏ Vannas scissors
  - ❏ Corneoscleral scissors (right and left)
  - ❏ McPherson tying forceps
  - ❏ Air cannula
- ❏ Anterior capsule stain (e.g., ICG or methylene blue)
- ❏ Posterior or anterior chamber intraocular lens (PCIOL or ACIOL)

Operative Procedure

Preferred technique of traumatic cataract removal in cases where there is moderate zonular dialysis.

1. Anesthesia: Peri- or retrobulbar blocks; topical anesthesia may also be used in select cases.
2. Prep and drape.
   a. Povidone iodide 5% on a cotton-tipped applicator to gently clean eyelashes and lid margin.
   b. Place one or two drops of povidone iodide in the conjunctival fornix.
3. Gently insert lid speculum.
4. Repair cornea and scleral lacerations using interrupted 10–0 (cornea) and 8–0 (sclera) nylon sutures (see section on Conjunctival Lacerations in Chapter 28).

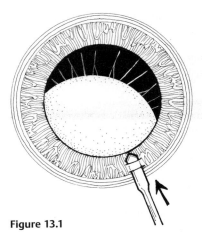

Figure 13.1

5. Create a paracentesis through clear cornea using a MicroSharp blade; place 2 to 3 clock hours from site of future incision (**Fig. 13.1**).
6. Inject a highly retentive viscoelastic (e.g., Viscoat) into anterior chamber and over any areas of zonular weakness or vitreous prolapse.
7. Reposit any viable iris tissue (see section on Conjunctival Lacerations in Chapter 28).
8. Reinflate anterior chamber with viscoelastic placing generous amount over areas of zonular dialysis.
9. Use keratome to create a limbal, clear corneal, or scleral tunnel incision (may require localized peritomy)
   a. Place the incision away from areas of cornea damage.
   b. Place the incision away from area of greatest zonular instability.
   c. Make a biplanar, self-sealing incision (see Chapter 8).

10. Correct for poor pupillary dilation and/or poor anterior capsule visibility (see Chapter 8).

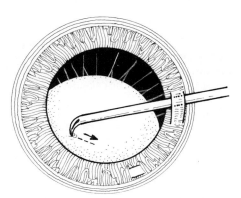

Figure 13.2

11. Perform anterior capsulotomy (**Fig. 13.2**).
    a. Use cystotome to initiate the capsulorhexis in an area remote from the zonular dialysis (thereby using the stronger remaining zonules for countertraction).
    b. Use cystotome needle or forceps (e.g., Utrata) to complete the curvilinear rhexis.
    c. Capsulotomy should be large enough (e.g., 6 to 7 mm) to allow easy nucleus manipulation.
    d. If necessary, stabilize the capsular bag with a blunt instrument or iris retractor to complete the rhexis.
12. If necessary, insert 1 to 4 iris retractors (disposable nylon or titanium) to stabilize the capsular bag.
    a. Create limbal stab incisions in one to four quadrants (Microsharp blade).

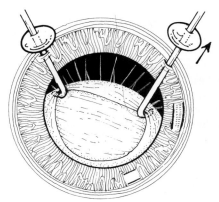

Figure 13.3

b. Insert retractor through wound and engage anterior capsule border (**Fig. 13.3**).

13. Hydro dissect gently with balanced salt solution (BSS) or viscoelastic (irrigating cannula).

Optional: Place the CTR inside the bag at this stage of the procedure; however, the bulk of the nuclear material makes this maneuver difficult and often traps epinuclear and cortical material in the bag, which inhibits removal.

Note: If the nucleus is soft and the capsulorrhexis is large enough, prolapsing the nucleus into the anterior chamber will markedly reduce zonular stress during phacoemulsification.

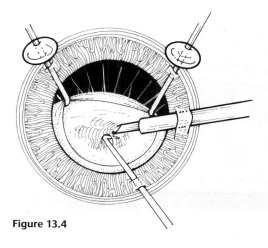

Figure 13.4

14. Nucleus emulsification (so-called slow-motion phacoemulsification) (**Fig. 13.4**).
    a. Use low aspiration and vacuum settings.
    b. Set a low bottle height to avoid hydrating the vitreous.
    c. Use chopping techniques with equal opposing forces to diminish zonular stress.
    d. Inject viscoelastic between nuclear halves or quadrants and the peripheral capsular bag to "lift" fragments out of the bag to emulsify them.
    e. Avoid vigorous cracking and lens manipulation.

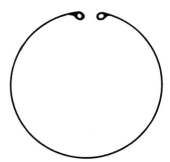

Figure 13.5

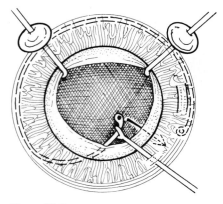

Figure 13.6

15. Insertion of the CTR (**Figs. 13.5–13.6**).
    a. Place viscoelastic under the surface of the anterior capsule rim to create space for the ring.
    b. Use viscoelastic to dissect away residual cortex from the capsule periphery, making entrapment by the CTR less likely.
    c. Use smooth forceps to grasp one end of the CTR (**Fig. 13.6**).
    d. Insert the CTR through the main limbal incision and into the capsular bag.

Note: Enter the bag in the area of greatest zonular weakness, which puts stress on the strong zonules 180 degrees away.

    e. Dial the CTR into the capsular bag with countertraction from a second instrument (e.g., Y-hook) (**Figs. 13.5 and 13.6**).
    f. Watch for the anterior capsulorrhexis to ovalize, indicating the CTR is in the capsular bag.

Note: Alternatively, use the capsular ring injector (Geuder).

Note: Inserting the CTR can traumatize the zonules further.

16. Cortex removal
    a. Fill the capsular bag with viscoelastic.
    b. Use 24 gauge cannula to manually remove cortical material.
    c. Pull cortex along the wall of the capsular bag instead of directly away (reduces zonular stress).
    d. Avoid automated irrigation/aspiration if possible.

17. If vitreous presents due to posterior capsule rupture or zonular dehiscence:
    a. Cellulose sponge removal of vitreous at wound site.
    b. Fill anterior chamber with viscoelastic.
    c. Use automated vitrector in a "dry" technique to remove all vitreous material and any remaining lens material from the anterior chamber.
    d. Use pars plana approach to retrieve lens fragments that have dropped posterior to the capsular bag (see Chapter 66).
18. Intraocular lens placement
    a. Capsular *bag placement*—preferred technique if capsule support is adequate.
        i. Fill the bag with viscoelastic.
        ii. Using an injector, insert foldable acrylic lens directly into the bag. (e.g., AcrySof SA60 and Monarch II delivery system, Alcon, Inc.) (see Chapter 8).
    b. *Ciliary sulcus placement*—make sure haptics are placed in areas of good capsule and zonule support.
    c. *Anterior chamber lens placement*—risk of long-term inflammation and corneal compromise (especially if significant corneal injury from initial trauma).
    d. *Transscleral sutured posterior chamber lens*—risks of retinal injury and displacement.
19. Carefully remove any iris hooks that were placed.
    a. Initially push forward to disengage capsule edge.
    b. Pull hook gently through stab incisions.
20. Aspirate viscoelastic from anterior chamber and capsular bag.
21. Instill Miochol into the anterior chamber to constrict the pupil.
    a. If the pupil peaks in one area, sweep away vitreous with cyclodialysis spatula.
    b. Use automated vitrectomy hand piece to further remove all vitreous from anterior chamber.
22. Hydrate the corneal wounds with balanced salt solution.
23. Check wounds for integrity and place interrupted 10–0 nylon sutures if necessary.
24. Perform subconjunctival injections of antibiotic (e.g., gentamicin 20–40 mg) and steroid (e.g., Decadron 4–8 mg).
25. Remove lid speculum.
26. Apply topical antibiotic and steroid ointment.
27. Patch eye and place fox shield.

Postoperative Procedure

1. Keep patch and shield in place until the patient is examined on postoperative day 1.
2. Topical antibiotic drops (e.g., moxifloxacin 0.5% [Vigamox, Alcon, Inc.], gatifloxacin 0.3% [Zymar, Allergan, Inc.]) 4 times per day for one week.
3. Steroid drops (e.g., prednisolone acetate 1%) 4 to 6 times per day, tapered over ~2 to 4 weeks, as inflammation subsides.
4. Intraocular pressure-lowering medications if necessary.
5. Patient may gradually increase activity level.

Follow-up Schedule

1. Postoperative day 1
2. Postoperative day 3 or 4
3. One, 2, and 4 weeks postoperatively and then as needed.

Complications

1. Lens or lens fragment dislocation into vitreous cavity.
2. CTR dislocation into the vitreous cavity.
3. Extension of zonular dialysis or weakness.
4. Entrapment of leading CTR eyelet within capsular fornix causing capsule rupture.
5. Endophthalmitis.
6. Increased intraocular pressure.
7. Hypotony or wound leak.
8. Vitreous or uveal incarceration in wound.
9. Retinal detachment.
10. Surgical damage to cornea or iris.
11. Persistent iritis.
12. Cystoid macular edema.
13. Uveitis-glaucoma-hyphema syndrome (after ACIOL placement).
14. PCIOL displacement.
15. Rotation of PCIOL or suture breakage (transscleral fixated PCIOL).

14

Nd:YAG Laser Posterior Capsulotomy

Indications

Posterior capsular opacification, fibrosis, or wrinkling of posterior capsule causing a decrease in visual acuity after cataract extraction.

Preoperative Procedure

Examine patient to determine degree of visual loss caused by posterior capsule.

For example:

1. Judge clarity of fundus view with direct ophthalmoscope.
2. Measure acuity with potential acuity meter or brightness acuity test if needed.
3. Optional: Perform fluorescein angiography to rule out cystoid macular edema.
4. If pupil is small, dilate with tropicamide 1%. Before dilating eye, examine posterior capsule carefully, identifying and diagramming landmarks for reference when centering the capsulotomy.
5. Measure baseline intraocular pressure. In glaucoma patients, may pretreat with a topical β-blocker (e.g., Timoptic 0.5%) or α agonist (Iopidine 1% or brimonidine tartrate 0.15%) to blunt any postlaser spike in intraocular pressure (IOP).

Instrumentation

- Nd:YAG laser
- Contact lens (e.g., Abraham-YAG lens)

Operative Procedure

1. Apply topical anesthetic (e.g., proparacaine).
2. Place contact lens to stabilize eye, magnify view, and decrease total energy needed.
3. Laser parameters:
   a. Power: Start with ~1 mJ.
   b. Adjust laser to give minimum power that will achieve effective cutting.
4. Focus Helium-Neon laser aiming beam directly on posterior capsule. If an intraocular lens (IOL) is closely apposed to the capsule, focus Helium-Neon laser slightly posteriorly to avoid pitting the lens).
5. Perform capsulotomy.

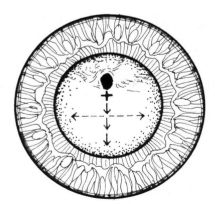

Figure 14.1

   a. Begin treatment superiorly and proceed inferiorly, "unzipping" capsule (**Fig. 14.1**).

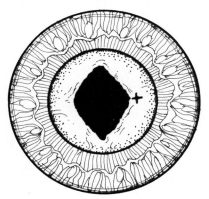

Figure 14.2

b. If necessary, perform cruciate incisions at 3 and 9 o'clock to increase the capsulotomy diameter (**Fig. 14.2**).

c. If an IOL is closely apposed to the capsule, start the treatment where there is adequate clearance, avoiding applications directly along the visual axis.

d. Final size of capsulotomy should approximate that of undilated pupil.

Postoperative Procedure

1. Nonsteroidal (e.g., nepafenac 0.1% [Nevanac, Alcon, Inc., Forth Worth, TX, US], ketorolac tromethamine [Acular, Allergan, Inc., Irvine, CA, US]) or corticosteroid (e.g., prednisolone acetate 1%) 4 times per day for 1 week to treat inflammation.

2. Optional: For prophylaxis against intraocular pressure elevation, use topical β−blocker (e.g., Timoptic 0.5% twice daily for 1 week) or α agonist (Iopidine 1% or brimonidine tartrate 0.15% twice daily for 1 week).

3. Treat any acute increase in intraocular pressure (IOP) with β-blockers, carbonic anhydrase inhibitors, and hyperosmotic agents as needed. (Transient elevations in IOP are found in 50 to 75% of patients; peak pressures are found ~1 to 3 hours after surgery).

Follow-up Schedule

1. Measure IOP 1 hour postlaser.
2. Measure IOP in 3 to 4 hours in:
   a. Patients with greater than 5 mm rise in IOP at 1 hour check.
   b. Glaucoma patients.
3. Optional: check IOP in 24 hours.
4. Follow up in 1 week postlaser.

Complications

1. Transient elevation in IOP.
2. Marking of IOLs.
3. Ocular inflammation.
4. Corneal endothelial cell loss or damage.
5. Hyphema in patients with rubeosis (e.g., diabetics, vein occlusion).
6. Retinal breaks and detachment.
7. Cystoid macular edema.
8. Forward movement of vitreous into anterior chamber.

Cornea

15

Penetrating Keratoplasty

Indications

- Replacement of optically inadequate cornea for visual rehabilitation (e.g., scarring, edema, dystrophy, degeneration)
- Tectonic support in cases of severe corneal melting, thinning, and impending or frank perforation
- Removal of infected cornea in certain cases of recalcitrant microbial keratitis
- Select traumatic corneal injuries
- Select cases of disfiguring corneal opacity for cosmesis

Preoperative Procedure

See Chapter 3.

Pupil Management

1. Phakic eye

Pilocarpine 1% every 15 minutes beginning 1 hour before surgery for a total of three drops to produce miosis, which protects lens during surgery. Alternatively, intraoperative acetylcholine (Miochol) may be used.

2. Aphakic eye
   a. If anterior vitrectomy is anticipated, it may be facilitated by preoperative pupil dilatation (e.g., tropicamide 1%, cyclopentolate 1% and phenylephrine 2.5% every 15 minutes beginning 1 hour before surgery).
   b. If a vitrectomy is not planned, preoperative dilation or constriction is unnecessary.

Instrumentation

- Honan balloon
- Mannitol 20% solution
- Speculum (Lieberman or Barraquer)
- Fine tissue forceps (e.g., 0.12 mm straight Castroviejo, 0.12 Colibri, Pierse)
- Bishop-Harmon forceps
- Teflon cutting block
- Cellulose sponges
- Disposable trephine (e.g., Katena, Storz, Weck)
- Vacuum trephine (e.g., Hessburg-Barron)
- Sutures (7–0 Vicryl, 4–0 silk, 10–0 nylon)
- Kalt or other strong needle holder
- Fine nonlocking needle holder
- Radial keratotomy (RK) marker
- Marking pen (e.g., methylene blue, gentian violet)
- Cautery
- Microsurgical knife (e.g., Superblade, 15 degree, Beaver #75M)
- Viscoelastic substance (e.g., Healon, Amvisc, Viscoat)
- Corneal scissors (right and left)
- Paton corneal spatula
- Vannas scissors
- Westcott scissors
- Intraocular lens (IOL) scissors
- McPherson tying forceps
- Cyclodialysis spatula
- Flieringa scleral ring
- Hemostats
- Jeweler's forceps
- Microvitrectomy suction/cutting instrumentation
- Acetylcholine solution (e.g., Miochol)

Operative Procedure

Phakic Penetrating Keratoplasty

1. Anesthesia: Retrobulbar or peribulbar injection plus lid block. May use general anesthesia if preferred, and for younger or uncooperative patients, hearing or mentally impaired patients, those with language obstacles, or patients with ruptured globes.
2. Decompress eye to avoid positive vitreous pressure.
   a. Mannitol 20% solution, 250 ml intravenous (slow drip over 1 hour) given 1 hour preoperatively.
   b. Patient to void before entering operating room.
   c. Secure Honan balloon in position for ~15 minutes (except in cases with globe perforation).
3. Prep and drape.
   a. Use povidone-iodide 5% on a cotton-tipped applicator to gently clean eyelashes and lid margins.
   b. Place one or two drops of povidone-iodide in the conjunctival fornix.

Note: There are many different trephines and corneal punches. The system used is based on surgeon preference.

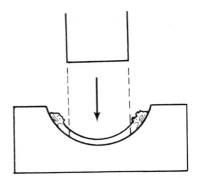

Figure 15.1

4. Trephine donor button from corneoscleral rim (**Fig. 15.1**).

Note: Secure a sterile work area with comfortable surgeon access and adequate lighting, away from the surgical instruments and patient (e.g., work table with stool)

   a. Hold corneoscleral rim with toothed forceps (e.g., Bishop-Harmon).
   b. Remove residual fluid from epithelial side of donor to avoid sliding during trephination (cellulose sponges).
   c. Place donor tissue epithelial side down (endothelial side up) and center on Teflon cutting block.
   d. Trephine appropriately sized button (disposable trephine on universal handle).

Note: An 8.0 mm donor button placed into a 7.5 mm recipient bed is a standard size differential.

   i. Keep trephine perpendicular to cornea.
   ii. Punch button in one fluid motion through entire donor thickness to avoid beveling the edge (listen for "crunch" sound).
   iii. May use guillotine-style trephine to better control trephination.
   e. Before removing trephine, ensure that the cut is through full-thickness cornea by gently raising the remaining scleral rim from the cutting block with toothed forceps, leaving the donor button behind.
   f. Remove trephine.
   g. Place a few drops of storage medium on the endothelial side of the button and cover the block to prevent drying of the donor.
   h. Keep corneal donor on work table in secure location and inform all operating room staff.
   i. Send corneoscleral rim and storage media for culture.
5. Return attention to the patient's eye.
6. Insert lid speculum, attempting to minimize pressure against globe from lid speculum.
   a. Optional: Place 4–0 silk bridle sutures.

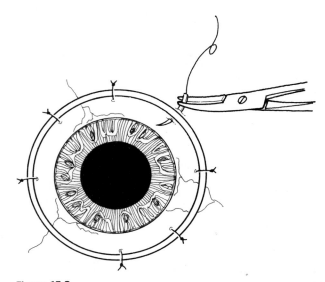

Figure 15.2

7. Secure Flieringa ring (**Fig. 15.2**).
   a. Choose ring size to leave ~2–3 mm between the ring and limbus.
   b. Secure globe with toothed forceps.
   c. Secure ring using four to eight equally spaced interrupted 7–0 Vicryl sutures.
   d. Place sutures through conjunctiva and episclera.
   e. Tie all sutures to equal tension to avoid distortion of globe.

Note: A Flieringa ring is not necessary in phakic keratoplasty, unless there is a possibility of lens removal at the time of surgery.

8. Optional: Mark cardinal positions and center of trephination on the recipient with a radial keratotomy marker and dye (gentian violet or methylene blue).
   a. Stain the corneal indentations with methylene-blue or gentian-violet marking pen or
   b. Use cautery at limbus to more permanently mark the cardinal positions.
9. Dry host corneal surface using Weck cell sponges.
10. Perform recipient trephination.

Note: Trephine system is based on surgeon preference. Systems include Hessburg-Barron, Storz, Hanna, and Krumeich.

   a. Storz or Weck handheld trephine:
      i. Preset at ~0.6 mm depth, depending on measurement of corneal thickness.
      ii. Stabilize globe by using 0.12 forceps to grasp limbal episclera without distorting the eye.
      iii. Center trephine on cornea, press down gently to mark the cornea, then remove trephine to verify central placement.
      iv. Once centration is verified, place trephine on corneal markings, and rotate back and forth (in circular fashion) between thumb and finger (middle finger or pointer) to perform trephination.
          I. Keep trephine perpendicular to eye.
          II. Apply equal, gentle, pressure to all areas of the trephination wound to ensure even cutting.

Note: Graft may need to be decentered or oversized based on pathology present.

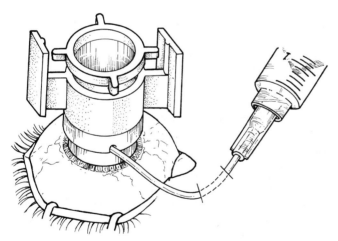

Figure 15.3

   b. Hessburg-Barron suction trephine (**Fig. 15.3**).
      i. Zero trephine blade under microscope.
      ii. Center trephine on cornea, press gently to mark cornea, then remove trephine to verify central placement.
      iii. Back up trephine three quarter-turns counterclockwise.

      iv. Place firmly on eye (center under microscope using crossbars to align).
      v. Apply suction. (May remove irregular epithelium with cellulose sponge if suction cannot be obtained or trephine slips.)
      vi. Turn three quarter-turns clockwise back to zero point and then additional turns depending on host corneal thickness.
          Each quarter-turn = 0.0625 mm.
      vii. Turn clockwise eight quarter-turns and enter anterior chamber in controlled manner with a microsurgical knife.

Note: Some surgeons advance trephine until anterior chamber is entered (aqueous gush noted)

      viii. Once anterior chamber is entered, do not advance trephine.
      ix. Release suction and remove trephine.
11. If bleeding is noted from corneal neovascularization, apply a cellulose sponge soaked in 2.5% neosynephrine. (May attempt to cauterize vessels before trephination to prevent excessive bleeding.)
12. Inspect trephination groove for 360 degrees using 0.12 straight forceps.
13. If anterior chamber has not been entered with trephine, enter slowly with a microsurgical knife (e.g., 15 degree blade, Superblade, Beaver #75M).
14. Irrigate viscoelastic into anterior chamber.
15. Raise edge of corneal button using 0.12 mm Colibri forceps.

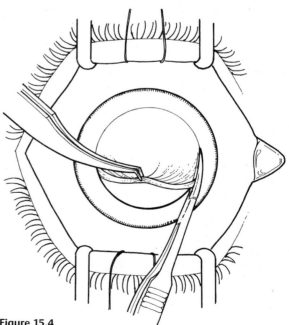

Figure 15.4

16. Excise corneal button with corneal scissors (right and left) parallel to iris plane; keep tips of scissors up to avoid cutting iris (**Fig. 15.4**).

a. Scissor blades should cut perpendicular to the cornea to create a vertical incision, avoiding formation of a wide, beveled internal lip.
b. Fine tissue forceps should be used to tangentially "pull" the host cornea away from the cut edge, allowing the scissors to fall into the groove created by the trephine.

Note: Some surgeons prefer to bevel the posterior wound slightly to form a two-step incision.

17. Remove excess posterior bevel and any residual tags of Descemet membrane or stroma with Vannas or corneal scissors.
18. Send host corneal button for laboratory testing.
19. Perform peripheral iridectomy in eyes prone to inflammation or aqueous misdirection (Vannas scissors, 0.12 forceps), or if anterior chamber lens placement is anticipated.
20. Irrigate viscoelastic over lens and into anterior chamber angle to keep chamber formed and to protect lens and donor endothelium.
21. Use Paton corneal spatula on epithelial surface to transfer donor button from the block to the recipient site (irrigate viscoelastic over donor button endothelium before placing it on recipient site).

Note: Keep fellow unused hand under cornea during transfer.

22. Use Colibri forceps to anchor donor with eight interrupted 10–0 nylon sutures (may use only four cardinal sutures in 24-bite running suture technique).

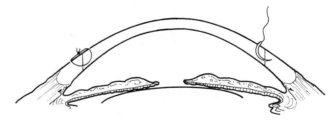

Figure 15.5

a. Sutures should be ~0.75–1 mm long on each side of the graft–host junction and with a depth of 90% thickness (**Fig. 15.5**).
b. For the first suture (12 o'clock), the assistant may stabilize the donor with 0.12 mm forceps at 6 o'clock to facilitate suture placement
c. Place and tie second suture at 6 o'clock, 180 degrees opposite the first.

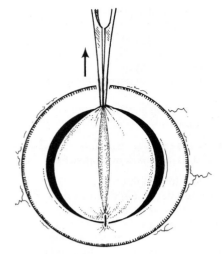

Figure 15.6

Ensure correct placement by grasping the 6 o'clock position with 0.12 mm forceps and noting the corneal fold radiating from the first suture to the 6 o'clock position. This should bisect the donor (**Fig. 15.6**).
d. Place and tie 3 and 9 o'clock sutures.
e. For the remaining four sutures, split the distance between each suture pair.

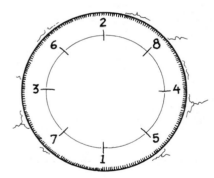

Figure 15.7

f. Ensure all sutures are radial and of similar length (**Fig. 15.7**).
g. Check to see that each suture is secure and of equal tension.
h. Replace any loose, tight, or nonradial sutures.

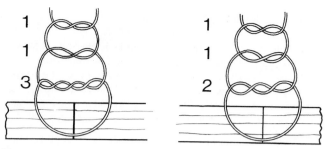

Figure 15.8

i. Suture tying techniques (**Fig. 15.8**).
   i. Surgeon's knot with 3–1-1 throws.
   ii. Surgeon's knot with 2–1-1 throws (need to cinch first throw to maintain tension while completing knot).
   iii. Slip knot with 1-1-1 throws (technically more difficult and may untie more easily if not properly performed).
23. Add balanced salt solution (BSS) (using an air canula) or viscoelastic as needed to reform the anterior chamber.
24. Trim knot ends using microsurgical blade or Vannas scissors.
25. Coat knot ends with viscoelastic, then irrigate (facilitates burying).

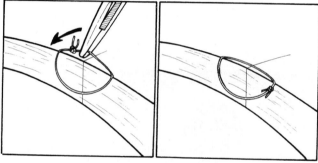

Figure 15.9

26. Bury knots on recipient side with tying forceps (**Fig. 15.9**).
   a. Knot should be placed just below surface of cornea.
   b. Cut ends of knot should be directed away from the surface to facilitate subsequent suture removal.
   c. Maintaining intraocular pressure (e.g., instilling BSS into anterior chamber) will facilitate suture burial.

27. Complete suturing: three techniques.
   a. Technique 1: 16 interrupted sutures.
      i. Add eight more 10–0 nylon interrupted sutures for a total of 16.
   May be advantageous for vascularized or inflamed recipient or other recipients for whom wound healing may vary in different parts of the graft–host junction.
      ii. Trim and bury sutures.
   b. Technique 2: eight interrupted and 16-bite running sutures.
      i. Use double-armed 10–0 nylon suture.
      ii. Place two radial throws between each pair of interrupted sutures.
   Each throw should be one quarter the distance from the neighboring interrupted suture to make the running suture bites evenly spaced.
      iii. When finished, tighten the suture.

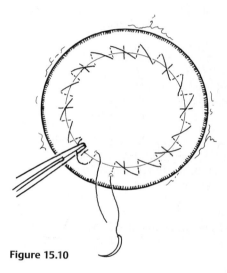

Figure 15.10

   I. Pull up on individual loops with tying forceps starting at 6 o'clock and finishing at 12 o'clock and repeat for other side of suture (**Fig. 15.10**).
   II. Cut off one needle.
   III. Secure suture with one double-looped throw.
   IV. Reform anterior chamber with BSS.
   V. Retighten the running suture
      iv. Tie 2–1-1 knot at recipient side of wound for easy burial.

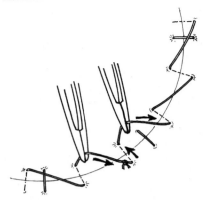

Figure 15.11

    v. Trim knot.
    vi. Bury knot: Again retighten one half the suture as in (I). This will give enough slack to bury the knot on the recipient side (**Fig. 15.11**).
    vii. Redistribute the suture to equalize tension over the entire graft–host junction.
    viii. Check for astigmatism by using hand-held keratometer or circular end of safety pin. Adjust suture using tying forceps to achieve corneal sphericity.
  c. Technique 3: 24-bite running suture (cornea should be initially marked with 12 bladed RK marker).
    i. Use double-armed 10–0 nylon suture.
    ii. Place radial throws at and between the guide marks for total of 24 bites
    iii. When finished, tighten the suture and adjust as described above.
    iv. Tie 2-1-1 knot at recipient side of wound for easy burial.
    v. Trim knot.
    vi. Bury knot.
    vii. Redistribute the suture to equalize tension over the entire graft–host junction.
    viii. Check for astigmatism by using hand-held keratometer or circular end of safety pin. Adjust suture using tying forceps to achieve corneal sphericity.
28. Reform the anterior chamber with BSS, irrigating out residual viscoelastic from opposite side of graft.
29. Ensure that no iris is incarcerated in the wound (if so, reposit iris with viscoelastic, BSS, or cyclodialysis spatula).
30. Check wound for watertightness (cellulose sponge or fluorescein strip).
31. Administer subconjunctival injections of dexamethasone (2 mg/0.5 ml) and cefazolin (100 mg/0.5 ml).
32. Remove lid speculum carefully.
33. Apply topical antibiotic and steroid ointment.
34. Patch and place Fox shield.

Aphakic Penetrating Keratoplasty

Note: Penetrating keratoplasty in an aphakic eye is essentially the procedure as described for the phakic eye. Additional maneuvers, however, facilitate surgery and improve the prognosis of corneal transplantation in the aphake. Frequently, anterior lens exchange with removal of an older style anterior chamber intraocular lens (ACIOL) is included in the procedure.

1. Prepare the patient and donor tissue as in steps 1 to 6, above.
2. Optional: Place Flieringa ring to prevent scleral collapse (see **Fig. 15.2**).
  a. Choose ring size to leave ~2–3 mm between the ring and limbus.
  b. Secure globe with toothed forceps.
  c. Secure ring using four to eight equally spaced interrupted 7-0 Vicryl sutures.
  d. Place sutures through conjunctiva and episclera.
  e. Tie all sutures to equal tension to avoid distortion of globe.
3. Remove recipient button as in steps 10 to 18 above.
4. Removal of anterior chamber IOL:
  a. Indications for removal
    i. Old style closed loop or rigid ACIOL
    ii. Lens malposition
    iii. Incarcerated lens haptics

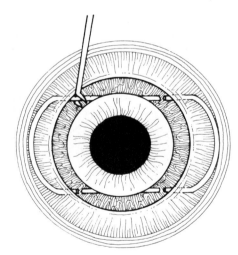

Figure 15.12

  b. Cut optic–haptic junction with lens scissors (**Fig. 15.12**).
  c. Remove optic with McPherson forceps
    i. Proceed carefully
    ii. Cut any adherent vitreous
  d. Spin remaining haptics in clockwise or counterclockwise fashion from angle

i. Haptics are frequently incarcerated in a fibrous cocoon in the angle.

ii. If unable to remove atraumatically, cut the haptic short and leave the adherent portion in situ.

5. Determine necessity of anterior vitrectomy.

a. Eyes with intact posterior capsule do not need vitrectomy.

b. Eyes with an absent or disrupted posterior capsule, but with vitreous behind iris plane do not always require vitrectomy. (Perform vitrectomy only if it appears that formed vitreous will enter the anterior chamber postoperatively.)

c. If vitreous is in the anterior chamber, an anterior vitrectomy should always be performed.

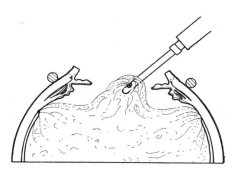

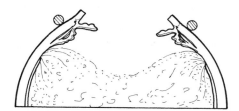

Figure 15.13

6. Perform open sky anterior vitrectomy (if indicated) (**Fig. 15.13**).

a. Use microvitrectomy suction/cutting instrument. (Infusion is not necessary in open sky procedure).

b. Vitrectomy instrument parameters.

i. Cutting rate: ~400 cps.

ii. Suction: start at 75–100 mm Hg and increase as necessary.

iii. If membranes (e.g., pupillary membranes) need to be removed with vitrectomy probe, increase suction (~150 mm Hg) and decrease cutting rate (~100 cps) (see Chapter 12).

c. Perform subtotal anterior vitrectomy.

i. Keep vitrectomy probe near center of pupil with port up.

ii. Do not make abrupt movements with instrument.

iii. Remove all vitreous from anterior chamber.

iv. At conclusion of vitrectomy, anterior surface of vitreous should be concave to prevent vitreous from entering anterior chamber or adhering to posterior iris surface postoperatively.

7. Use cellulose sponges to check for any residual vitreous in the anterior chamber.

8. Irrigate anterior chamber with Miochol to constrict pupil.

9. Perform peripheral iridectomy (0.12 forceps, Vannas scissors).

10. Irrigate viscoelastic into anterior chamber and angle to keep chamber formed and protect donor endothelium.

11. Optional: Place anterior chamber IOL

a. A flexible, one-piece, all-polymethyl methacrylate IOL is preferred.

b. Ensure pupil is round without iris capture.

12. Place and secure donor tissue as in steps 21–30, above.

13. Remove Flieringa ring.

Postoperative Procedure

Note: The success of penetrating keratoplasty depends on thorough and energetic postoperative care. The medications used and follow-up required will vary depending on the patient's underlying problems and the speed and efficacy of recovery. The following are suggestions for a routine, uncomplicated case.

1. Topical antibiotic drops (e.g., moxifloxacin 0.5% [Vigamox, Alcon Laboratories, Inc., Fort Worth, TX, US], gatifloxacin 0.3% [Zymar, Allergan, Inc., Irvine, CA, US]) 4 times per day for the first 2–3 weeks.

2. Steroid drops (e.g., prednisolone acetate 1%) from 4 times per day up to every hour, depending on degree of inflammation.

Note: Topical immunomodulators such as cyclosporine may be beneficial in eyes that are pressure-sensitive to steroids or have a high chance of graft rejection (e.g., repeat grafts, grafts of patients with immunologic diseases).

3. Cycloplegia as necessary for inflammation.

Note: Do not use a long-acting cycloplegic in a keratoconic eye, as it may remain tonically dilated.

4. Control intraocular pressure as necessary with β blockers and carbonic anhydrase inhibitors. (Elevated intraocular pressure is a leading cause of early graft failure.) Avoid epinephrine, prostaglandin analogues, and pilocarpine if possible since these may increase inflammation, which may lead to cystoid macular edema.

5. Discharge patient when stable (patient may be discharged home on the same day as the procedure if there are no medical or anesthesia-related contraindications).

6. For protection, patient should wear Fox shield or glasses during day and Fox shield at night for 6 weeks.

Suture Removal

1. Remove loose, vascularized, or infiltrated sutures as they present.
2. May selectively remove interrupted sutures for astigmatism control in ~3 months. (Do this judiciously, as overzealous suture removal may compromise wound, cause irregular astigmatism, or produce an overcorrection).
3. May remove sutures when wound is healed. Evidence of healing includes new vessels at the wound margin and a gray, fibrotic appearance of the wound.

Note: Adequate wound healing may take more than 1 year. Moreover, different areas of the wound may heal at different rates. Therefore, because quiescent sutures will not cause a problem, leave them in place unless necessary to remove.

4. Treat eye with steroid *and* antibiotic drops after removing suture (e.g., 4 times daily for 1 week; if patient is off steroids, may use steroid/antibiotic combination and taper over 1 to 2 weeks).
5. Technique of suture removal.
   a. Interrupted sutures.
      i. Place one drop of topical anesthetic (e.g., proparacaine 0.5%) in eye.
      ii. Cut suture over recipient with knife (e.g., #11 Bard-Parker blade or tip of 25 G needle).
      iii. Tease suture end up through epithelium.
      v. Remove with jeweler's forceps.

Note: Attempt to remove knot through the host side, if possible (less damage to graft endothelium and less chance of rejection). If unable to remove entire suture, suture remnant may be left in place, as long as no part protrudes past the epithelial surface.

   b. Running suture.
      i. Cut suture at every other loop.
      ii. Remove each segment with jeweler's forceps, grasping central segment of the suture.

When possible, may begin contact lens fitting in uncomplicated cases 1 month after suture removal.

Complications

1. Wound leak
2. Hypotony
3. Shallow anterior chamber
4. Peripheral anterior synechiae
5. Choroidal detachment
6. Glaucoma
7. Epithelial ingrowth
8. Suture loosening or breakage
9. Infection
10. Persistent epithelial defect
11. Persistent inflammation
12. Severe astigmatism
13. Primary graft failure
14. Graft rejection

16

Combined Penetrating Keratoplasty/Extracapsular Cataract Extraction/Posterior Chamber Intraocular Lens

Indications

- Patient requiring penetrating keratoplasty for visual rehabilitation of an eye which also has a visually significant cataract
- Patient with symptomatic corneal endothelial dystrophy (e.g., Fuchs) who requires cataract surgery

Preoperative Procedure

See Chapters 3 and 9.

Calculate intraocular lens (IOL) power using Sanders-Retzlaff-Kraff (SRK II) formula:

$$\text{Power of IOL} = A - 2.5(AL) - 0.9(K), \text{ where:}$$

- A-constant (A) is determined by the manufacturer for a specific lens. A typical value for a posterior chamber lens is 118.4.
- Axial length (AL) of eye in millimeters.
- Keratometry measurement (K) cannot be directly determined preoperatively.
  - ❑ The surgeon may use past postoperative keratometry results obtained with a specific technique as an approximate K reading.
  - ❑ The curvature of the normal fellow cornea may be measured and used in the SRK formula. When using a 0.5 mm oversized graft, however, subtract 1 to 2 diopters from the SRK result as the graft is typically steeper than the original cornea.

Dilate Pupil

1. Cyclopentolate 1%, phenylephrine 2.5%, and tropicamide 1% every 15 minutes beginning 1 hour before surgery.
2. Optional: Topical nonsteroidal anti-inflammatory agent (e.g., flurbiprofen 0.3% [Ocufen, Allergan, Inc., Irvine, CA,

US]) every 30 minutes beginning 2 hours before surgery to minimize intraoperative miosis.
3. Optional: Preoperative antibiotic drops (e.g., moxifloxacin 0.5% [Vigamox, Alcon Laboratories, Inc., Fort Worth, TX, US], gatifloxacin 0.3% [Zymar, Allergan, Inc.]) every 15 minutes for a total of 3 drops may be used as prophylaxis.

Instrumentation

- Honan balloon
- Mannitol 20% solution
- 0.12 mm straight Castroviejo forceps
- 0.12 mm Colibri forceps
- Bishop-Harmon forceps
- Teflon cutting block
- Marking pen (e.g., methylene blue, gentian violet)
- Cellulose sponges
- Speculum (e.g., Lieberman or Barraquer)
- Kalt or other strong needle holder
- Fine nonlocking needle holder
- Flieringa ring
- Sutures (7–0 Vicryl, 4–0 silk, 10–0 nylon)
- Hemostats
- Radial keratotomy marker
- Disposable trephine (e.g., Storz, Weck)
- Vacuum trephine (e.g., Hessburg-Barron)
- Cautery
- Microsurgical knife (e.g., Superblade, 15 degree, Beaver #75M)
- Viscoelastic substance (e.g., Healon, Amvisc, Viscoat)
- Corneal scissors (right and left)
- Cystotome
- Cyclodialysis spatula
- Lens loop
- Kuglen hook
- IOL forceps
- Muscle hook

- Sinskey hook
- Acetylcholine solution (e.g., Miochol)
- Jeweler's forceps
- Paton corneal spatula
- Vannas scissors
- McPherson tying forceps

Operative Procedure

1. Anesthesia: Retrobulbar or peribulbar injection plus lid block. May use general anesthesia for younger or uncooperative patients, hearing or mentally impaired patients, those with language obstacles, or patients with ruptured globes.
2. Decompress eye to avoid positive vitreous pressure.
   a. Mannitol 20% solution, 250 ml intravenous (slow drip over 1 hour) 1 hour preoperatively.
   b. Patient to void before entering operating room.
   c. Secure Honan balloon in position for ~15 minutes (except in cases with globe perforation).
3. Prep and drape.
   a. Use povidone-iodide 5% on a cotton-tipped applicator to gently clean eyelashes and lid margins.
   b. Place 1 or 2 drops of povidone-iodide in the conjunctival fornix.

Note: There are many types of trephines and corneal punches. The system used is based on surgeon preference.

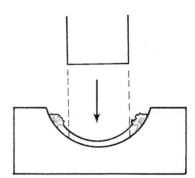

Figure 16.1

4. Trephine donor button from corneoscleral rim (**Fig. 16.1**).

Note: Secure a sterile work area with comfortable surgeon access and adequate lighting, away from the surgical instruments and patient (e.g., work table with stool).

a. Hold corneoscleral rim with toothed forceps (e.g., Bishop-Harmon).
b. Remove residual fluid from epithelial side of donor to avoid sliding during the trephination (cellulose sponges).
c. Place donor tissue epithelial side down (endothelial side up), on Teflon cutting block.
d. Trephine appropriately sized button (disposable trephine on universal handle).

Note: An 8.0 mm button placed into a 7.5 mm recipient bed is a standard size differential.

    i. Keep trephine perpendicular to cornea.
    ii. Punch button in one motion through the entire donor thickness to avoid beveling the edge (listen for "crunch" sound).
    iii. May use guillotine-style trephine to better control trephination.

e. Before removing trephine, ensure that the cut is through full-thickness cornea by gently raising the remaining scleral rim from the cutting block with toothed forceps, leaving the donor button behind.
f. Remove trephine.
g. Place a few drops of storage medium over the endothelial side of the button and cover the block to prevent drying of the donor.
h. Keep donor tissue on work table in secure location and inform all operating room staff.
i. Send corneoscleral rim and storage media for culture.

5. Return attention to the patient's eye.
6. Insert lid speculum atraumatically. Minimize pressure against globe.
   a. Optional: Place 4–0 silk bridle sutures.

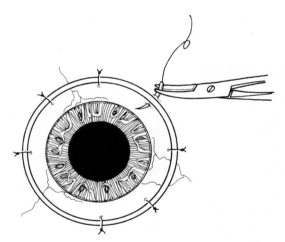

Figure 16.2

7. Affix Flieringa ring to prevent scleral collapse (**Fig. 16.2**).
   a. Choose ring size to leave ~2–3 mm between the ring and limbus.
   b. Secure globe with toothed forceps.
   c. Affix ring to globe using four to eight equally-spaced interrupted 7–0 Vicryl sutures (spatulated needle).
   d. Place sutures through conjunctiva and episclera. (May perform conjunctival peritomy to facilitate proper depth of sutures through episclera).
   e. Tie all sutures to equal tension to avoid distortion of globe.
8. Optional: Mark cardinal positions and center of trephination on the recipient with a radial keratotomy marker.

a. Stain the corneal indentations with methylene-blue or gentian-violet marking pen or

b. May use light cautery at limbus to mark the cardinal positions.

9. Dry host corneal surface using cellulose sponges.

10. Perform recipient trephination.

a. Storz or Weck handheld trephine:

  i. Preset at ~0.6-mm depth, depending on measurement of corneal thickness.

  ii. Stabilize globe by using 0.12 forceps to grasp limbal episclera without distorting the eye.

  iii. Center trephine on cornea, press down gently to mark the cornea, then remove trephine to verify central placement.

  iv. Once centration is verified, place trephine on corneal marking and rotate back and forth (in circular fashion) between thumb and finger (middle finger or pointer) to perform trephination.

    I. Keep trephine perpendicular to eye.

    II. Apply equal gentle pressure to all areas of the trephination wound to ensure even cutting.

Note: Graft may need to be decentered or oversized based on pathology.

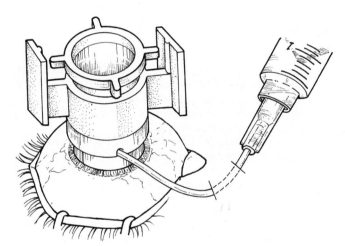

Figure 16.3

b. Hessburg-Barron suction trephine (**Fig. 16.3**).

  i. Zero trephine blade under microscope.

  ii. Center trephine on cornea, press gently to mark cornea, then remove trephine to verify central placement.

  iii. Back up trephine three quarter-turns counterclockwise.

  iv. Place firmly on eye (center under microscope, using crossbars to align).

  v. Apply suction (may remove irregular epithelium with cellulose sponge if suction cannot be obtained or trephine slips).

  vi. Turn three quarter-turns clockwise back to zero point and then additional turns depending on host corneal thickness. Each quarter-turn = 0.0625 mm.

vii. Turn clockwise eight quarter-turns and enter anterior chamber in controlled manner with a microsurgical knife.

Note: Some surgeons advance trephine until anterior chamber is entered (aqueous gush noted).

viii. Once anterior chamber is entered, do not advance trephine.

  ix. Release suction and remove trephine.

11. If bleeding is noted from corneal neovascularization, apply a cellulose sponge soaked in 2.5% neosynephrine. (May attempt to cauterize vessels before trephination to prevent excessive bleeding.)

12. Inspect trephination groove for 360 degrees using 0.12 straight forceps.

13. If anterior chamber has not been entered with trephine, enter slowly with a microsurgical knife (e.g., 15 degree blade, Superblade, Beaver #75M).

14. Irrigate viscoelastic into anterior chamber.

15. Raise edge of corneal button using 0.12 Colibri forceps.

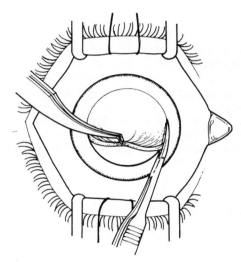

Figure 16.4

16. Excise corneal button with corneal scissors (right and left) parallel to iris plane; keep tips of scissors up to avoid cutting iris or nicking anterior capsule (**Fig. 16.4**).

a. Scissor blades should cut perpendicular to the cornea to create a vertical incision, avoiding formation of a wide, beveled internal lip.

b. Fine tissue forceps should be used to tangentially "pull" the host cornea away from the cut edge, allowing the scissors to fall into the groove created by the trephine.

Note: Some surgeons prefer to bevel the posterior wound slightly to form a two-step incision.

17. Remove excess posterior bevel and any residual tags of Descemet membrane or stroma with Vannas or corneal scissors.

18. Send host corneal button for laboratory testing.

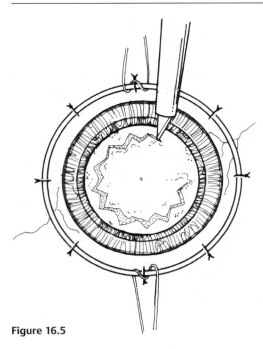

Figure 16.5

19. Perform an anterior capsulotomy (**Fig. 16.5**).
    a. May use a microsurgical knife or cystotome to perform punctures in the capsule in beer can fashion.
    b. May use Vannas scissors to cut anterior capsule.
20. Remove anterior capsular flap (McPherson forceps).
21. Remove lens nucleus (**Figs. 16.6A and 16.6B**).
    a. Gently rock nucleus horizontally to break nuclear-cortical adhesions (cyclodialysis spatula or irrigating cannula) (**Fig. 16.6A**).

A

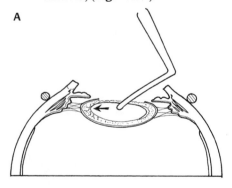

B

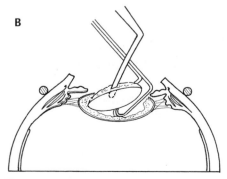

Figure 16.6

b. Use cyclodialysis spatula and lens loop to gently rotate and lift nucleus out of eye (**Fig. 16.6B**).
c. May apply gentle pressure at limbus to facilitate nucleus delivery (e.g., muscle hook).

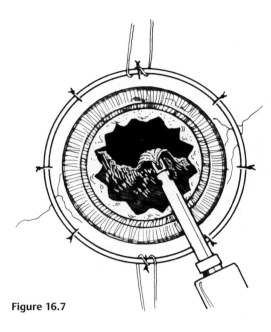

Figure 16.7

22. Remove residual cortical material with an automated or manual irrigation/aspiration device (**Fig. 16.7**) (may use Kuglen hook to retract iris to visualize cortex).
23. Irrigate viscoelastic into fornices of capsular bag.
24. Implant posterior chamber IOL
    a. Grasp superior portion of optic with IOL forceps.
    b. Place inferior haptic into capsular bag or ciliary sulcus, depending on status of posterior capsule.
    c. Place superior haptic (**Fig. 16.8**).

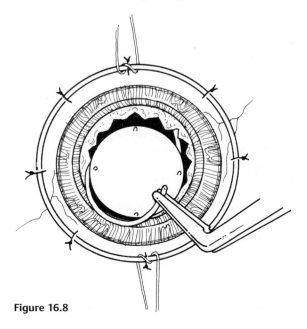

Figure 16.8

i. Grasp with angled McPherson forceps.
ii. Pronate hand to flex knee of superior haptic into position

d. Center intraocular lens (Sinskey hook).

25. Irrigate Miochol into anterior chamber to constrict pupil.
26. Optional: Perform peripheral iridectomy (jeweler's forceps, Vannas scissors).
27. Irrigate viscoelastic over lens and into anterior chamber angle to keep chamber formed and protect donor endothelium.
28. Use Paton corneal spatula on epithelial side to transfer donor button from block to the recipient site (irrigate viscoelastic over donor button endothelium before placing it on recipient site).

Note: Keep fellow unused hand under cornea during transfer.

29. Using Colibri forceps, anchor donor with eight interrupted 10–0 nylon sutures.

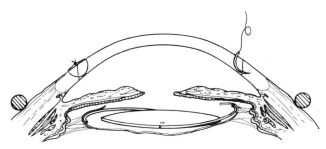

Figure 16.9

a. Sutures should be ~0.75–1 mm in length on both sides of the graft-host junction and with a depth of 90% (**Fig. 16.9**).
b. For the first suture (12 o'clock), the assistant may stabilize the donor with 0.12 mm forceps at 6 o'clock to facilitate suture placement.
c. Place and tie second suture at 6 o'clock, 180 degrees opposite the first.

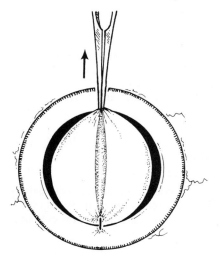

Figure 16.10

(Ensure correct placement by grasping the 6 o'clock position with 0. 12 mm forceps and noting the corneal fold radiating from the first suture to the 6 o'clock position. This should bisect the donor) (**Fig. 16.10**).

d. Place and tie 3 and 9 o'clock sutures.
e. For the remaining four sutures, split the distance between each suture pair.

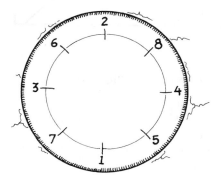

Figure 16.11

f. Ensure that all sutures are radial and are of similar length (**Fig. 16.11**).
g. Check to see that each suture is secure and of equal tension.
h. Replace any loose, tight, or nonradial sutures.

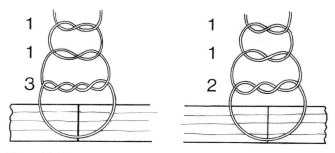

Figure 16.12

i. Suture tying techniques: (**Fig. 16.12**)
    i. Surgeon's knot with 3–1–1 throws (may be more difficult to bury at completion of case).
    ii. Surgeon's knot with 2–1–1 throws (must cinch first throw to maintain tension while completing knot).
    iii. Slip knot with 1–1–1 throws (technically more difficult and may untie more readily if not properly performed).
30. Trim knots using microsurgical blade or Vannas scissors.
31. Coat knot ends with viscoelastic, then irrigate (facilitates burying).

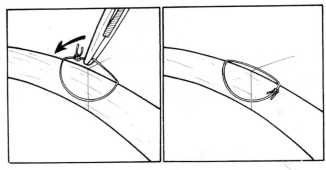

Figure 16.13

32. Bury knots on recipient side with tying forceps (**Fig. 16.13**).
    a. Knot should be placed just below surface of cornea.
    b. Cut ends of knot should be directed away from the surface to facilitate subsequent suture removal.
    c. Maintaining intraocular pressure (e.g., instilling balanced salt solution [BSS] into anterior chamber) will facilitate suture burial.
33. Complete suturing: two techniques:
    a. Interrupted suture technique
        i. Add eight more 10–0 nylon interrupted sutures for a total of 16 may be advantageous for vascularized recipient or other recipients in which wound healing may vary in different parts of the graft-host junction).
        ii. Trim and bury sutures.
    b. Running suture technique.
        i. Use double-armed 10–0 nylon suture.
        ii. Place two radial throws between each pair of interrupted sutures. (each throw should be one-quarter the distance from the neighboring interrupted suture to make the running suture bites evenly spaced).

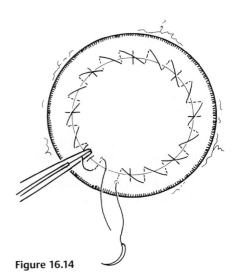

Figure 16.14

iii. When finished, tighten the suture.
    I. Pull up on individual loops with tying forceps starting at 6 o'clock and finishing at 12 o'clock and repeat for other side of suture (**Fig. 16.14**).
    II. Remove one needle.
    III. Secure suture with one double-looped throw.
    IV. Reform anterior chamber with BSS.
    V. Retighten the running suture as in (I), above.
iv. Tie 2–1–1 knot at recipient side of wound for easy burial.
v. Trim knot.

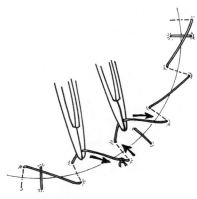

Figure 16.15

vi. Bury knot: Again retighten one half of the suture as in (I), above. This will give enough slack to bury the knot on the recipient side (**Fig. 16.15**).
vii. Redistribute the suture to equalize tension over the entire graft–host junction.

34. Reform the anterior chamber with BSS, irrigating out residual viscoelastic if necessary.
35. Ensure that no iris is incarcerated in the wound (if so, reposit iris with viscoelastic, balanced salt solution, or cyclodialysis spatula).
36. Check wound for watertightness (cellulose sponge or fluorescein).
37. Remove Flieringa ring.
38. Administer subconjunctival injections of dexamethasone (2 mg/0.5 ml) and cefazolin (100 mg/0.5 ml).
39. Remove lid speculum atraumatically.
40. Apply topical antibiotic and steroid ointment.
41. Patch eye and place Fox shield.

Postoperative Procedure

Note: The success of penetrating keratoplasty depends on thorough and energetic postoperative care. The medications used and the follow-up required will vary depending on the patient's underlying problems and the speed and efficacy of recovery. The following are suggestions for a routine, uncomplicated case.

1. Topical antibiotics (e.g., moxifloxacin 0.5% [Vigamox, Alcon Laboratories, Inc.], gatifloxacin 0.3% [Zymar, Allergan, Inc.] 4 times per day for the first 2 to 3 weeks.
2. Steroid drops (e.g., prednisolone acetate 1%) from 4 times per day up to every hour, depending on degree of inflammation.
3. Topical immunomodulators such as cyclosporine may be beneficial in eyes that are pressure-sensitive to steroids or have a high chance of graft rejection (e.g., repeat grafts, grafts of patients with immunologic diseases).
4. Cycloplegia as necessary for inflammation.
5. Intraocular pressure control as necessary with β–blockers and carbonic anhydrase inhibitors. (Elevated intraocular pressure is a leading cause of early graft failure.) Avoid epinephrine, prostaglandin analogues, and pilocarpine if possible, as these may increase inflammation.
6. Discharge patient when stable. (Patient may be discharged home on the same day as the procedure if there are no medical or anesthesia-related contraindications.)
7. For protection, patient should wear Fox shield or glasses during day and Fox shield at night for 6 weeks (see Chapter 6).

Suture Removal

See Chapter 15.

Complications

1. Posterior capsule rupture
2. Vitreous loss
3. Hyphema
4. Wound leak
5. Hypotony
6. Shallow anterior chamber
7. Peripheral anterior synechiae
8. Glaucoma
9. Infection
10. Persistent epithelial defect
11. Severe astigmatism
12. Primary graft failure
13. Graft rejection
14. Persistent inflammation
15. Choroidal detachment
16. Cystoid macular edema
17. Posterior capsule opacification
18. Suture loosening/breakage

17

Pterygium Excision

Indications

- Reduced vision secondary to:
  - ❑ Pterygium advancing toward or already impinging upon visual axis
  - ❑ Induced astigmatism
- Cosmesis
- Significant discomfort that is not relieved by medical therapy
- Limited ocular motility secondary to muscle restriction

Note: the free conjunctival graft or amniotic membrane technique is preferred for treating advanced and recurrent pterygium. This technique has been shown to decrease the rate and severity of pterygium recurrence. The primary disadvantage of the graft technique is prolonged operative time.

Preoperative Procedure

Treat any significant inflammation with topical steroids, as it is best to operate on the least inflamed tissue possible. Optional: Prophylactic antibiotics (see Chapter 3).

Instrumentation

- Lid speculum (e.g., Lieberman or Barraquer)
- Bishop-Harmon forceps
- Tissue forceps (e.g., 0.12 mm and 0.3 mm Castroviejo)
- Anatomic forceps
- Disposable cautery
- Sutures (6–0 silk, 10–0 nylon, 10–0 Vicryl)
- Scarifier (e.g., Grieshaber #681.01 or Beaver #57)
- Cellulose sponges
- Cotton-tipped applicators
- Westcott scissors
- Diamond burr
- Castroviejo calipers
- Needle holder
- Clamp

Operative Procedure

Bare Sclera Pterygium Excision

Note: Primary bare sclera pterygium excision has a high recurrence rate.

1. Anesthesia:
   a. Topical anesthetic (e.g., proparacaine).
   b. Peribulbar or retrobulbar plus lid block in uncooperative patient or when surgical time is anticipated to be long.
2. Prep and drape.
   a. Use povidone-iodide 5% on a cotton-tipped applicator to gently clean eyelashes and lid margins.
   b. Place one or two drops of povidone-iodide in the conjunctival fornix.
3. Insert lid speculum.
4. Perform forced duction testing to rule out any restriction of rectus muscles secondary to involvement with the pterygium (0.3 forceps).
5. Optional: Place a double-armed 6–0 silk episcleral limbal stay suture at the 6 or 12 o'clock meridian, or both.
6. Position eye with stay sutures and clamp.

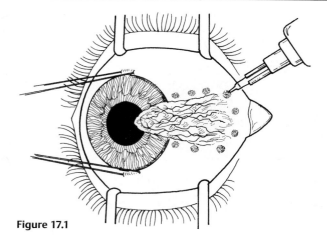

Figure 17.1

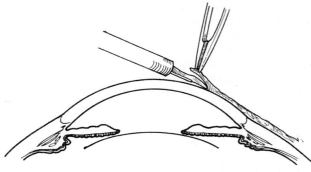

Figure 17.3

7. Demarcate the body of the pterygium with cautery (**Fig. 17.1**).
   a. Place spots on normal conjunctiva along the area to be resected.
   b. **Note:** If administering subconjunctival lidocaine under the body of the pterygium, do so after placing demarcation spots.

Alternatively, grasp the head of the pterygium using a 0.3 or 0.12 forceps and lift while using a Beaver #57 blade to perform a lamellar dissection (**Fig. 17.3**).

9. If necessary, perform lamellar dissection of the head of the pterygium from the cornea using a scarifier (Beaver #57 blade). Stay in one plane.

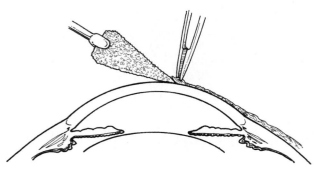

Figure 17.2

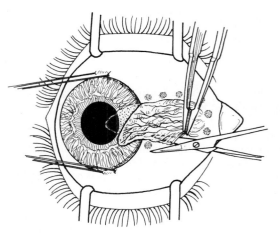

Figure 17.4

8. Use the tip of a dry cellulose sponge to bluntly undermine the head of the pterygium (the part on the cornea as opposed to the tail, which is on the sclera) while applying counter traction (lifting pterygium) with tissue forceps (**Fig. 17.2**).

Note: Remove as much as the pterygium as possible from corneal surface using cellulose sponges. Sponges will need to be changed constantly.

10. Excise the episcleral portion of the pterygium (**Fig. 17.4**).
    a. Use Westcott scissors to cut along previously placed cautery marks ("connect-the-dots").
    b. Undermine pterygium with scissors.
    c. Remove all pterygium and underlying tissue (including Tenon capsule) down to bare sclera.

   d. If necessary, identify horizontal rectus muscle and isolate with a muscle hook to avoid inadvertent damage while removing overlying pterygium and accompanying tissue (Chapter 37).
11. Remove the pterygium at the limbus using sharp and blunt dissection with scissors.
12. Send excised tissue for pathologic evaluation.
13. Obtain adequate hemostasis with disposable cautery.

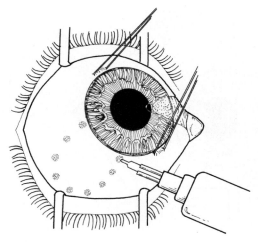

Figure 17.6

10. Demarcate donor site with light cautery or marking pen (**Fig. 17.6**).

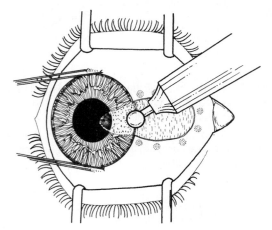

Figure 17.5

14. Smooth limbus to achieve normal contour (**Fig. 17.5**).
   a. May use diamond burr to polish limbus (preferable), or
   b. Scrape with back edge of scarifier blade.
15. Apply topical combination antibiotic and steroid ointment (e.g., tobramycin 0.3% and dexamethasone 0.1% [Tobradex, Alcon Laboratories, Inc., Fort Worth, TX, US])
16. Place light pressure patch and Fox shield.

Pterygium Excision with Free Autogenous Conjunctival Transplantation

Note: The use of a free conjunctival graft in conjunction with pterygium excision has been shown to reduce the recurrence rater significantly.

1. Anesthesia: Peribulbar or retrobulbar plus lid block.
2. Prep and drape.
3. Insert lid speculum.
4. Perform forced duction testing to rule out any restriction of rectus muscles secondary to involvement with the pterygium (0.3 forceps).
5. Place a double-armed 6–0 silk episcleral limbal stay suture at the 6 or 12 o'clock meridian, or both.
6. Position eye with stay sutures and clamp.
7. Remove pterygium as described above; see section "Bare Sclera Pterygium Excision" (steps 7–14) earlier in this chapter.
8. Measure horizontal and vertical dimensions of bare sclera with calipers.
9. Choose donor site (usually superotemporal bulbar conjunctival) and rotate eye into position with stay suture(s) and clamp.

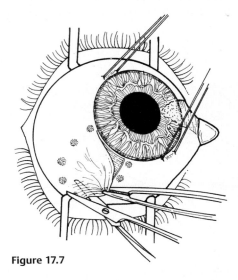

Figure 17.7

11. Dissect a thin conjunctival flap along cautery marks using anatomic forceps and blunt Westcott scissors (**Fig. 17.7**).
   a. Remove all Tenon capsule and other subconjunctival tissue from donor.

   Optional: Inject 2% lidocaine subconjunctivally at the donor site to create a plane between Tenon and conjunctiva.

   b. Handle tissue very gently (an assistant may be helpful in "tenting up" conjunctiva with two smooth forceps as Tenon is freed by gently snipping with Westcott scissors). Do not buttonhole conjunctiva.
   c. Maintain orientation of tissue, keeping limbal donor conjunctiva aligned so that it will be placed at limbal host site.

Note: Limbal site on graft will not have any cautery burns

d. Donor site does not require suturing.

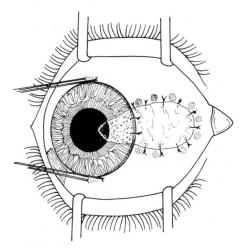

Figure 17.8

13. Secure transplant to scleral bed with interrupted 10–0 nylon and 10–0 Vicryl sutures (**Fig. 17.8**).
    a. Suture two limbal corners, two posterior corners, and middle of posterior flap edge using 10–0 nylon.

    Optional: place central limbal sutures.

    b. Suture the remaining graft using 10–0 Vicryl or 10–0 nylon, closing and gapes.
14. Rotate knots to the conjunctival host side. If it is difficult to rotate the knots, cut the sutures slightly long so they lie flat (this may help relieve patient discomfort).
15. Apply topical combination antibiotic and steroid ointment (e.g., tobramycin 0.3% and dexamethasone 0.1% [Tobradex, Alcon Laboratories, Inc.]).
16. Apply light pressure patch and Fox shield.

Adjunctive Therapy with Mitomycin C

Antimetabolites such as mitomycin C (MMC) prevent the proliferation of fibroblasts, thereby reducing the incidence and severity of pterygium recurrence. Due to the possibility of significant complications—including scleral melting, glaucoma, and delayed epithelial healing—associated with using topical MMC and bare sclera technique, many surgeons use a single intraoperative MMC application in conjunction with a free conjunctival graft. Use of MMC should be limited to cases that involve recurrent pterygium, pterygium that have significant fibrous and vascular patterns, and to patients who have had pterygium recurrence in their fellow eye after conjunctival autograft procedures.

Intraoperative Mitomycin C Application

1. Remove pterygium as described above; see section "Bare Sclera Pterygium Excision" (steps 1–14) earlier in this chapter.
2. Measure bare sclera area with calipers

3. Cut cellulose sponge into slightly smaller size than bare scleral area. Undersize sponge area by 1 mm vertically and 1 mm horizontally to minimize MMC application to the viable conjunctival edges of the host tissue.
4. Soak sponge in MMC 0.02% solution.
5. Place MMC-soaked sponge onto the bare sclera for 2 minutes.
6. Remove sponge and irrigate entire area (including fornices) well with balanced salt solution.

Use of Amniotic Membrane with or without Fibrin Glue (e.g., Tisseal Glue)

Note: Current formulations of fibrin glue require at least 30 minutes of preparation time; plan accordingly. Future formulations may not require such preparation time.

1. Remove pterygium as described above; see section "Bare Sclera Pterygium Excision" (steps 1–14) earlier in this chapter.
2. Measure bare sclera area with calipers.
3. Apply MMC if indicated as noted above.
4. If MMC is used, apply vigorous irrigation.
5. Dry bare sclera and surrounding conjunctiva. Obtain full hemostasis of the bed.

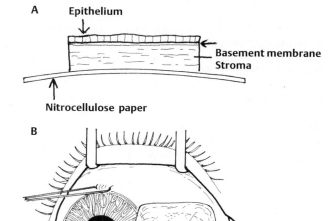

Figure 17.9

6. Cut amniotic membrane with a blunt Westcott, keeping the basement membrane side down. Oversize the amniotic membrane graft by at least 1 mm on all sides (**Figs. 17.9A and 17.9B**).

7. Using fibrin glue
   a. Apply fibrin glue over bare sclera and surrounding conjunctiva.
   b. Directly place amniotic membrane over bare sclera and allow overlap onto surrounding conjunctiva.
   c. Ask nurse to time 1 minute on the clock. Be sure there are no gaps between the amniotic membrane and surrounding conjunctiva.
   d. Allow 2–4 minutes for the glue to fix.
   e. Carefully check fornix and lid speculum for strands of attached fibrin glue. Remove the strands gently in a way that does not affect the amniotic membrane.
8. Using sutures:
   a. Secure transplant to scleral bed with interrupted 10–0 Vicryl or 10–0 nylon sutures.
   b. Suture two limbal corners, two posterior corners, and middle of posterior flap edge using 10–0 nylon.
   Optional: Central limbal sutures.
   c. A running or interrupted technique may be used; interrupted sutures usually take more time.
9. Carefully lift the lid speculum to prepare for removing the lid drape underneath. Again examine lid speculum to ensure no attachments if using fibrin glue.
10. Carefully remove lid drapes and then lid speculum as speculum is lifted to avoid touching the cornea.
11. Place a drop of antibiotic (e.g., moxifloxacin 0.5% [Vigamox, Alcon Laboratories, Inc.], gatifloxacin 0.3% [Zymar, Allergan, Inc., Irvine, CA, US]) in fornix.
12. Carefully close eyelids and apply an antibiotic–steroid ointment over the eyelids.
13. Patch eye.
14. Postoperative day 1: Be careful as the patch is removed that there is no attachment of the graft to the patch.
15. **Note:** If there are any gaps between the amniotic membrane and surrounding conjunctival surface intraoperatively or postoperatively, or if the fibrin glue is unable to properly glue the graft in place, interrupted 9–0 or 10–0 Vicryl or nylon sutures should be placed.

Postoperative Procedure

1. Pain control may be needed (e.g., acetaminophen with codeine, Vicodin, Percocet).
2. Steroid drops (e.g., prednisolone acetate 1%) 4 times per day; slowly taper over 6–8 weeks.
3. Antibiotic drops (e.g., moxifloxacin 0.5% [Vigamox, Alcon Laboratories, Inc.], gatifloxacin 0.3% [Zymar, Allergan, Inc.]) 4 times per day for 1 week.

Note: Should continue antibiotic longer if persistent corneal or conjunctival epithelial defects are present.

4. Alternatively, an antibiotic and steroid ointment (e.g., Tobradex, Alcon Laboratories, Inc.) 4 times per day can be used for the first week if compliance is a concern. After the first week, a steroid drop can be used and tapered over 6–8 weeks.
5. Remove nylon sutures after 1 month.
6. If recurrence is noted in the postoperative period, subconjunctival injection of steroid in the area of the recurrence may be beneficial in preventing further growth.

Complications

1. Epithelial defect in area of superficial keratectomy
2. Inflammation/edema of conjunctival graft
3. Infection
4. Donor graft retraction
5. Corneoscleral dellen in area adjacent to conjunctival closure
6. Damage to rectus muscle
7. Corneal scarring
8. Recurrence of pterygium

18

Conjunctival Flap

Indications

- Indolent corneal epithelial defects with sterile stromal ulceration
- Painful bullous keratopathy or other surface abnormalities eyes with little or no visual potential
- Recalcitrant fungal keratitis
- Blind eyes to allow comfortable placement of prosthetic shell
- Other progressive corneal thinning disorders

Contraindications

- Active bacterial keratitis
- Corneal perforation

Preoperative Procedure

See Chapter 3.

1. Intensive topical or systemic treatment of any infectious process.
2. Ensure that there is no active wound leak or corneal perforation (Seidel test).

Instrumentation

- Lid speculum (e.g., Lieberman)
- Fine-toothed tissue forceps (e.g., 0.12 mm Castroviejo)
- Westcott scissors
- Sutures (6–0 silk, 10–0 nylon)
- Smooth forceps (e.g., Chandler, Bracken, anatomic forceps)
- Cellulose sponges
- Calipers
- Diluted alcohol (20%)
- Lidocaine 1–2% with epinephrine
- Scarifier (e.g., Beaver #57 blade, or Grieshaber #681.01)
- Disposable cautery
- Clamp

Operative Procedure

Total "Gunderson" Flap

1. Anesthesia: Retrobulbar or peribulbar plus lid block. May use general anesthesia for younger, hearing or mentally impaired, or uncooperative patient.
2. Prep and drape.
   a. Use povidone-iodide 5% on a cotton-tipped applicator to gently clean eyelashes and lid margins.
   b. Place one or two drops of povidone-iodide in the conjunctival fornix.
3. Insert lid speculum.
4. Perform 360 degree conjunctival peritomy at the limbus (Westcott scissors).
5. Place a 6–0 silk traction suture at the 12 o'clock limbus, just inside clear cornea.
6. Use the traction suture to rotate the eye inferiorly (clamp to drape).
7. Optional: Slowly inject 1–2 ml of 2% lidocaine epinephrine (on a 30 gauge needle) subconjunctivally at the medial or lateral canthus, away from site of eventual flap, to dissect conjunctiva from Tenon capsule.

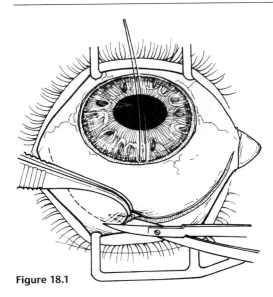

Figure 18.1

8. Incise the superior bulbar conjunctiva, leaving Tenon capsule intact (smooth forceps, Westcott scissors). The incision should be curvilinear and begun as superiorly as possible (close to 12 mm from limbus) without involving the forniceal conjunctiva (**Fig. 18.1**).
9. Extend the conjunctival incision ~180 degrees.

Note: Try to make the incision as wide as possible (from 15 to 20 mm).

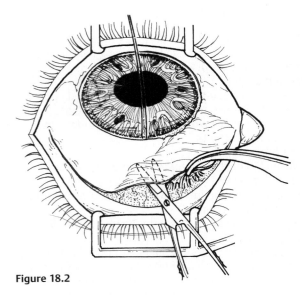

Figure 18.2

10. Undermine the conjunctival flap, carefully separating it from the underlying Tenon capsule with blunt and sharp dissection (smooth forceps, cellulose sponges, and Westcott scissors) (**Fig. 18.2**).
    a. Surgical assistant may help tent up the conjunctival flap as it is being created.
    b. Take precautions not to buttonhole the conjunctiva.

11. Extend the dissection as inferiorly as possible and then free the flap at the limbus. Leave flap attached at the hinges, medially and laterally.
12. Remove corneal epithelium.
    a. 20% alcohol may be applied to loosen the epithelium.
    b. Debride corneal epithelium with dry cellulose sponges and back edge of scalpel or a 57 blade.
13. Remove traction suture.
14. Bring flap into position over the denuded cornea. Make sure that there is no tension or stretch to the tissue.

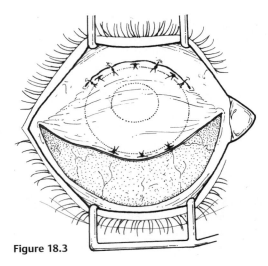

Figure 18.3

15. Secure the superior border of the flap to the episclera at the superior peritomy site with 3 or 4, 10–0 nylon horizontal mattress sutures, passing suture from flap through episclera and back through flap (**Fig. 18.3**).
16. Secure the inferior border of the flap to the episclera at the inferior peritomy site with four to six horizontal mattress 10–0 nylon sutures.
17. Place two or three, 10–0 nylon interrupted sutures from the conjunctival flap to the edge of host bulbar conjunctiva.
18. Inspect flap tissue carefully.
    a. If any buttonholed areas are present, repair with interrupted 10–0 nylon sutures
    b. If any areas of the flap-to-limbus attachments are gaping, add interrupted 10–0 nylon as needed.
19. Remove lid speculum.
20. Apply topical antibiotic or steroid ointment (e.g., tobramycin 0.3% and dexamethasone 0.1% [Tobradex, Alcon Laboratories, Inc., Fort Worth, TX, US]) and a light pressure patch.

Partial Conjunctival Flap

Small peripheral ulcerations or perforations may be treated with a localized pedunculated conjunctival flap.

Obtaining a flap that maintains a good vascular supply and positions easily without significant tension (which may cause displacement) is key to a successful outcome. This type of flap is especially useful if a view of the anterior chamber is necessary immediately postoperatively or a subsequent corneal transplant is planned.

1. Anesthesia: Retrobulbar or peribulbar injection plus lid block. May use general anesthesia for younger, hearing or mentally impaired, or uncooperative patient.
2. Prep and drape.
   a. Use povidone-iodide 5% on a cotton-tipped applicator to gently clean eyelashes and lid margins.
   b. Place one or two drops of povidone-iodide in the conjunctival fornix.
3. Insert lid speculum
4. Debride corneal epithelium over affected area plus an extra 1 mm surrounding area using Beaver 57 blade or back edge of scalpel.
5. Measure total area to be covered by flap with calipers.
6. Delineate area to be mobilized with disposable cautery or marking pen.

Note: Do not underestimate the size of the partial flap; if in doubt make it slightly larger than necessary.

7. Undermine the conjunctival flap, carefully separating it from the underlying Tenon capsule with blunt and sharp dissection (smooth forceps, cellulose sponges, and Westcott scissors).
8. Position pedicle flap over the affected area on the cornea. The tissue should be able to stay in position without tension.

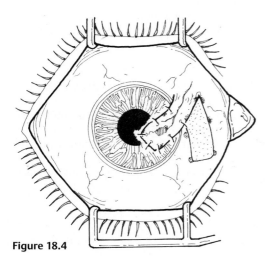

Figure 18.4

9. Suture flap into position with interrupted 10–0 nylon suture. Sutures should pass through edge of flap and be approximately two thirds corneal thickness (**Fig. 18.4**).

Postoperative Procedure

1. Avoid a tight pressure patch to avoid strangulating flap.
2. Steroid drops (e.g., prednisolone acetate 1%) 4 times per day and slowly taper over 4–6 weeks.
3. Antibiotic (e.g., moxifloxacin 0.5% [Vigamox, Alcon Laboratories, Inc.], gatifloxacin 0.3% [Zymar, Allergan, Inc., Irvine, CA, US]) 4 times per day for the first week or two.

Postoperative Course

1. Gradual thinning of the conjunctival flap will take place over the first 3–6 months, providing some anterior segment visualization.
2. Specific sutures should be removed if suture abscesses or localized granulomatous reactions take place.
3. Otherwise, nylon sutures should be left in place for at least 6 months, if not indefinitely.

Complications

1. Buttonhole in flap
2. Excessive tension on flap and subsequent retraction
3. Hemorrhage under flap
4. Corneal perforation under the flap
5. Suture abscess
6. Epithelial inclusion cysts (when epithelial cells are allowed to remain under the flap)
7. Ptosis

19

Superficial Keratectomy/Phototherapeutic Keratectomy

Indications

Superficial keratectomy and/or phototherapeutic keratectomy is suitable for removal of pathologic epithelial and subepithelial tissue in selected patients with:

- Recurrent erosion syndrome or decreased vision caused by anterior basement membrane dystrophy
- Anterior stromal or Bowman layer corneal dystrophies (e.g., Reis-Bucklers dystrophy)
- Band keratopathy
- Superficial pannus
- Other superficial opacities or irregularities (e.g., Salzmann nodules)

Preoperative Procedure

1. Slit lamp examination with attention to the level and nature of corneal pathology.
2. **Note:** Slit beam analysis is best for assessing the depth of abnormality; postdilation transillumination viewing is helpful for establishing the horizontal and vertical borders of pathology.

Instrumentation

- Lid speculum (e.g., Lieberman)
- Fine toothed tissue forceps (e.g., 0. 12 mm Castroviejo or Colibri)
- Jeweler's forceps
- Diluted alcohol (20%)
- Cellulose sponges
- Scarifier (e.g., Beaver #57 or Grieshaber #681.01)
- Cyclodialysis spatula
- Excimer laser
- Bandage soft contact lens

Operative Procedure

Superficial Keratectomy

1. Anesthesia
   a. Topical proparacaine
   b. Peribulbar or retrobulbar block plus lid block in uncooperative patient
2. Prep and drape
   a. Use povidone-iodide 5% on a cotton-tipped applicator to gently clean eyelashes and lid margins.
   b. Place one or two drops of povidone-iodide in the conjunctival fornix.
3. Insert lid speculum.
4. Remove epithelium overlying the involved area.
   a. Apply 20% alcohol on pledget to loosen epithelial adhesion.
   b. Scrape epithelium with dry cellulose sponge or scarifier, avoiding sharp dissection.
   c. Preserve as much of the limbal epithelium as possible (necessary for reepithelialization).
5. Keep cornea dry with cellulose sponges (facilitates visualization and manipulation of the abnormal tissue).

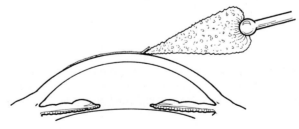

Figure 19.1

6. Identify cleavage plane between abnormal tissue and Bowman layer or stroma using dry cellulose sponges, Beaver #57 blade, or scarifier (**Fig. 19.1**).

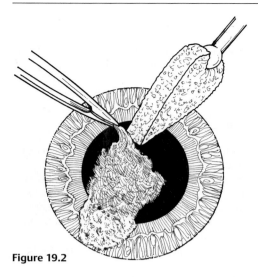

Figure 19.2

7. Apply countertraction with 0. 12 mm forceps and strip the abnormal material along its cleavage plane (**Fig. 19.2**).
   a. The tip of a dry cellulose sponge may be used as a dissecting instrument.
   b. In some cases (Salzmann nodules), adherent tissue can be directly peeled away with jeweler's forceps.
   c. A scarifier may be carefully used to scrape or dissect abnormal tissue.

Note: Use caution to remain in cleavage plane, thus avoiding excessive damage to Bowman membrane, which will promote corneal scarring.

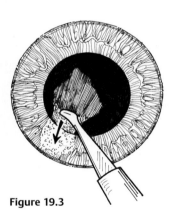

Figure 19.3

8. Smooth corneal surface by scrubbing with cellulose sponges or gently scraping with back edge of scarifier (**Fig. 19.3**).
9. Optional: May use diamond burr to polish irregular surface or smooth out resilient tissue—for peripheral pathology only.
10. Optional: Apply bandage contact lens to facilitate re-epithelialization.
11. Use topical antibiotic and anti-inflammatory drops if contact lens is used. Otherwise, ointments can be used.

12. Apply pressure patch with ointment if contact lens is not used.

Phototherapeutic Keratectomy

1. Anesthesia: Topical proparacaine.
2. Prep and drape.
   a. Use povidone-iodide 5% on a cotton-tipped applicator to gently clean eyelashes and lid margins.
   b. Place one or two drops of povidone-iodide in the conjunctival fornix.
3. Insert lid speculum.
4. Epithelial removal.
   a. Manual technique
      i. Apply 20% ethanol on pledget to loosen epithelial adhesion.

Note: Some surgeons use an optical zone marker as a "well" to hold fluid against cornea for allotted time (30 seconds for 20% ethanol).

Note: Avoid placing ethanol on the peripheral (limbal) epithelium (necessary for reepithelialization).

      ii. Debride epithelium with dry cellulose sponge or scarifier, avoiding sharp dissection.
   b. Transepithelial ablation technique
      i. Planar ablation or "phototherapeutic keratectomy (PTK) mode" selected on excimer laser platform
      ii. Select optical zone for epithelial removal that is slightly larger than planned optical ablation

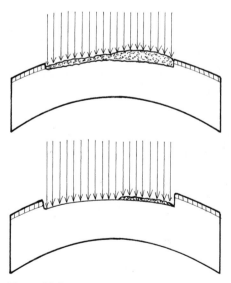

Figure 19.4

      iii. With 50 um ablation depth programmed, perform transepithelial ablation (**Fig. 19.4**).

Note: Epithelium fluoresces with a cobalt blue color when ablated with the excimer laser. When the ablation passes through the epithelium, islands of black (corresponding to the nonfluorescent stroma) can be seen.

    iv. Use a manual technique (cellulose sponges) to remove residual epithelium once ablation is terminated (when the initial break through epithelium is encountered).

    v. Alternatively, transepithelial ablation can be used to remove all epithelium, and PTK can proceed without manipulating the base of the ablation (so-called no-touch technique).

5. Dry cornea with cellulose sponges.

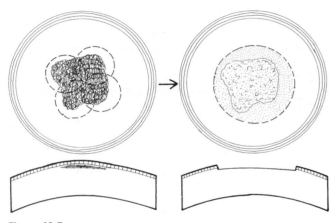

Figure 19.5

6. Program the excimer laser for an ablation depth that will remove most anterior stromal opacities and apply treatment (**Fig. 19.5**).

Note: Do not be over aggressive with ablation treatment. Stop ablation when ~50% of pathology is removed.

7. For a central elevated nodule, a masking agent (methylcellulose) to fill in the area surrounding the lesion helps create a smooth leveling of the tissue.

8. Recheck patient at slit lamp to ensure adequate removal of opacities and scars. Return to excimer laser if additional treatment is necessary.

9. Optional: Apply bandage contact lens to facilitate reepithelialization.

10. Use topical antibiotic and anti-inflammatory drops if contact lens is used, or apply pressure patch with ointment if contact lens is not used.

Postoperative Procedure

1. Bandage soft contact lens or pressure patch until cornea is reepithelialized.

2. Antibiotic drops (e.g., moxifloxacin 0.5% [Vigamox, Alcon Laboratories, Inc., Fort Worth, TX, US], gatifloxacin 0.3% [Zymar, Allergan, Inc., Irvine, CA, US]) 4 times per day (may use ointment if bandage contact lens not used) until epithelial defect closed.

3. Steroid drops (e.g., prednisolone acetate 1%) 4 times per day.

4. Nonsteroidal anti-inflammatory agent (NSAID) drops (e.g., diclofenac sodium 0.1%, [Voltaren, Novartis Pharmaceuticals, Co., East Hanover, NJ, US]) 4 times per day.

5. Taper NSAID and steroid drops according to patient healing.

6. Oral pain medications as necessary.

Complications

1. Persistent epithelial defect
2. Anterior stromal scarring and loss of best corrected visual acuity
3. Infection
4. Recurrence of dystrophic condition
5. Sterile infiltrates*
6. Corneal graft rejection*
7. Hyperopia*
8. Reactivation of herpes simplex keratitis*
   Complication of PTK only

20

Lamellar Keratoplasty

Indications

- Tectonic support in selected cases of corneal melting, thinning, and perforation
- Select cases in which anterior stromal scarring precludes good vision
- Select cases of keratoconus and keratoglobus
- Select traumatic corneal injuries with loss of tissue

Preoperative Procedure

See Chapter 3.

Ensure that the cornea is not perforated. Treat any infectious process as necessary. Either viable (fresh) or nonviable (frozen or glycerin-preserved) donor tissue may be used.

Instrumentation

- Donor eye (fresh, frozen, or glycerin-preserved)
  It is often helpful to have a second eye available if there is difficulty in preparing the first donor button. Moreover, tissue adhesive should be available and viable full-thickness donor tissue on standby if intraoperative perforation of the cornea is a possibility.
- Lid speculum (e.g., Lieberman)
- Sutures (4–0 silk, 10–0 nylon)
- Fine tissue forceps (e.g., 0.12 mm Castroviejo or Colibri, Pierse forceps)

- Scalpel (e.g., #15 Bard-Parker blade)
- Martinez dissector
- Scarifier (e.g., Grieshaber #681.01 or Beaver #57)
- Disposable trephine (e.g., Storz, Weck)
- Vacuum trephine (e.g., Hessburg-Barron)
- Vannas scissors
- Kalt needle holder
- Fine nonlocking needle holder
- Elschnig forceps
- Cellulose sponges
- Paufique knife
- Suarez spreader

Operative Procedure

1. Anesthesia: Peribulbar or retrobulbar injection plus lid block. May use general anesthesia if preferred for younger or uncooperative patients, hearing or mentally impaired patients, or those with language obstacles.
2. Prep and drape.
   a. Use povidone-iodide 5% on a cotton-tipped applicator to gently clean eyelashes and lid margins.
   b. Place one or two drops of povidone-iodide in the conjunctival fornix.
3. Donor preparation.
   a. Use fresh or frozen whole donor eye.
   b. For ease of manipulation, wrap eye in gauze, leaving cornea visible.
   c. If donor epithelium is nonviable, remove it by scraping with a dry cellulose sponge.

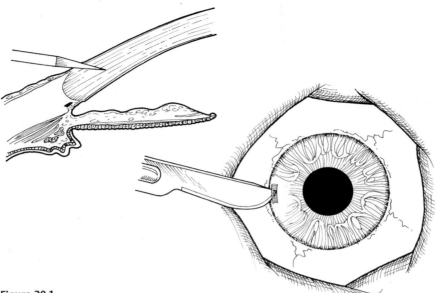

Figure 20.1

d. Incise cornea starting just inside limbus to depth of desired dissection (**Fig. 20.1**).
   i. Hold blade nearly parallel to cornea.
   ii. Dissect anteriorly until desired depth is reached (usually approximately one half to two thirds corneal thickness and slightly thicker than recipient bed).

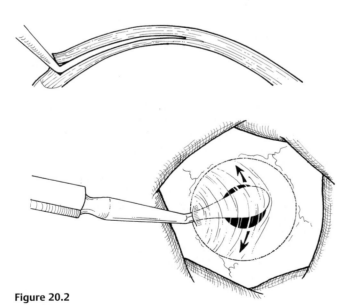

Figure 20.2

e. Use Martinez dissector to gently separate cornea along a lamellar cleavage plane (**Fig. 20.2**).
   i. Do not force the dissector, or the plane of dissection might be lost.
   ii. Extend dissection plane along the entire extent of the donor cornea.

f. Move trephine button directly from donor globe (handheld corneal trephine). Donor button should be ~0.5 mm larger than recipient bed.

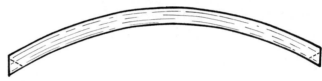

Figure 20.3

g. Bevel the posterior edge of the donor button with Vannas scissors (**Fig. 20.3**).
4. Place lid speculum.
5. Place 4–0 silk bridle sutures (Kalt needle holder, Elschnig forceps).
6. Preparation of recipient bed.
   a. Place trephine cornea to required depth (handheld or vacuum trephine).
      i. Attempt to encompass entire depth of pathology.
      ii. Avoid perforating the globe.
         I. Estimate corneal thickness before setting trephine depth.
         II. 0.4 mm is a common depth when performing a lamellar keratoplasty on a cornea of normal thickness.

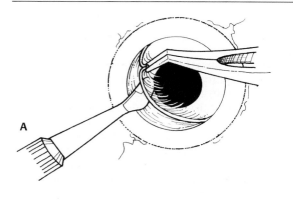

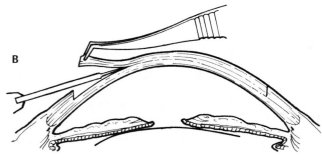

Figure 20.4

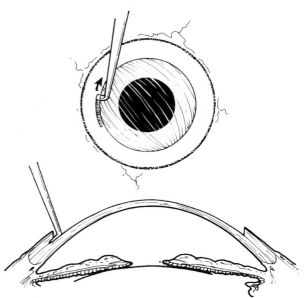

Figure 20.5

c. Undermine the edge of the bed for 360 degrees to create a horizontal groove through which to guide the sutures and enhance graft–host apposition (**Fig. 20.5**).
  i. Groove should extend ~0.5–1 mm into the host.
  ii. Use Paufique knife or Suarez spreader.
7. Irrigate bed with balanced salt solution and swab with a cellulose sponge to remove any epithelial cells or foreign bodies before placing the donor button.
8. Place donor button onto recipient bed.
9. Secure button with 16 interrupted 10–0 nylon sutures or eight interrupted plus a running 10–0 nylon suture.

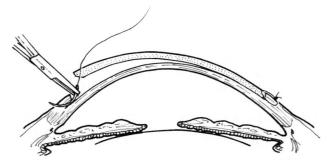

Figure 20.6

b. Perform lamellar dissection with scarifier or Martinez dissector (**Fig. 20.4**).
  i. Hold blade almost parallel to cornea.
  ii. Keep bed dry to facilitate visualization of the cleavage plane (cellulose sponges).
  iii. If inadvertent perforation of cornea occurs, the following interventions may be performed:
    I. Carefully suture perforation with interrupted or mattress 10–0 nylon, placing the knot in the graft–host interface.
    II. Convert to penetrating keratoplasty (see Chapter 15).

a. Pass suture through partial thickness (~90%) donor button and out through groove in recipient bed (**Fig. 20.6**).
b. For the first suture (12 o'clock), the assistant may stabilize the donor with 0.12 mm forceps at 6 o'clock to facilitate suture placement.
c. Place and tie the second suture at 6 o'clock, 180 degrees opposite the first.
  i. Ensure correct placement by grasping the 6 o'clock position with 0.12 mm forceps and noting the corneal fold radiating from the 12 o'clock suture to the 6 o'clock position. This should hemisect the donor (see Chapter 15).
  ii. If graft and host margins cannot be easily apposed, an anterior chamber paracentesis may be performed to soften the globe.
d. Place and tie 3 and 9 o'clock sutures.
e. For the remaining interrupted sutures, split the distance between each suture pair, making certain that all sutures are evenly spaced and radial.

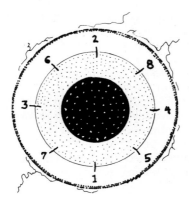

Figure 20.7

f. Ensure that the button is properly nestled in the host bed (**Fig. 20.7**).

g. Ensure all sutures are secure (slightly tighter than for penetrating keratoplasty).

h. Trim and bury interrupted sutures.
   i. Place knot just below surface of recipient cornea.
   ii. Direct cut ends of knot away from the surface to facilitate subsequent suture removal.

i. If using a running suture, tighten, tie, and bury it as described in Chapter 15.

10. Remove bridle sutures.
11. Perform subconjunctival injections of gentamicin (20–40 mg and Decadron 4–8 mg) if indicated.
12. Remove lid speculum.
13. Apply topical antibiotic and steroid ointment.
14. Patch and place Fox shield.

Postoperative Procedure

Note: The following are suggestions for a routine case. The postoperative regimens will vary depending upon the initial indications for lamellar keratoplasty as well as the patient's speed and efficacy of recovery.

1. Topical antibiotics (e.g., moxifloxacin 0.5% [Vigamox, Alcon Laboratories, Inc., Fort Worth, TX, US], gatifloxacin 0.3% [Zymar, Allergan, Inc., Irvine, CA, US]) or ciprofloxacin ointment [Ciloxan, Alcon Laboratories, Inc.] 4 times per day).
2. Steroid drops (e.g., prednisolone acetate 1%) 4 times per day. Taper as indicated.
3. Keep eye patched until graft has reepithelialized.

Suture Removal
1. Remove loose, vascularized, or infiltrated sutures as they appear.
2. May selectively remove interrupted sutures for astigmatism control in approximately 6 weeks.
3. May remove sutures when wound is secure. (This will vary depending on the original indication for surgery. In an uncomplicated case for visual rehabilitation, it may be safe to remove sutures as early as 4–8 weeks. Usually, however, the lamellar graft is for tectonic support of a thinned cornea. Sutures in such cases may be left in place for prolonged periods if they do not loosen or cause reaction.

Complications

1. Perforation of recipient cornea
2. Poor lamellar dissection, resulting in increased interface scarring
3. Persistent epithelial defect and graft melting
4. Infection
5. Graft rejection
6. Astigmatism

21

Tissue Adhesive Application

Actions of Tissue Adhesive

Cyanoacrylate tissue adhesive acts by:

- Directly sealing corneal perforations
- Providing tectonic support to a weakened cornea
- Excluding inflammatory cells from an area of corneal melting
- Promoting vascularization
- Possible antibacterial action

Indications

- Corneal perforations smaller than 1 mm in diameter. (Larger perforations are unlikely to seal with tissue adhesive alone and have a higher risk of inadvertent anterior chamber instillation and subsequent toxicity.)
- Sterile corneal ulceration with progressive thinning, descemetocele formation, or frank perforation.
- Select infected corneal ulcers with progressive thinning and impending perforation.
- Traumatic corneal injuries
  - Puncture wounds
  - Small corneal lacerations (< 1 mm)
  - As an adjunct to corneal suturing in poorly apposed wounds (e.g., stellate wounds)
  - Small wounds that would otherwise require suture placement in the visual axis.

Preoperative Procedure

1. Perform procedure under slit lamp or operating microscope.
2. Culture the base of corneal thinning or margins of perforation if infection is suspected.

Instrumentation

- Lid speculum
- Cellulose sponges
- Scarifier (e.g., Beaver #57, Grieshaber #681.01)
- Capillary tube-type applicator
- Sterile polyethylene or silicone disc
- Cyanoacrylate tissue adhesive (e.g., Histoacryl, Nexacryl)
- Vannas scissors
- Jeweler's forceps

Operative Procedure

1. Apply topical anesthetic (e.g., proparacaine). Lid block may be used for an uncooperative patient.
2. Gently insert lid speculum.
3. Debride loose epithelium and necrotic tissue from the planned site of adhesive application (cellulose sponges, jeweler's forceps, scarifier).
4. Deepithelialize a 1 to 2 mm rim around the application site (cellulose sponges, jeweler's forceps, scarifier).

Note: Tissue adhesive will adhere poorly to an epithelialized or wet surface.

5. Optional: If iris is incarcerated in the perforation and deemed viable, it may be carefully swept back into position with a spatula or irrigation cannula. Alternatively, air or a viscoelastic may be irrigated into the anterior chamber in an attempt to reposit and hold the iris back during adhesive application. Any necrotic iris tissue should be excised (Vannas scissors).
6. Optional: In select cases, a hand-created patch of lamellar corneal or scleral tissue (fresh or preserved) may be used to first plug the perforation before adhesive application.

7. Carefully dry the application site again with cellulose sponges. Adhesive will not stick well to a wet surface.
   a. If a perforation persistently leaks, a cellulose sponge may be used to carefully drain some aqueous to prevent vigorous leakage when area is again dried.
   b. Alternatively, a small air bubble can be introduced into the anterior chamber through a paracentesis and the patient positioned so the perforation is occluded posteriorly.
8. Apply tissue adhesive

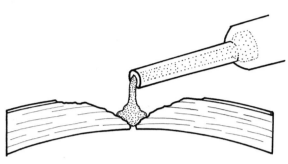

Figure 21.1

Technique 1 (**Fig. 21.1**)
   a. Load tissue adhesive into capillary tube–type applicator. Adhesive will enter thin end of applicator tube by capillary action.
   b. Apply adhesive.
      i. Initiate flow by applying gentle finger pressure over top of applicator.
      ii. If tip of tube clogs with polymerized glue, remove with scissors.

Note: Apply only a very thin film over site, as tissue adhesive will expand significantly as it dries.

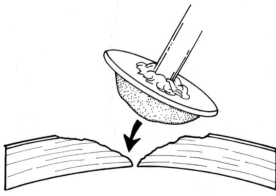

Figure 21.2

Technique 2 (**Fig. 21.2**)
   a. Assemble applicator: Using sterile ophthalmic ointment as an adhesive, affix a sterile 2–4 mm (can be cut to appropriate size) polyethylene or silicone disc to a stick (e.g., back end of a cotton-tip swab).

   b. Place small drop of tissue adhesive on applicator face.
   c. Apply to cornea in "mortarboard" fashion.
   d. The disc may be left in place or carefully removed.

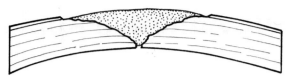

Figure 21.3

9. Allow adhesive to polymerize for 3–5 minutes. Keep area dry and prevent patient from squeezing or moving during this time period. When glue settles, it should not protrude anterior to the epithelial plane surrounding it (**Fig. 21.3**).
10. Check for persistent leakage with cellulose sponge or perform Seidel test with 2% fluorescein strip. (Alternatively, await spontaneous reformation of the anterior chamber, which should occur within 30 minutes.)
11. If seal is not adequate, remove tissue adhesive with forceps (gently rock adhesive until it dislodges) and reapply as described in Step 8.
12. Apply bandage soft contact lens (prevents eyelid irritation and dislocation of glue).

Postoperative Procedure

1. Apply topical antibiotics as indicated.
   a. Intensive fortified antibiotic regimen if infection is suspected (or previous culture results indicate).
   b. Administer prophylactic antibiotics if infection is not likely (e.g., moxifloxacin 0.5% [Vigamox, Alcon Laboratories, Inc., Fort Worth, TX, US], gatifloxacin 0.3% [Zymar, Allergan, Inc., Irvine, CA, US]) four times per day. Continue antibiotic drops until epithelial defect has closed.
2. Steroid drops (e.g., prednisolone acetate 1%) may be used for sterile perforations once the epithelial defect closes.
3. Removing tissue adhesive.
   a. Tissue adhesive will often spontaneously dislodge several weeks—often sooner—after application as the surface reepithelializes.
   b. May remove adhesive when the stroma appears tectonically stable (e.g., scar formation or vascular ingrowth). *Method:* Gently rock adhesive with jeweler's forceps until it dislodges from stroma. (Have additional adhesive on hand in case the perforation reopens.)

Complications

1. Inability to close wound
2. Persistent infection causing reopening of tissue defect
3. Premature loosening of tissue adhesive
4. Corneal vascularization
5. Corneal endothelial and lens toxicity

IV

Refractive Surgery

22

Laser in Situ Keratomileusis (LASIK)

Indications

- Surgical correction of natural myopia, hyperopia, and astigmatism
- Select cases of postsurgical myopia, hyperopia, and astigmatism
- Select cases of presbyopia management with a monovision goal

Contraindications

- Keratoconus and forme fruste keratoconus
- Collagen vascular diseases and inflammatory ocular diseases
- Herpes keratitis
- Epithelial basement membrane dystrophy
- Pregnancy

Preoperative Procedure

1. Discontinue soft contact lens wear at least 1–2 weeks and rigid contact lens wear 2–4 weeks preoperatively. Confirm stability and regularity of corneal topography.
2. Patient should not wear eye makeup on day of procedure.
3. Treat preexisting dry eye and blepharitis. Consider non-preserved lubricants, lid hygiene, punctual plugs, topical cyclosporine, and oral doxycycline for blepharitis.
4. Ensure appropriate corneal thickness with ultrasonic pachymeter.

Note: Corneal thickness minus flap thickness minus ablation depth should be > 250 μm to minimize risk of corneal ectasia.

Instrumentation

- Lid speculum
- Gentian violet marking pen (± 3 mm optical zone marker or Sinskey hook)
- Cellulose sponges
- Microkeratome or femtosecond laser
- LASIK or cyclodialysis spatula
- LASIK irrigating cannula

Operative Procedure

1. For lasers requiring pupil dilation, administer tropicamide 1% ± phenylephrine 2.5%. Otherwise, no dilation.
2. Prep and drape operative eye.
3. Place lid speculum.
4. Create LASIK flap.
   a. For mechanical microkeratomes:
      i. Choose proper ring size and nominal thickness of microkeratome head, depending on corneal thickness, keratometric steepness, corneal width, and expected ablation depth.
      ii. Optional: Premark cornea at anticipated junction of flap and cornea using 3 mm optical zone marker and gentian violet in two or three positions.
      iii. Place suction ring, centered on patient's pupil or geometric center of cornea.
      iv. Engage suction.
      v. Ensure proper suction pressure with handheld tonometer.
      vi. For translational microkeratomes, ensure full engagement of head on ring. For rotational microkeratomes, ensure engagement of head on vertical post.
      vii. Ensure there are no impediments to the translational path of the microkeratome head.

viii. Engage foot pedal for complete microkeratome pass.
ix. Reverse microkeratome pass.
x. Discontinue suction.
xi. Remove microkeratome assembly from cornea.

b. For femtosecond laser flap creation:
i. Choose flap diameter and thickness, hinge width, and side cut angle. Typical settings:
(a) Diameter: 8.5–9 mm.
(b) Flap thickness: 100–120 μm.
(c) Hinge width: 45–55 degrees.
(d) Side cut angle: 70 degrees.
ii. Confirm energy settings.
iii. Choose hinge placement (superior, nasal, temporal).
iv. Optional: Mark cornea over pupil center with 3 mm OZ marker or Sinskey hook impregnated with gentian violet.
v. Place suction ring centered on pupil.
vi. Engage suction.
vii. Dock applanation cone into suction ring.
I. Maintain centration.
II. Ensure size of meniscus is larger than flap width.
viii. Perform laser application.

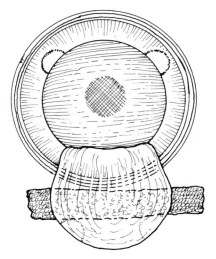

Figure 22.2

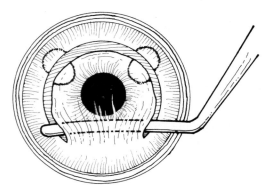

Figure 22.1

5. Lift LASIK flap with LASIK or cyclodialysis spatula (**Fig. 22.1**). For laser flap procedures, use cyclodialysis spatula to break flap adhesions.
a. Enter edge of dissection with spatula near hinge.
b. Release flap edge using edge of spatula or Sinsky hook starting from hinge and proceeding around edge for ~180–270 degrees.
c. Advance spatula across cornea at hinge.
d. Sweep approximately one third to one half of cornea from hinge to opposite end of flap.
e. Repeat spatula entry at hinge and sweep gently to break all lamellar and edge adhesions.

6. Retract flap and place on moistened section of cellulose sponge (**Fig. 22.2**).
7. Optional:
a. Perform intraocular pachymetry to ensure postoperative corneal bed will be > 250 μm to minimize risk of corneal ectasia.
b. May perform "bubble" pachymetry before lifting flap in laser-flap procedures.
8. Gently wipe bed with cellulose sponge to remove residual fluids.
9. Engage laser eye tracker and align laser as necessary
a. Alignment technique varies with laser platform.
b. Center over pupil.
10. Encourage patient to maintain gaze at fixation target.
11. Perform laser ablation with laser focused at corneal plane.
12. Replace flap.
a. Use irrigating cannula or spatula.
b. Float flap into proper position using modest irrigation.

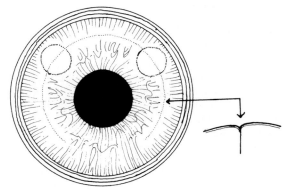

Figure 22.3

c. Align gutter with preplaced gentian violet positioning marks (**Fig. 22.3**).

d. Ensure there are no flap striae or interface debris. Irrigate, reposition, or gently smooth with spatula as necessary.
13. Administer corticosteroid and antibiotic drops.
14. Administer nonpreserved lubricant.
15. Remove lid speculum carefully so as not to disrupt flap position.

Postoperative Procedure

1. Place protective shields or goggles until patient is examined on postoperative day 1. Continue eye protection for 2 additional nights when sleeping.
2. Corticosteroid drops 4 times per day for 1 week.
3. Topical antibiotic 4 times per day for 1 week.
4. Nonpreserved lubricants as needed.
5. Continue dry eye/blepharitis management as needed.
6. Explain postoperative management to patient.

Follow-up Schedule

1. Postoperative day 1: General examination with attention to flap striae. If significant striae are present, reposition flap in operating room.
2. Postoperative week 1: General examination with attention to flap, assess for any infection of diffuse lamellar keratitis
3. Month 1
4. Month 3 (full exam to assess status and consider retreatment if necessary)
5. Months 6, 12 as necessary

Complications

Intraoperative Flap Problems

1. Short flap
2. Thin flap
3. Buttonhole in flap
4. Free flap

Early Postoperative Complications

1. Slipped flap or flap macrostriae
2. Epithelial defects or sloughing
3. Iris tuck by the intraocular lens

Intermediate-Term Complications

1. Diffuse lamellar keratitis (DLK)
2. Microbial keratitis
3. Microstriae
4. Epithelial ingrowth

Late-Term Complications

1. Over- and undercorrections
2. Induced astigmatism
3. Induced topography irregularities
4. Corneal ectasia and keratoconus

23

Photorefractive Keratectomy (PAK)/ Laser Epithelial Keratomileusis (LASEK)

Indications

- Surgical correction of natural myopia, hyperopia, and astigmatism
- Select cases of postsurgical myopia, hyperopia, and astigmatism
- Select cases of presbyopia management with a monovision outcome
- Select cases of thinner corneas in which LASIK contraindicated
- Select cases of epithelial basement membrane dystrophy
- Vocational needs (occupations in which LASIK flap not allowed)

Contraindications

- Keratoconus and forme fruste keratoconus
- Collagen vascular diseases and inflammatory ocular diseases
- Herpes keratitis
- Pregnancy

Preoperative Procedure

1. Discontinue soft contact lens wear at least 1–2 weeks and rigid contact lens wear 2–4 weeks preoperatively. Confirm stability and regularity of corneal topography.
2. Patient should not wear eye makeup on day of procedure.
3. Treat pre-existing dry eye and blepharitis. Consider non-preserved lubricants, lid hygiene, punctual plugs, topical cyclosporine, and oral doxycycline for blepharitis.

4. Optional: Administer oral corticosteroid on day of procedure and taper thereafter to decrease postoperative discomfort.
5. Ensure appropriate corneal thickness with ultrasonic pachymeter.

Note: The corneal thickness minus the ablation depth should leave > 350 μm to minimize risk of corneal ectasia. This number is a suggestion and has not been validated.

Instrumentation

- Lid speculum
- Cellulose sponges
- Spatula
- Amoils epithelial brush
- 20% ethanol with 8–9 mm optical zone marker bath
- Epithelial microkeratome
- Mitomycin C 0.02% (optional)
- Therapeutic soft contact lens

Operative Procedure

1. For lasers requiring pupil dilation, administer tropicamide 1% ± phenylephrine 2.5%. Otherwise, no dilation.
2. Prep and drape operative eye.
3. Place lid speculum.
4. Remove corneal epithelium over a 8–9 mm area using one of following techniques:
   a. Mechanically scrape with spatula.
   b. Mechanically remove with Amoils epithelial brush.

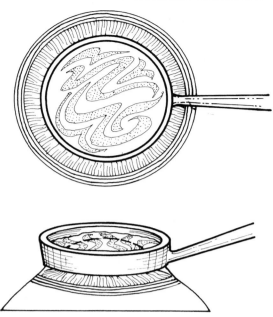

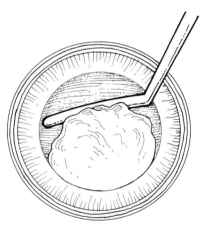

Figure 23.1

d. Elevate epithelial flap with an epithelial micro-keratome. For techniques (c) and (d), the flap may be discarded or repositioned after the laser ablation.
5. Gently wipe bed with cellulose sponge or spatula to remove residual fluids.
6. Engage laser eye tracker and align laser as necessary.
   a. Alignment technique varies with laser platform.
   b. Center over pupil.
7. Encourage patient to maintain gaze at fixation target.

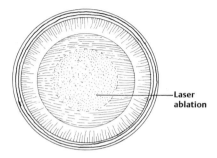

Laser ablation

Figure 23.3

c. Place 20% ethanol for ~20 seconds in 8–9 mm optical zone marker bath (**Fig. 23.1**).
   i. Irrigate residual ethanol with chilled balanced salt solution (BSS).
   ii. Loosen epithelium with cellulose sponge.

8. Perform laser ablation (**Fig. 23.3**).
9. Irrigate surface with chilled balanced salt solution or lactated Ringer solution (chilled solution aids in minimizing discomfort postoperatively).
10. Optional: To minimize postoperative haze formation, apply mitomycin C 0.02% on cellulose pledget for 12–30 seconds. Copiously irrigate with chilled BSS after application.
11. Reposition epithelial flap if desired.
12. Apply therapeutic contact lens.
13. Administer corticosteroid and antibiotic drops.
14. Remove lid speculum.

Postoperative Procedure

1. Corticosteroid drops 4 times per day for 1 week and taper to 2 times daily for one week and one time daily for one week
2. Topical antibiotic 4 times per day for 1 week.
3. Nonpreserved lubricants as needed.
4. Taper oral corticosteroid if used.
5. Topical and oral nonsteroidal anti-inflammatory agent for pain control as needed.
6. Oral narcotics for pain as needed.
7. Optional: Vitamin C 1000 mg daily (may aid in corneal haze prevention).
8. Continue dry eye/blepharitis management as needed.
9. Explain postoperative management to patient.

Figure 23.2

iii. Remove epithelial sheet with cellulose sponge or spatula (**Fig. 23.2**).

Follow-up Schedule

1. Postoperative day 1.
2. Postoperative day 3–5 (general examination with attention to epithelial healing and contact lens removal).
3. Month 1.
4. Month 3 (full exam to assess status and consider retreatment if necessary).
5. Months 6, 12 as necessary.

Complications

Early Postoperative Complications

1. Poor epithelialization.

Intermediate-Term Complications

1. Epitheliopathy.
2. Corneal haze.
3. Microbial keratitis.

Late-Term Complications

1. Over- and undercorrections.
2. Induced astigmatism.
3. Induced topography irregularities.
4. Corneal haze.

24

Conductive Keratoplasty

Indications

- Surgical correction of hyperopia (1–3 D).
- Surgical management of presbyopia via monovision/ multifocal approach.
- Selected cases of postsurgical hyperopia and astigmatism. Non-FDA approved "off-label" application.

Preoperative Procedure

1. Discontinue soft contact lens wear at least 1 week and rigid contact lens wear 2 weeks preoperatively. Confirm stability and regularity of corneal topography.
2. Patient should not wear eye makeup on day of procedure.
3. Treat preexisting dry eye and blepharitis. Consider non-preserved lubricants, lid hygiene, punctual plugs, topical cyclosporine, and oral doxycycline for blepharitis.
4. Determine treatment plan. Consult recent nomograms for application pattern and expected effect. In general, concentric rings of 8 spots are placed at optical zones of 7 or 8 mm, or both.
5. Perform preoperative keratometry.

Instrumentation

1. Integrated conductive keratoplasty (CK) lid speculum.
2. Cellulose sponges.
3. CK corneal marking template.
4. CK console.
5. Sinskey hook.
6. Gentian violet marking pen or pad.

Operative Procedure

1. Mark center of entrance pupil either at slit lamp or under coaxial microscope. Mark axis of astigmatism if astigmatism to be treated.

   a. Sinskey hook.
   b. Gentian violet.
2. Prep operative eye.
   a. Do not use lid drape.
   b. Speculum need direct contact with lid and conjunctiva for proper instrument function.
3. Place integrated CK lid speculum (supplies return path for electric current).
4. Mark spot placement using CK marking template. Center over pupil.

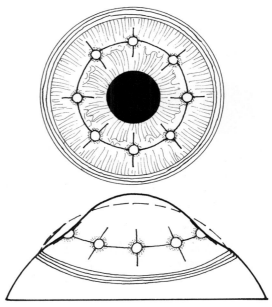

Figure 24.1

5. Apply CK spots:
   a. CK effect is consequent to midperipheral collagen contracture from circumferential applications leading to secondary central corneal steepening (**Fig. 24.1**).

b. Place probe perpendicular to cornea at area of placement.
  i. Probe is 90×450 μm.
  ii. Penetration depth is restricted by insulated Teflon-coated governor.
c. Insert probe over positioning mark. Ensure complete depth of penetration by noting dimple in cornea.

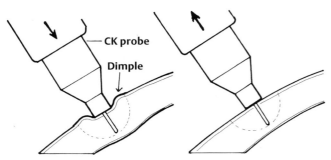

Figure 24.2

d. For light touch CK technique, gently elevate probe until dimple disappears and corneal contour regains normal configuration (**Fig. 24.2**).
e. Apply CK spot
  i. 0.6 seconds
  ii. 0.6 Watts
  iii. Follow cornea inward with probe as the surface retracts.
  iv. After spot, wait 1 second before probe removal.

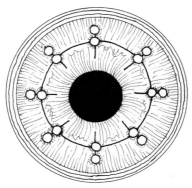

Figure 24.3

f. Continue CK application to conclude rings (**Fig. 24.3**). Place spots consecutively 180 degrees away from previously placed spot.

6. Alternative template method
  a. Proceed with steps 1–3.
  b. Place CK template over pupil center mark.
  c. Secure with suction via integrated syringe.
  d. Place probe into template holes and activate application.
  e. Proceed with placement of spots for one or two, eight-spot rings as planned.
  f. Release suction and remove template.
7. At conclusion of procedure, check intraoperative keratometry.
  a. May reapply application to previous spot or add one spot if > 1 D of induced astigmatism.
  b. Place in flat meridian.
8. Optional: Administer corticosteroid and antibiotic drops.
9. Administer nonpreserved lubricant.
10. Remove lid speculum.

Postoperative Procedure

1. Optional: Corticosteroid drops 4 times per day for 1 week.
2. Topical antibiotic 4 times per day for 1 week.
3. Nonpreserved lubricants as needed.
4. Topical and oral nonsteroidal anti-inflammatory agent for pain control as needed.
5. Explain postoperative management to patient.

Follow-up Schedule

1. Postoperative day 1.
2. Week 1.
3. Month 1.
4. Month 3 (full exam to assess status and consider retreatment if necessary).
5. Months 6, 12 as necessary.

Complications

1. Over- and undercorrections.
2. Induced astigmatism.
3. Induced topography irregularities.

25

Intracorneal Ring Segments (INTACS)

Indications

- Surgical management of keratoconus in patient intolerant of contact lens treatment.
- Primary goal to restore contact lens tolerance and prevent need for penetrating keratoplasty.
- Secondary goal to improve spectacle and uncorrected visual acuity.
- Surgical management of post-LASIK ectasia.
- Mild to moderate natural myopia.

Contraindications

- Visually significant corneal scar.
- Corneal thickness at Intacs entry site < 450 μm; thinnest pachymetry < 350.

Preoperative Procedure

1. Patient should not wear eye makeup on day of procedure.
2. Treat preexisting dry eye and blepharitis. Consider non-preserved lubricants, lid hygiene, punctual plugs, topical cyclosporine, and oral doxycycline for blepharitis.
3. Assess refraction, keratometry, and corneal topography for axis of Intacs placement and proper size of Intacs segments:
   Nominal expected correction:
   250 μm segments: -1.3 diopters
   300 μm segments: -2.0 diopters
   350 μm segments: -2.7 diopters
   400 μm segments: -3.4 diopters
   450 μm segments: -4.1 diopters

Note: Segments may be placed asymmetrically for noncentered cones. For peripherally displaced cones, one segment may be considered to improve asymmetry in corneal topography.

Instrumentation

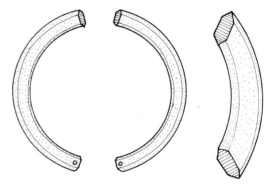

Figure 25.1

- Intacs specifications (**Fig. 25.1**):
  - Hexagonal cross section
  - 6.8 mm inner diameter; 8.1 mm outer diameter
  - 150 degree arc length
  - Available thickness: 250, 300, 350 μm; 400, 450 μm pending FDA approval
- Lid speculum
- Gentian violet marking pen or pad
- Cellulose sponges
- Intacs console
- Incision and placement marker
- Pocketing hook
- Symmetric glide
- Clockwise and counterclockwise dissector
- 11 mm centration marker
- Sinskey hook
- Calibrated diamond knife
- Ultrasonic pachymeter
- Lamellar spreader
- Combined left and right handed spreader
- Intacs forceps

- 0.12 mm forceps
- Needle holder
- 10–0 nylon suture
- Optional: Femtosecond laser

Operative Procedure

1. Prep and drape operative eye.
2. Place lid speculum.
3. Mark geometric center of cornea with 11 mm centration marker.
4. Mark geometric center with Sinskey hook and gentian violet. Some surgeons center procedure on entrance pupil or between geometric center and pupil center.

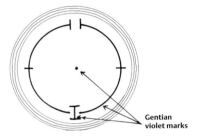

Figure 25.2

5. Place incision and placement marker with gentian violet on centration mark, and mark incision spot at desired meridian (**Fig. 25.2**).
6. Take pachymetry measurement over entry site.
7. Calculate 70–75% depth at entry site.
8. Set calibrated diamond knife to 70–75% depth.

9. Incise entry site for 1.2 mm to full depth of blade.
10. Place pocketing hook to base of incision.
    a. Create a box-shaped lamellar entry to begin the Intacs channel.
    b. Create similar dissection for second Intacs segment.
11. Extend lamellar dissection in both directions with symmetric glide (**Fig. 25.3**).
    a. Enter deep in incision.
    b. Maintain spreader parallel to deep corneal lamellae.
12. Place suction ring centered on limbus.
13. Engage suction ring to suction level 1.
14. Ensure suction, and raise to level 2.
15. Reinsert symmetric glide to depth of previously created dissection.
16. Place lamellar dissector into suction ring and beneath symmetric glide to start tunneling.
17. Remove spreader from atop dissector.
18. Gently rotate dissector completely until hub reached.
19. Carefully remove dissector.
20. Repeat steps 15–18 in other direction.
21. Stop suction and remove ring.
22. For Intralase procedures, skip steps 7–21. Instead:
    a. Choose inner and outer channel diameter (typically 6.6–6.8 × 7.4–7.8 mm), depth (typically 400 μm or 70–75% entry site depth), and meridian of entry site.
    b. Confirm energy settings.
    c. ±Mark cornea over pupil center with 3 mm optical zone (OZ) marker or Sinskey hook impregnated with gentian violet.
    d. Place suction ring centered on pupil.
    e. Engage suction.
    f. Dock applanation cone into suction ring.
       i. Maintain centration.
       ii. Ensure size of meniscus is larger that flap width.
       iii. Center channel ring using video display.
    g. Perform laser application.
    h. Break proximal tunnel adhesions with symmetric glide.

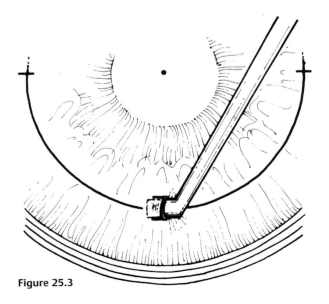

Figure 25.3

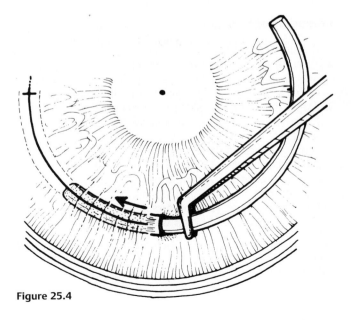

Figure 25.4

i. Enter deep in incision
ii. Maintain spreader parallel to deep corneal lamellae
23. Irrigate Intacs segment with antibiotic drop.
24. Grasp Intacs with Intacs forceps.
25. Enter site with segment at acute angle to bring its head to base of incision.
26. Turn segment parallel to dissection channel.
27. Slowly advance segment (**Fig. 25.4**).
    a. Irrigate cornea during procedure.
    b. Counter pressure with cellulose sponge or forceps may help to expand channel and facilitate entry.
28. Repeat steps 23–27 for second segment.

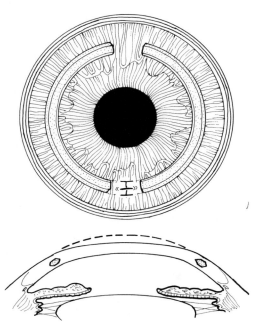

Figure 25.5

29. Place 10–0 nylon suture to secure incision (**Fig. 25.5**).
    a. Place deep to base of incision for good closure.
    b. Tie securely.
    c. **Note:** Some surgeons do not use suture and apply bandage soft contact lens instead.
30. Administer corticosteroid and antibiotic drops.
31. Remove lid speculum.

Postoperative Procedure

1. Corticosteroid drops 4 times per day for 1 week.
2. Topical antibiotic 4 times per day for 1 week.
3. Nonpreserved lubricants as needed.
4. Explain postoperative management to patient.
5. Optional: Bandage soft contact lens.

Follow-up Schedule

1. Postoperative day 1.
2. Postoperative week 1.
3. Month 1 (may remove suture here on myopia and LASIK ectasia patients).
4. Month 3 (may remove suture here on keratoconus patients).
5. Months 6, 12 as necessary.

Complications

1. Segment migration.
2. Segment extrusion.
3. Optical side effects such as glare and halo.
4. Induced astigmatism.
5. Microbial keratitis.

V

Eye Trauma

26

Corneal Foreign Body Removal

Indications

- Superficial foreign bodies that are easily accessible
- Stromal foreign bodies such as wood that have a high likelihood of harboring infections
- Embedded foreign bodies in the anterior corneal stroma
- Any foreign body that has an associated infiltrate
- Iron foreign bodies with rust ring formation

Note: Any corneal or limbal foreign body that has penetrated into the anterior chamber must be removed under controlled sterile conditions under magnification (see Chapter 28).

Note: Substances such as glass and certain minerals are inert, and rarely cause an inflammatory response. If the foreign body has been present for a few days, is not exposed to the surface (the epithelium has covered the area in a smooth plane), and it has not induced an inflammatory response, it may be left in place, especially if it is near the visual axis, where overzealous removal or burring may cause scarring. Close follow-up is warranted in these cases. If the foreign body is an unknown material, it should be removed.

Preoperative Procedure

1. Perform a careful, slit lamp examination, paying particular attention to the depth and nature of the foreign body.
2. If the foreign body is deep, perform Seidel test to rule out penetration into the anterior chamber.
3. If an intraocular foreign body is considered, check angle and lens carefully, measure intraocular pressure, and perform dilated ophthalmoscopy.
4. Diagnostic imaging (B-scan ultrasonography, computerized tomography, and magnetic resonance imaging) may be indicated to rule out an occult foreign body.

Ultrasound biomicroscopy may be useful for assessing foreign bodies in the angle.

Instrumentation

- Lid speculum (optional)
- Cotton tipped applicators or cellulose sponges
- 25 or 27 gauge needle or hockey stick
- Jeweler's forceps
- Motorized corneal burr
- Topical anesthetic (e.g., proparacaine)

Operative Procedure

1. Anesthesia:
   a. Topical proparacaine.
   b. Peribulbar or retrobulbar block in very uncooperative patient.
2. Insert lid speculum (optional).

Note: It is preferable to remove the foreign without a speculum if possible. This allows the patient to blink between operative steps to lubricate the corneal surface, allowing for better visualization and, often, mobilization of an already loosened foreign body.

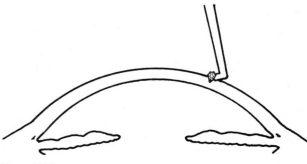

Figure 26.1

3. Undermine the foreign body from the cornea (25 gauge needle tip).
   a. Place tip of needle (bevel up) under edge of foreign body and dislodge outward. May use hockey stick (**Fig. 26.1**).
   b. Avoid repeated stabs at material, which may damage surrounding Bowman and stroma, and lead to scarring and delayed healing.

Note: When performing this procedure at the slit lamp, make sure the patient's head is fully pressed in against the headband and the examiners arm is stabilized as to prevent the needle from penetrating the cornea should the patient move.

4. Once the foreign body is loosened, it may be removed in whole with a moistened cotton swab or cellulose sponge.

   Optional: If there is any suspicion of infectious material, culture the foreign body as well as the corneal bed.

5. Remove residual debris using steps 3 and 4.
6. If a rust ring is noted once the foreign body is removed:
   a. Remove the rust ring with a corneal motorized burr.
   b. If the ring cannot be removed easily or it is in deep stroma, consider waiting 24–48 hours *for the rust to rise to the anterior stroma.*

Note: Small specks of rust material may be left if they cannot be removed.

7. Debride any loose and nonviable epithelium (cotton tipped applicator, jeweler's forceps).

Postoperative Procedure

1. Close follow-up is required. The patient should be reexamined 24 hours after foreign body removal, and every 24–48 hours until the area reepithelializes. Careful attention should be paid to possible early infection or stromal necrosis.
2. Cycloplegic drops (e.g., cyclopentolate 1%).

3. Antibiotic drops (e.g., moxifloxacin 0.5% [Vigamox, Alcon Laboratories, Inc., Fort Worth, TX, US], gatifloxacin 0.3% [Zymar, Allergan, Inc., Irvine, CA, US]) 4–8 times per day, or ointment (e.g., ciprofloxacin, [Ciloxan, Alcon Laboratories, Inc.).
4. Fortified antibiotics (e.g., tobramycin, cefazolin) should be considered in cases of organic foreign bodies with a large inflammatory/infectious response even before cultures results are confirmed.
5. Oral pain medications as necessary.
6. Once epitheliazation is complete, topical steroid medications (e.g., prednisolone acetate 1%) may be administered to reduce scarring and inflammatory consequences of foreign body removal.

Note: We prefer to avoid bandage contact lenses and pressure patches after foreign body removal, even in cases where inert, supposedly noninfectious material is embedded. It may be difficult to truly ascertain the infectious risk in such cases.

Complications

1. Persistent epithelial defect (usually with retained material and/or rust ring)
2. Persistent inflammation or iritis
3. Anterior stromal scarring or loss of best corrected visual acuity
4. Iatrogenic perforation into anterior chamber
5. Infection
6. Recurrent corneal erosion

27

Hyphema Evacuation

Indications

- First sign of corneal stromal blood staining
- Total or near-total hyphemas that do not resolve by day 5
- Sickle cell trait or disease patients with intraocular pressure (IOP) greater than 25 for more than 24 hours
- Progressively worsening visual acuity
- Persistent blood clot in angle for longer than 10 days
- Increase in IOP despite maximum medical therapy (IOP greater than 50 mm Hg for 5 days or greater than 35 mm Hg for 7 days)

Preoperative Procedure

1. Perform a complete ocular examination to rule out a ruptured globe.
2. Document the size (percentage of anterior chamber) of the hyphema, as well as any other anterior segment abnormalities.
3. Measure the IOP and perform a dilated fundus exam (avoid scleral depression).
4. B-scan ultrasonography, computerized tomography magnetic resonance imaging, and ultrasound biomicroscopy may be useful in assessing the anterior segment and posterior segment.
5. Patients of African and Mediterranean descent must be screened for sickle cell trait or sickle cell disease (Sickledex prep; hemoglobin electrophoresis if necessary).

Supportive Treatment

1. Shield the affected eye with metal or plastic at all times.
2. Confine patient to bed rest, or to very limited activity.
3. Elevate head 30 degrees while resting and sleeping.
4. Prescribe mild analgesia (e.g., acetaminophen).
5. Avoid aspirin-containing products, nonsteroidal anti-inflammatory agents, or anticoagulants.

Medical Treatment

1. Cycloplegia (e.g., Atropine 1% drops 2–3 times per day).
2. Steroid drops (e.g., prednisolone acetate 1% 4–8 times per day), based on inflammation.
3. Management of IOP.
   a. β-blockers should be used if IOP > 30 mm Hg (lower threshold for sickle cell and previous glaucoma patients).
   b. Add α-agonist or topical carbonic anhydrase inhibitor, or both if needed.
   c. Consider oral acetazolamide or intravenous mannitol if drops are unsuccessful.

Note: Sickle cell patients may use β-blockers, but all other medicines must be used with caution. Topical and systemic carbonic anhydrase inhibitors may induce sickling. α-agonists may affect iris vessels. Prostaglandin-analogs and miotics may promote inflammation.

4. In hospitalized patients, oral or topical aminocaproic acid may be administered to reduce rebleeding, if not medically contraindicated.

Instrumentation

- Lid speculum (e.g., Lieberman)
- 21 gauge infusion cannula
- Irrigation/aspiration device (bimanual preferred)
- Intraocular diathermy
- Viscoelastic substance (e.g., Healon, Amvisc)
- Microvitrectomy suction/cutting instrument
- Microsharp blade
- Keratome
- Fine-toothed tissue forceps (e.g., 0. 12 mm Castroviejo, Colibri)
- Vannas scissors
- Cellulose sponges
- Cyclodialysis spatula

- 10–0 nylon suture
- 7–0 Vicryl suture
- Needle holder
- Muscle hook
- Lens loop

Operative Procedure

Hyphema Evacuation Procedures

Anterior chamber washout is the simplest and safest method of clearing blood from the anterior chamber. For large clots, a "hyphemectomy" using a vitrectomy cutting device or limbal clot delivery through a large incision may be useful.

Anterior Chamber Washout

1. Anesthesia:
   a. Topical anesthetic (e.g., proparacaine).
   b. Peribulbar or retrobulbar plus lid block for an un-cooperative patient or when surgical time is antici-pated to be prolonged.
2. Prep and drape.
   a. Use povidone-iodide 5% on a cotton-tipped applica-tor to gently clean eyelashes and lid margins.
   b. Place one or two drops of povidone-iodide in the conjunctival fornix.
3. Gently insert lid speculum.
4. Create two paracentesis ports through clear cornea.
   a. Place incisions at 1 and 10 o'clock.
   b. Internal openings should be 2 mm.
   c. Use a MicroSharp blade.

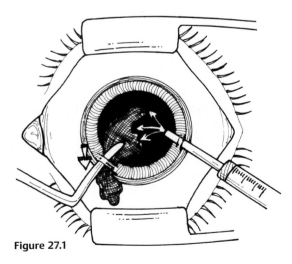

Figure 27.1

5. Irrigate the anterior chamber (**Fig. 27.1**).
   a. Use balanced salt solution (BSS) on a 21 gauge irriga-tion cannula.
   b. Depress the posterior lip of the fellow paracentesis with a cyclodialysis spatula.

6. Anterior chamber fluid, including red blood cells and possibly small free-floating clots should be seen exiting the wound (**Fig. 27.1**).
7. Reverse the irrigation cannula and spatula sites and ir-rigate again.

Note: Extra care should be taken in phakic individuals to avoid capsule or lens damage during these maneuvers.

8. Repeat steps 5 and 6 as necessary until good anterior segment visualization is achieved.
9. Hydrate the wounds with BSS and test for integrity
10. Place 10–0 nylon interrupted sutures.

Note: It is not necessary to remove the entire clot with this technique. Evacuation of suspended red blood cells and de-bris is the goal. Removal of larger clots should be approached through limbal clot expression or a microvitrectomy cutting device

Limbal Clot Delivery

Hyphema clots reach their maximal consolidation and re-traction by day 4 to 7, which is the optimal time to perform this technique.

1. Perform steps 1–3 as above.
2. Create limbal clear corneal incision of at least 6 mm in length with a keratome.

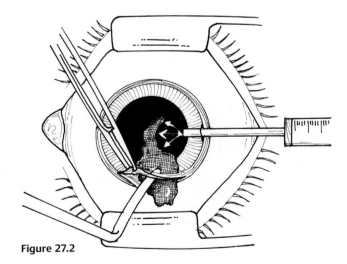

Figure 27.2

3. If clot does not spontaneously prolapse from wound, ir-rigate through paracentesis with BSS on cannula (**Fig. 27.2**).
4. Gently place a muscle hook or cyclodialysis spatula at the inferior limbus and roll upward toward the superior lim-bus to help manually express the clotted blood.
5. An assistant may elevate the anterior lip of the wound with 0.12 forceps.

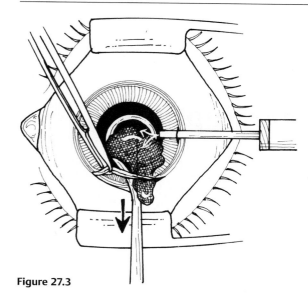

Figure 27.3

Optional: Place a lens loop through the superior incision to engage the blood clot. Mobilize the clot through the wound in a controlled manner, as in extracapsular cataract extraction (**Fig. 27.3**).

6. Perform a peripheral iridectomy (Vannas scissors, 0.12 forceps).
7. Close the wound with interrupted 10–0 nylon sutures.
8. Reposition the conjunctiva and secure with 7–0 Vicryl sutures (0.12 forceps, needle holder).

Microvitrectomy Cutting/Aspiration Removal (Automated Hyphemectomy)

1. Perform steps 1–4 as in anterior chamber washout.

Note: The same ports that are used in anterior chamber washout may be used for this technique. Many surgeons begin with a washout and proceed with hyphemectomy only if a persistent clot cannot be sufficiently removed.

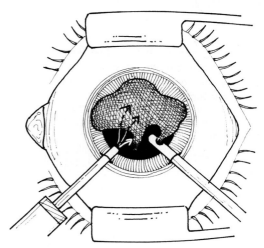

Figure 27.4

2. Remove clot using the vitrectomy cutting device in one hand and the irrigation device in the other (**Fig. 27.4**).
3. Avoid trauma to lens, iris, and corneal endothelium by keeping instrument tip in view at all times.
4. Tamponade any active bleeding that may arise when the clot is pulled away from the fragile iris vessels by using the pressure of the infusion cannula.

Note: Viscoelastic placed over these active areas may help; bimanual diathermy should be reserved for recalcitrant bleeding.

5. Hydrate wounds with BSS.
6. Close wound with 10–0 nylon interrupted sutures.

Postoperative Procedure

Immediate Follow-up Schedule

1. Keep patch and shield in place until the patient is examined on postoperative day 1.
2. The medical treatment instituted prior to surgery should be continued in the postoperative period (see "Medical Treatment").
3. Topical antibiotic drops (e.g., moxifloxacin 0.5% [Vigamox, Alcon Laboratories, Inc., Fort Worth, TX, US], gatifloxacin 0.3% [Zymar, Allergan, Inc., Irvine, CA, US]) 4 times per day for 1 week.
4. Steroid drops (e.g., prednisolone acetate 1%) 4 to 6 times per day, tapered over ~4 to 6 weeks, as inflammation improves.
5. Cycloplegia (e.g., cyclopentolate 1%) 3 times per day, tapered as the inflammation subsides.
6. IOP-lowering medications may be systematically eliminated if the pressure remains controlled (this may take weeks or longer in some patients)
7. Patient may gradually increase activity level.

Follow-up Schedule

1. Postoperative day 1.
2. Postoperative day 2 or 3, then every few days.
3. Two, 4, and 6 weeks postoperatively and then as necessary.

Long-Term Follow-up Schedule

1. Perform gonioscopy and dilated fundus examination with scleral depression 2–6 weeks after initial trauma.
2. Complete yearly checkups to rule out angle recession glaucoma.

Complications

1. Surgical damage to cornea, iris, or lens
2. Inadvertent damage to iris
3. Rebleeding (most frequently 2–5 days after injury).
4. Synechiae formation
5. Glaucoma

28

Corneoscleral Lacerations and Ruptured Globe Repair

Indications

- Partial-thickness wounds with significant override or gape
- Specific partial-thickness wounds that are at a higher risk of perforation (e.g., children)
- Full-thickness wounds larger than 3 mm that do not self-seal
- Full-thickness wounds that do not close adequately with bandage lens or tissue glue placement
- Wounds with loss of corneal tissue
- All full-thickness wounds with iris incarceration
- All full-thickness wounds with vitreous incarceration
- All posterior scleral lacerations (and any suspected posterior lacerations based on exam)

Objectives

Primary Objective

To obtain complete watertight closure of the globe with restoration of structural integrity.

Secondary Objectives

- Remove disrupted tissues (e.g., lens, vitreous).
- Remove intraocular foreign bodies.
- Prevent infection.
- Prepare for future reconstruction and rehabilitation strategies.

Preoperative Procedure

Overall goals for treating a patient with a possible corneal or scleral laceration include:

1. Recognize and address any life-threatening systemic conditions.
2. Obtain a detailed history.
   a. Specifically address the possibility of an intraocular foreign body.
   b. Determine if previous eye surgery took place (e.g., radial keratotomy or RK incisions and cataract wound predispose to rupture: LASIK scars predispose to flap dehisence).
3. Carefully evaluate the eye and adnexa.
   a. Eyelid irregularities may be a foreign body entrance site.
   b. Assess pupillary function and inspect pupil at slit lamp.
   c. Severe subconjunctival hemorrhage and shallow or unusually deep anterior chamber are strong indicators of ruptured globe.
   d. Document hyphema size, lens or iris injury, and optic nerve or retinal damage.

Note: Avoid intraocular pressure measurements when there is a possibility of globe rupture.

4. Obtain imaging studies as necessary (plain film, computed tomographic scan).
   a. Magnetic resonance imaging should be avoided in any case where a metallic foreign body is possible.
   b. A- and B-scans should be avoided in cases of globe rupture until the globe is watertight.

Supportive Treatment

1. Shield (metal or plastic) the affected eye at all times.
2. Reduce pain and nausea to prevent lid squeezing.
3. Confine patient to bed rest and fasting until time of surgery.

4. Administer prophylactic intravenous broad spectrum antibiotics.
   a. Cefazolin (1 g IV every 8 hours) and ciprofloxacin (400 mg IV 2 times per day) are a typical combination.
   b. Clindamycin is added when an intraocular foreign body is suspected (for *Bacillus* coverage).
5. Tetanus toxoid as needed.

Nonsurgical Management

Self-Sealing or Partial-Thickness Wounds

1. A Seidel test should be conducted to rule out occult perforation.
2. Provocation with gentle finger pressure at the slit lamp may be done.

   If either (1) or (2) above are positive, broad spectrum antibiotic coverage should be initiated and patient should be followed closely.

Soft contact lens

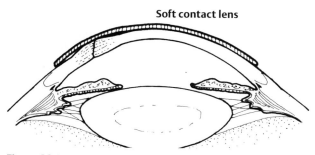

Figure 28.1

3. If minimal wound gape is present, the edges do not override, and the anterior chamber remains formed—usually in lacerations smaller than 3 mm—a bandage contact lens may be used (**Fig. 28.1**).
4. Alternatively, a pressure patch may be used.
5. A cycloplegic agent (e.g., homatropine 5%) and antibiotic drop (e.g., moxifloxacin 0.5% [Vigamox, Alcon Laboratories, Inc., Fort Worth, TX, US], gatifloxacin 0.3% [Zymar, Allergan, Inc., Irvine, CA, US]) 6 times per day should be used.
6. Bandage lens should be left on for 2–4 weeks, or when the stromal wound appears to be stabilized.
7. A plastic or metal shield should be placed over affected eye each evening and protective daytime eyewear should be worn until wound is sufficiently healed.

Puncture Wounds or Small Tissue-Loss Wounds

1. Cyanoacrylate glue may be useful in these situations (see Chapter 21).
2. For children and uncooperative patients, and those who may have difficulty keeping follow-up exams, definitive surgical closure is more appropriate.

   The surgeon should remember that the best way to ensure good tissue closure is with suture placement. Any wound with significant override or gape—whether partial or full thickness—should be repaired with sutures.

Conjunctival Laceration Repair

Any case of traumatic conjunctival laceration should be suspected to be a ruptured globe. If any examination findings are suggestive of scleral laceration, the patient should be taken to the operating room for exploration. Exploration of the sclera with cotton-tipped applicator under topical anesthesia (e.g., proparacaine) may be useful.

If the injury involves only the conjunctiva, treatment is as follows:

1. Conjunctival lacerations less than 1.0 cm, with minimal exposed Tenon capsule:
   a. Antibiotic ointment (e.g., erythromycin) or drops (e.g., moxifloxacin 0.5% [Vigamox, Alcon Laboratories, Inc.], gatifloxacin 0.3% [Zymar, Allergan, Inc.]) 4–6 times per day.
   b. Consider pressure patching for the first 24 hours.
2. For conjunctival lacerations larger than 1 cm, or irregular wounds with exposed Tenon capsule or muscle sheath:
   a. Carefully inspect tissue edges to excise Tenon capsule (blunt Westcott scissors).
   b. Perform interrupted suture closure with absorbable sutures (e.g., 8–0 Vicryl).
      i. Avoid burying edge of conjunctiva when closing wound.
      ii. Avoid suturing directly to the plica semilunaris or caruncle.

Instrumentation

- Lid speculum (e.g., Lieberman)
- Fine-toothed tissue forceps (e.g., 0.12 mm forceps)
- Westcott scissors
- Sutures (4–0 silk, 8–0 nylon, 10–0, and 11–0 nylon with spatulated needle, 8–0 Vicryl)
- Needle holder
- Smooth forceps (e.g., Chandler or Bracken forceps)
- Viscoelastic material (e.g., Amvisc, Viscoat)
- Cyclodialysis spatula
- Vannas scissors
- Muscle hook
- MicroSharp blade
- Cellulose sponges
- Cotton-tipped applicator
- Fluorescein strip
- Culture materials

Operative Procedure

1. Anesthesia: Many cases can be repaired using peribulbar anesthesia with a lid block or topical anesthesia. General anesthesia is an option in certain cases, unless medically contraindicated.
2. Prep and drape with minimal pressure on globe.
3. Gently insert lid speculum (in a severely traumatized globe, 4–0 silk traction sutures through the upper and lower lids or Steri-Strips can be used to retract the lids to avoid speculum pressure).

4. Culture the wound edges on blood, chocolate, thioglyco-late, and Sabouraud's agar. Culture any foreign bodies or excised tissuet.

Simple Full-Thickness Corneal Lacerations

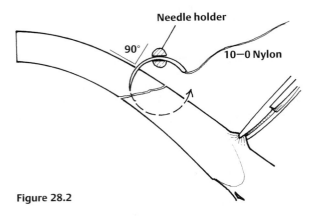

Figure 28.2

1. If the wound is watertight and the anterior chamber remains formed, direct suturing is advisable, using a minimal-touch or no-touch technique.
2. Gently irrigate wound with balanced salt solution (BSS).
3. Fixate globe using 0.12 forceps.
4. Place a 10–0 nylon suture (spatulated needle) through midpoint of laceration length, using a one-handed technique.
   a. Direct needle into cornea at a 90 degree angle, and rotate hand to pass through stroma following the needle curve (**Fig. 28.2**).
   b. Corneal sutures should be ~1.5 mm in length and 90% deep in the stroma.

Note: Full-thickness bites should be avoided as the suture may act as a conduit for microorganisms.

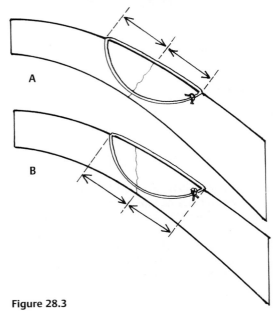

Figure 28.3

c. Linear lacerations: Suture pass should be equidistant on both sides of the wound (**Fig. 28.3A**).
   d. Oblique lacerations: Needle pass should be equidistant to the deepest part of the wound to prevent override (**Fig. 28.3B**).
5. Place subsequent sutures by progressively halving the length of the corneal wound.
6. If the wound is not stable, irrigate viscoelastic into the anterior chamber through a limbal paracentesis (avoids disruption of wound edges, and allows better access for instruments).

Note: If the anterior chamber is flat, may irrigate viscoelastic directly through wound to deepen chamber; a paracentesis may be placed secondarily.

7. Temporary superficial sutures may be used to help stabilize the eye in certain cases.

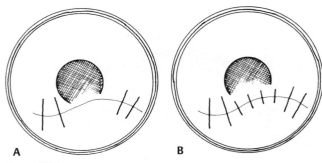

Figure 28.4

8. Typical corneal suture length should be 1.5 mm (equal length on both sides of wound).
   a. Longer sutures may be used near the limbus to induce central corneal steepening, thereby maintaining the pretrauma corneal contour (**Fig. 28.4A**); central support suture is removed after peripheral sutures are placed.
   b. Use longer suture bites in edematous or macerated wound edges to ensure closure.
   c. Shorter sutures (and finer sutures, e.g., 11–0 nylon) should be used in the visual axis to minimize scarring (may wish to straddle visual axis with sutures) (**Fig. 28.4B**).
   d. Each suture bite should be of moderate tension.
9. Tie suture knots with 3–1–1 throws and then cut ends (see Chapter 15).
10. Any loose or temporary sutures should be replaced, but avoid overzealous removal or replacement (increased manipulation compromises the wound).
11. Trim knot ends and bury knots away from the visual axis. Direct the ends of the knots away from the surface to facilitate subsequent removal (see Chapter 15).
12. Deepen the anterior chamber with BSS and check wound for leaks using a cellulose sponge and/or a fluorescein strip.

Stellate Lacerations with and without Tissue Avulsion

1. Simple interrupted suture closure of each wing of a stellate laceration may be performed if there is no tissue loss.
   a. Place 10–0 nylon sutures perpendicular to each linear laceration.
   b. Check with fluorescein strip to ensure watertight closure.

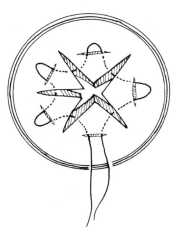

Figure 28.5

2. Close stellate lacerations that do not obtain watertight closure with a purse-string technique (**Fig. 28.5**).
   a. Use diamond or MicroSharp blade to create partial thickness stromal incisions in each wing of stellate wound.
   b. Pass needle through one stromal incision to the other, engaging each corneal laceration at 90% stromal depth.
   c. Once the continuous suture is passed back through the entrance incision, the needle is removed, the suture is drawn tight and then tied in 3–1–1 fashion.
   d. Additional interrupted sutures may be placed as needed
3. If the center of the laceration continues to leak, apply tissue adhesive and a bandage contact lens (see Chapter 21).
4. In cases where an avulsed piece of corneal tissue is present, suture the apex first, then proceed with additional sutures.

Corneal Lacerations with Iris Incarceration

1. Carefully inspect tissue for viability.
   a. Attempt to preserve as much iris tissue as possible.
   b. Obviously devitalized or macerated tissue should be excised by cutting flush to the cornea (Vannas scissors).
   c. Any iris tissue that appears epithelialized should be excised and sent for culture.
   d. If injury occurred more than 24 hours earlier, excise exposed iris to reduce infection risk.
2. Select cases with minimal iris incarceration may be managed pharmacologically

   a. Central wounds with iris incarceration may be treated with a dilating agent (e.g., intraocular epinephrine 1:10,000).
   b. Peripheral wounds with incarceration may be treated with a miotic agent (e.g., intraocular acetylcholine).
3. If pharmacologic therapy fails, create a paracentesis at the limbus furthest away from site of the corneal wound (MicroSharp blade).

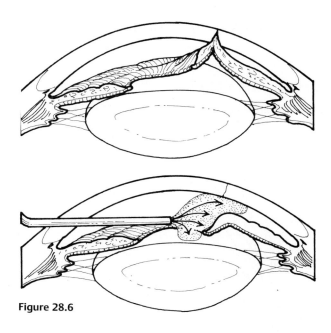

Figure 28.6

4. Instill viscoelastic through paracentesis to deepen anterior chamber (**Fig. 28.6**).

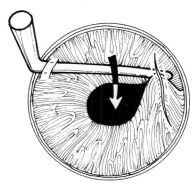

Figure 28.7

5. If the chamber is flat and the wound is unstable, a temporary nylon suture through the center of the laceration (placed superficially to avoid iris involvement) may facilitate chamber deepening.
6. If the iris remains incarcerated in wound after chamber deepening, sweep with a cyclodialysis spatula or irrigating cannula (**Fig. 28.7**).

a. Insert instrument through paracentesis.
b. Methodically sweep (e.g., windshield wiper) parallel to iris plane.
c. Avoid iatrogenic damage to cornea, iris, and lens.
7. Repair of iris damage is usually performed at a later date, in association with other reconstruction procedures, including lens removal, anterior vitrectomy, and intraocular lens implantation (see Chapter 29).

Corneal Lacerations with Lens Damage

See Chapter 13.

Simple Corneoscleral Lacerations

1. Large lacerations may require stabilization with temporary sutures to restore structural integrity.

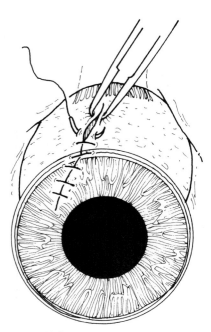

Figure 28.8

2. Realign the limbus with 8–0 nylon or silk sutures (**Fig. 28.8**).
3. Reposit prolapsed iris, if necessary.
4. Close corneal wound as discussed.
5. Create peritomy.
   a. If scleral portion of wound is small, a localized peritomy may be made over laceration area.
   b. For larger injuries, a 360 degree peritomy is made, and each quadrant is explored.
6. Place scleral sutures as soon as a new area of laceration is uncovered (**Fig. 28.8**).
   a. Surgical loupes may be helpful for posterior sutures.
   b. 8–0 nylon or 7–0 Vicryl sutures may be used.
   c. Pass needle completely through one end of wound before making the second pass.

7. Carefully examine areas near the laceration, as well as behind muscle insertions.
   a. Clean overlying Tenon capsule (0.12 forceps, Westcott scissors).
   b. Use muscle hook or retractor to explore behind muscle insertions.
   c. May use 4–0 silk traction suture to retract rectus muscle.
   d. If necessary, the muscle may be disinserted after securing with a 6–0 double-armed Vicryl suture and then reattached after the scleral laceration is repaired (see Chapter 37).

Posterior Scleral Lacerations

The posterior extent of lacerations that extend very far posteriorly (sometimes to the optic nerve) may be left unsutured. Significant globe distortion would occur with attempted posterior closure, often leading to expulsion of intraocular contents.

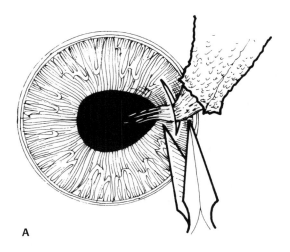

A

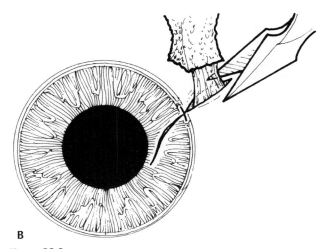

B

Figure 28.9

Corneoscleral Lacerations with Uveal and Vitreous Prolapse

1. Create a 360 degree peritomy and identify areas of globe rupture and uveal/vitreous loss.
2. Vitreous prolapsing through the wound can be secured with dry cellulose sponges and cut flush with the scleral surface. Avoid excess traction on the vitreous (**Figs. 28.9A and 28.9B**).
3. If the view is adequate, a vitreous cutting device may be used at the wound

Note: Posterior wounds with vitreous incarceration are likely to have accompanying retinal damage, which may require subsequent vitreous surgery. The overall goal of the initial surgery is watertight closure of the globe, which will facilitate any future procedures.

4. Reposit uvea prolapsing through the scleral wound, if possible.

Note: Excising uveal tissue leads to extensive bleeding and excising uvea in wounds posterior to the pars plana may damage the retina.

Note: In severe trauma cases, may excise prolapsed tissues to obtain closure (in such cases, the tissue should be identified by histopathologic examination).

5. Beginning at the anterior (limbal) edge, proceed posteriorly with interrupted 8–0 nylon or silk sutures in a zipper-like fashion.

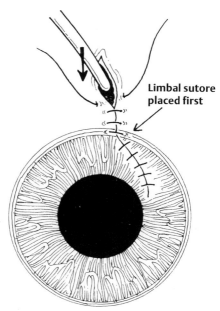

Limbal suture placed first

Figure 28.10

6. Reposit prolapsed uveal tissue by having an assistant gently push the uveal tissue into the wound using a cyclodialysis spatula as the surgeon sutures (**Fig. 28.10**).
7. Raise the wound edges with forceps to keep suture passage away from the underlying uvea.
8. Pass the needle completely through one end of the scleral gape before making the second pass.
9. Tighten each suture so the scleral edges appose well, with no uvea or vitreous in wound.

Corneoscleral Lacerations with Tissue Loss

1. Directly suture small puncture wounds and small avulsive injuries (though tissue distortion often leads to excessive scarring and astigmatism).
2. Small stellate lacerations may require closure with tissue adhesives if a central leak persists (see Chapter 21).
3. Replace tissue if necessary in cases with excessive tissue loss:
   a. Lamellar patch graft (see Chapter 20) with fresh or frozen corneal or scleral tissue.
   b. Full-thickness patch graft (requires healthy tissue "bed" to suture into).
   c. Penetrating keratoplasty (PK) (see Chapter 15) is rarely indicated in primary repair after trauma.
      i. Best to quiet inflammation and treat possible infection prior to a PK
      ii. In cases of extensive corneal tissue loss, a primary PK and anterior segment reconstruction procedure may be considered
      iii. Extreme care should be taken while trephinating an open globe

Irreparable Tissue Injury

Cases of severe globe disruption with loss of intraocular contents may be irreparable. If every attempt to restore the globe's integrity is unsuccessful, primary enucleation may be performed if proper informed consent was obtained before surgery. Consideration of sympathetic ophthalmia and anesthesia risks of a second procedure must be made. When possible, some restoration of globe integrity allows time for the patient and family to accept the necessity of a secondary enucleation

Postoperative Procedure

At Conclusion of Surgery

1. Administer subconjunctival injection of a broad-spectrum antibiotic (e.g., cefazolin 100 mg).
2. Subconjunctival gentamicin administration should be avoided due to potential retinal toxicity.
3. Administer subconjunctival steroids (e.g., dexamethasone 12 to 24 mg) in cases with a low suspicion of postoperative endophthalmitis.

Follow-up Schedule

1. Intravenous antibiotics (see Supportive Treatment section earlier in this chapter) should be continued for 3–4 days.
2. Topical fortified antibiotics (vancomycin 50 mg/ml and ceftazidime 50 mg/ml) administered every hour. Alternatively, topical fluoroquinolone drops (e.g., moxifloxacin 0.5% [Vigamox, Alcon Laboratories, Inc., Fort Worth, TX, US], gatifloxacin 0.3% [Zymar, Allergan, Inc., Irvine, CA, US]) 4 times per day for 1 week may be given hourly, then lowered in frequency as the eye heals.
3. Monitor culture results and adjust antibiotic regimen accordingly.
4. Cycloplegia (e.g., cyclopentolate 1%) 3 times per day, tapered as the inflammation subsides.
5. Topical steroid drops (e.g., prednisolone acetate 1%) 4–6 times per day, tapered over 4–6 weeks may be used to reduce postoperative scarring and prevent vessel ingrowth.

Note: Steroid drops increase the risk of infection, especially in wounds caused by vegetable matter or foreign bodies.

6. The injured eye should be shielded at all times (other than when drops are administered) for 6–8 weeks postoperatively.

Complications

1. Endophthalmitis
2. Hyphema
3. Increased intraocular pressure
4. Hypotony or wound leak
5. Vitreous or uveal incarceration in wound
6. Cystoid macular edema
7. Glaucoma
8. Retinal detachment
9. Epithelial downgrowth
10. Corneal scarring or edema
11. Irregular astigmatism
12. Sympathetic ophthalmia

29

Repair of Iris Trauma and Iris Suturing Techniques

Indications

Iridodialyses and iris sphincter tear, causing glare, photophobia, or cosmetically unacceptable anisocoria

Objectives

- Preserve as much iris tissue and maintain as normal ocular anatomy as possible.
- Reconstruct pupil to prevent glare and photophobia.
- Restore a firm iris structure to avoid synechia formation and glaucoma.
- Protect cornea (or corneal graft) from iridocorneal adhesions and glaucoma.
- Create a stable iris diaphragm for support of anterior or posterior intraocular lens.

Preoperative Procedure

The initial treatment of iris injury is conservative until initial trauma repair is complete and wound is stabilized.

1. Shield (metal or plastic) the affected eye at all times.
2. Reduce pain and nausea to prevent lid squeezing.
3. Confine patient to bed rest and keep fasting (NPO) until time of surgery.
4. Administer prophylactic intravenous broad-spectrum antibiotics if appropriate
   a. Cefazolin (1 g IV every 8 hours) and ciprofloxacin (400 mg IV 2 times per day) are a typical combination.
   b. Clindamycin is added when an intraocular foreign body is suspected (for *Bacillus* coverage).
5. Tetanus toxoid as needed.

Nonsurgical Management

- Sunglasses
- Tinted contact lenses
- Contact lenses with an artificial iris peripheral pigmentation
- Topical medications
  - Miotic agents (e.g., pilocarpine 1%) may reduce size of a traumatically dilated pupil.
  - Mydriatic agents (e.g., cyclopentolate 1%) may normalize a decentered pupil.

Laser Treatments

Note: This technique is most useful when dilating drops are ineffective, where adhesions and bands can be lysed, and a sphincterotomy can recenter an eccentric pupil.

1. Argon laser settings: 50 µ (micron) spot size, power 1000 mW (milliwatts) power, 0.1 second duration; low risk of lens capsule rupture (can use in phakic patients).
2. Neodymium:yttrium-aluminum-garnet (Nd:YAG) laser settings: 5 to 6 mJ and higher; higher rate of bleeding than argon laser.

Instrumentation

- Lid speculum (e.g., Lieberman)
- Fine-toothed tissue forceps (e.g., 0.12 mm forceps)
- Westcott scissors
- 10-0 polypropylene sutures (with a long needle e.g., Ethicon CIF-4 for closed-chamber cases; Short needle e.g., Ethicon BV 100-4 for open sky cases)
- Sutures (4-0 silk, 10-0 nylon, 8-10 Vicryl)
- Needle holder
- Smooth forceps (e.g., Chandler or Bracken forceps)
- Viscoelastic material (e.g., Amvisc, Viscoat)

- Cyclodialysis spatula
- Vannas scissors
- MicroSharp blade
- Cellulose sponges
- Kuglen hook
- Scalpel (e.g., #15 Bard-Parker blade)
- Handheld cautery
- Wheeler knife
- MVR blade

Operative Procedure

Iridodialysis Repair

1. Anesthesia: Peribulbar or retrobulbar block with or without lid block. Certain cases may require general anesthesia (extensive repair, medically unstable patient).
2. Prep and drape.
   a. Use povidone-iodide 5% on a cotton-tipped applicator to gently clean eyelashes and lid margins.
   b. Place one or two drops of povidone-iodide in the conjunctival fornix.
3. Gently insert lid speculum (in a severely traumatized globe, 4–0 silk traction sutures through the upper and lower lids or Steri-Strips can be used to retract the lids to avoid speculum pressure).
4. Using 0.12 forceps and Westcott scissors, create a localized conjunctival peritomy in the region of the dialysis.
5. Lightly cauterize the underlying scleral bed.

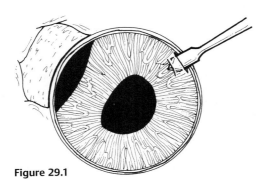

Figure 29.1

6. Create paracentesis using MicroSharp or MVR blade 4–5 clock hours away from area of dialysis (**Fig. 29.1**).
7. Instill viscoelastic into the anterior chamber through paracentesis port.
8. If necessary, use cyclodialysis spatula to break synechia and free as much iris tissue as possible.

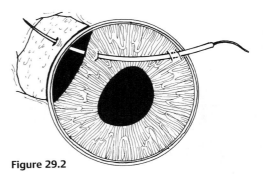

Figure 29.2

9. Introduce one arm of a double-armed 10–0 polypropylene suture through the paracentesis and engage the dialyzed edge of the iris (**Fig. 29.2**).

Note: Care must be taken not to allow the needle to pass through Descemet membrane and to avoid touching the lens.

10. Pass the needle through the adjacent sclera. Use second instrument (e.g., 0.12 forceps) to apply pressure behind needle exit point.

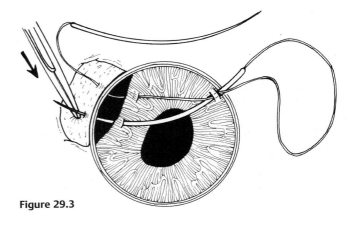

Figure 29.3

11. Pass the fellow arm of the same suture in similar fashion through the paracentesis, iris, and sclera, using forceps for countertraction (**Fig. 29.3**).

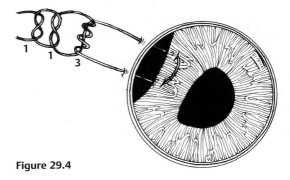

Figure 29.4

12. Cut the needles off and tie the suture securely in 3–1–1 fashion (**Fig. 29.4**).

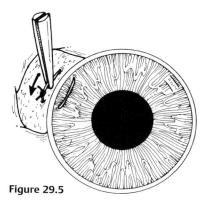

Figure 29.5

13. Cut the knot ends and rotate below the scleral surface (**Fig. 29.5**).
14. Close the conjunctival flap over the polypropylene suture with absorbable sutures (e.g., 8–0 Vicryl).
15. Hydrate the paracentesis with balanced salt solution and check integrity; place interrupted 10–0 nylon suture if necessary.

Pupil Repair (McCannel Suture Technique)

1. Anesthesia: Peribulbar or retrobulbar block with or without lid block
2. Prep and drape.
   a. Use povidone-iodide 5% on a cotton tipped applicator to gently clean eyelashes and lid margins.
   b. Place 1 or 2 drops of povidone-iodide in the conjunctival fornix.
3. Gently insert lid speculum (in a severely traumatized globe, 4–0 silk traction sutures through the upper and lower lids or Steri-Strips can be used to retract the lids to avoid speculum pressure).
4. Place a limbal paracentesis 2–3 clock hours from the iris defect (good position to suture iris ends easily).
5. Instill viscoelastic into the anterior chamber through paracentesis port.
6. If necessary, use cyclodialysis spatula to break synechia and mobilize iris tissue.

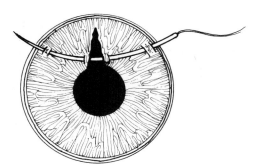

Figure 29.6

7. Pass 10–0 polypropylene suture through the paracentesis and engage two adjacent edges of the iris defect (**Fig. 29.6**).

8. Pass the suture through the opposite peripheral clear cornea (**Fig. 29.6**).

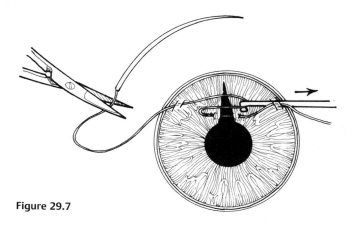

Figure 29.7

9. Cut the needle off (**Fig. 29.7**).
10. Introduce Kuglen hook through paracentesis and engage a loop of suture (**Fig. 29.7**).

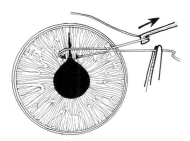

Figure 29.8

11. Retract Kuglen hook through paracentesis while holding opposite suture end with tying forceps (**Fig. 29.8**).

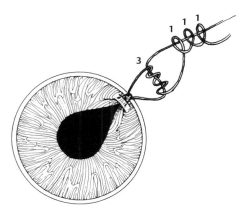

Figure 29.9

12. Pull iris to wound and tie the suture securely with four throws (3–1–1–1) (**Fig. 29.9**).

Note: If the iris is not flaccid enough to allow the knot to tie outside the paracentesis, make suture loops inside the anterior chamber and slide knot down to iris plane.

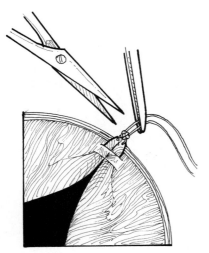

Figure 29.10

13. After knot is tightened, cut suture ends short by drawing knot through wound (**Fig. 29.10**).

Alternatively, introduce a sharp knife (e.g., Wheeler blade) through paracentesis to cut suture ends without putting traction on iris.

14. Hydrate the paracentesis with balanced salt solution and check integrity; place interrupted 10–0 nylon suture if necessary.

Postoperative Procedure

At Conclusion of Surgery

1. Administer subconjunctival injection of a broad-spectrum antibiotic (e.g., cefazolin 100 mg).

2. Administer subconjunctival steroids (e.g., dexamethasone 12 to 24 mg) in cases with a low suspicion of postoperative endophthalmitis.

Immediate Follow-up Schedule

1. Topical antibiotic drops (e.g., moxifloxacin 0.5% [Vigamox, Alcon Laboratories, Inc., Fort Worth, TX, US], gatifloxacin 0.3% [Zymar, Allergan, Inc., Irvine, CA, US]) 4 times per day for 1 week.
2. Topical steroid drops (e.g., prednisolone acetate 1%) 4–6 times per day, tapered over 2–4 weeks to reduce postoperative scarring and prevent vessel ingrowth.

Note: Steroid drops increase the risk of infection, especially in wounds caused by vegetable matter or foreign bodies.

3. The eye should be shielded at night for at least 1 week.

Complications

1. Polypropylene suture breakage or loosening
2. Irregular pupil shape
3. Synechia formation
4. Endophthalmitis
5. Hyphema
6. Increased intraocular pressure
7. Tonic pupil
8. Cystoid macular edema
9. Retinal detachment
10. Corneal scarring or edema
11. Sympathetic ophthalmia

VI

Glaucoma

30

Glaucoma Filtration Procedures

■ Trabeculectomy/Posterior Lip Sclerectomy

Indications

Glaucoma uncontrolled by maximally tolerated medical therapy and by laser trabeculoplasty.

Preoperative Procedure

See Chapter 3.

1. Preoperative intraocular pressure (IOP) should be < 30 mm Hg. If the IOP is too high, intravenous or oral osmotics may be used.
2. Some medications used to treat glaucoma can, theoretically, compromise the prognosis of the filtration bleb. Therefore, they may be discontinued preoperatively. This should only be done, however, if adequate IOP control can be maintained without these medications or with substitute medications. The following agents are listed in the order of priority in which they should be stopped.
   a. Discontinue cholinesterase inhibitors (e.g., phospholine iodide) 2 weeks preoperatively to decrease bleeding and postoperative inflammation.
   b. Discontinue carbonic anhydrase inhibitors 1–2 days preoperatively to increase aqueous flow through bleb.
   c. If IOP allows, discontinue β-blockers 1–2 weeks preoperatively, because decreased aqueous flow may compromise the bleb.
   d. Discontinue epinephrine, dipivefrin, apraclonidine, brimonidine, and latanoprost or other prostaglandin analogues 1 week preoperatively to decrease pre- and postoperative conjunctival injection and intraocular inflammation in the case of the prostaglandin analogues.

3. The eye should be as quiet as possible preoperatively to enhance the prognosis for successful filtration.
   a. *Optional:* Steroid drop 4 times per day to every hour preoperatively to decrease postoperative inflammation.
   b. *Optional:* Oral steroids (e.g., prednisone 80 mg) starting 1 day preoperatively.

Instrumentation

- Lid speculum (e.g., Lieberman)
- Sutures (4–0 silk or 7–0 Vicryl braided, 10–0 nylon or 10–0 Vicryl monofilament)
- Kalt needle holder
- Elschnig/tissue forceps
- 3 ml syringe with 30 gauge irrigating cannula
- Smooth forceps (Chandler or Bracken)
- Cautery (microdiathermy)
- Westcott scissors
- Iris spatula
- Castroviejo calipers
- Scalpel (e.g., #15 Bard-Parker blade)
- Cellulose sponges
- Fine tissue forceps (e.g., 0.12 mm Castroviejo, Pierse)
- Microsurgical knife (e.g., Beaver #75M, Superblade)
- Scarifier (e.g., Grieshaber #681.01, Beaver #57)
- Wheeler or 15-degree microsurgical knife
- Kelly Descemet membrane punch
- Jeweler's forceps
- Vannas scissors
- DeWecker scissors
- Tying forceps
- Needle holder

Operative Procedure

Trabeculectomy

1. Anesthesia: Retrobulbar or peribulbar injection plus lid block. May use general anesthesia if preferred, and for younger or uncooperative patients, hearing or mentally impaired patients, or those with language obstacles
2. Prep and drape.
   a. Use povidone-iodide 5% on a cotton-tipped applicator to gently clean eyelashes and lid margins.
   b. Place 1 or 2 drops of povidone-iodide in the conjunctival fornix.
3. Place lid speculum.
4. Place a 4–0 silk bridle suture under superior rectus tendon. Be careful not to injure conjunctiva (Kalt needle holder, Elschnig forceps). Alternatively place a 7–0 Vicryl braided suture through the peripheral cornea for traction.
5. Select position for filter placement, usually in superotemporal or superonasal quadrant in area of least inflamed or scarred conjunctiva. Superonasal placement leaves room for subsequent cataract surgery if necessary.
6. Prepare limbus-based conjunctival flap.

Note: Always handle conjunctiva gently and at the edges. Use nontoothed forceps.

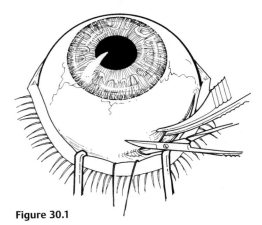

Figure 30.1

   a. Incise superior bulbar conjunctiva for ~90 degrees, 10 mm posterior to the limbus (Bracken or Chandler smooth forceps, Westcott scissors) (**Fig. 30.1**).

Note: Take caution to avoid the superior rectus muscle.

   b. Fashion a thin conjunctival flap down to the limbus, freeing the conjunctiva from subjacent adhesions

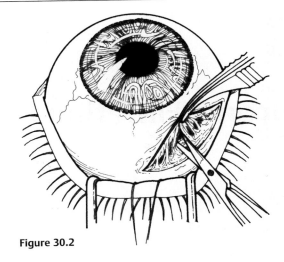

Figure 30.2

to Tenon capsule. Have assistant elevate flap while adhesions are lysed with sharp and blunt dissection (smooth forceps, Westcott scissors) (**Fig. 30.2**).

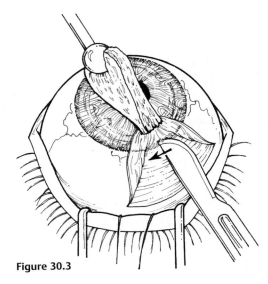

Figure 30.3

   c. Carefully free remaining adhesions anteriorly using an iris spatula, cellulose sponge, or the back of a scalpel (#15 Bard-Parker blade) (**Fig. 30.3**).
      i. Do not buttonhole conjunctiva.
      ii. Hold flap back with moistened cellulose sponges to avoid trauma to the conjunctiva.
      iii. Ascertain the anterior extent of the dissection by viewing the iris spatula or scissors blades through the flap (the flap should be dissected well up onto the limbus to avoid placing the sclerostomy too posteriorly).
7. Always keep the conjunctival flap moist with balanced salt solution (BSS).
8. Perform meticulous hemostasis (monopolar microdiathermy).

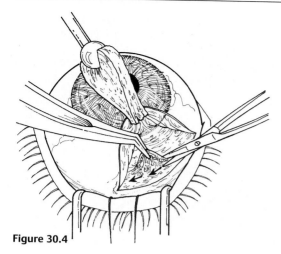

Figure 30.4

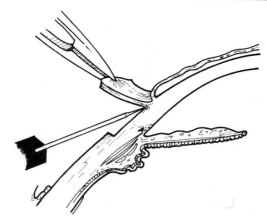

Figure 30.6

9. Remove residual Tenon capsule from the episclera (0.12 mm forceps, Westcott scissors).
   a. To avoid bleeding, do not cut too close to the episclera.
   b. Superiorly, cut Tenon off parallel to conjunctival incision (**Fig. 30.4**).
10. Use calipers to measure width of scleral flap (flap may be rectangular or triangular with an ~3–4 mm base and 3–4 mm posterior extent).
11. Outline edges of scleral flap with microdiathermy.

13. Perform a lamellar dissection of the scleral flap with a scarifier (**Fig. 30.6**).
   a. Flap should be ~50% deep.
   b. Apply counter traction with 0.12 mm or Pierse forceps to facilitate dissection.
   c. Remain in plane of dissection.
   d. Extend anteriorly over the limbus to the level of the conjunctival insertion.

   Optional: Apply mitomycin C (MMC) 0.2 to 0.5 mg/ml or 5-flurouracil 50 mg/ml soaked in a sponge and placed over the scleral dissection area for 1–5 minutes, depending on the desired effect to prevent postoperative fibrosis. Irrigate MMC off eye using BSS.
14. Cauterize planned entry site.

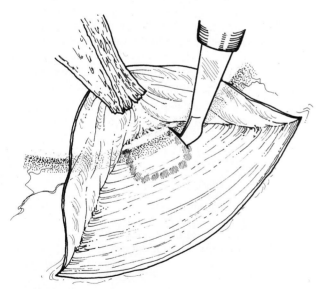

Figure 30.5

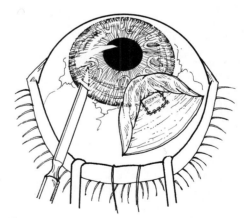

Figure 30.7

12. Make a partial-thickness scleral groove incision (approximately one half to two thirds) over the diathermy outline extending anteriorly to the conjunctival flap (Beaver #57 or Grieshaber #681.01) (**Fig. 30.5**).

15. Perform paracentesis through clear cornea just inside the limbus in a quadrant neighboring the filter site with a Wheeler or similar microsurgical knife (see Chapter 7). Note the surrounding landmarks to relocate site at end of case (**Fig. 30.7**).

Note: Temporal placement of paracentesis may facilitate office-based manipulation postoperatively, if necessary.

16. Verify the patency of the paracentesis with a 30 gauge cannula on a syringe.

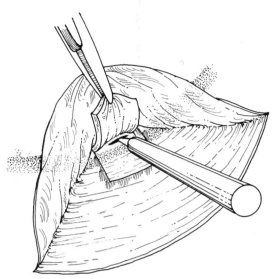

Figure 30.8

17. Enter the anterior chamber under the scleral flap with a microsurgical knife as anteriorly as possible (**Fig. 30.8**).
18. Extend the entry site horizontally for ~2 mm.

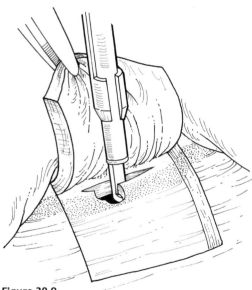

Figure 30.9

19. Perform sclerectomy with Kelly Descemet punch (**Fig. 30.9**).
    a. Hold the posterior lip of the wound with 0.12 mm forceps to facilitate placing the punch.
    b. The sclerostomy should be ~2–3 mm long and 1–2 mm wide, with its posterior extent at the level of the scleral spur.

c. Alternatively, the trabeculectomy block may be removed in one piece with a microsurgical knife (e.g., Beaver #75M) and Vannas scissors.
20. Cauterize the posterior lip of sclerostomy to expand the opening and prevent bleeding (microdiathermy).

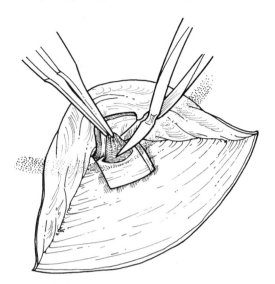

Figure 30.10

21. Perform a broad, basal iridectomy (Jeweler's forceps, Vannas or DeWecker scissors) (**Fig. 30.10**).
22. Secure the scleral flap with two interrupted 10–0 nylon sutures tied loosely at corners and bury knots (add additional sutures and/or tie more tightly if less filtration is desired).

    Optional: Postoperatively, indicate in chart which sutures are tight: (e.g., 1 is tightest; 4 loosest).

23. Reposition conjunctival flap.
24. Remove bridle suture or corneal traction suture.

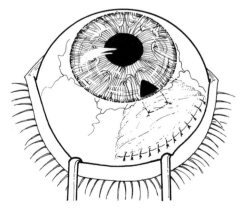

Figure 30.11

25. Suture conjunctival flap with either (**Fig. 30.11**):
    a. Interrupted 10–0 nylon sutures tied with a 2–1–1 surgeon's knot.

b. Running 9–0 or 10–0 nylon or Vicryl monofilament suture with vascular needle and the edge of Tenon capsule (created with the tenonectomy in Step 9).

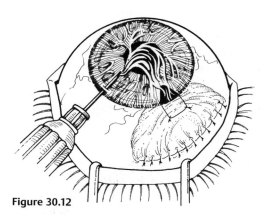

Figure 30.12

26. Check patency of sclerostomy site and security of conjunctival closure by irrigating BSS through the previously placed paracentesis (**Fig. 30.12**).
    a. Conjunctival bleb should form and anterior chamber should reform.
    b. Place 2% fluorescein solution over the suture line and bleb to check for leaks and add additional sutures as necessary.
    c. If a buttonhole is noted, close with an interrupted or mattress 10–0 nylon suture with a vascular needle.
    d. Paracentesis site usually does not need to be sutured.
27. Inject subconjunctival Decadron (4–8 mg) 180 degrees away from filter site into the conjunctival fornix.
28. Apply topical antibiotic, steroid ointment, and 1% atropine drops.
29. Apply light dressing and shield.

Posterior Lip Sclerectomy (Full-Thickness Filter)

Note: The technique of posterior lip sclerectomy is similar to that for trabeculectomy, except that in the former a full-thickness sclerotomy is formed without an overlying scleral flap.

1. Prepare conjunctival flap as in Steps 1 to 9 above.
2. Ensure that the planned sclerectomy site is free of any residual conjunctival adhesions (a site at least 5 mm in length should be prepared).
3. Cauterize limbus at base of conjunctival flap over the planned sclerectomy site (monopolar microdiathermy).
4. Perform paracentesis through clear cornea just inside limbus in quadrant neighboring filter site (Wheeler knife).

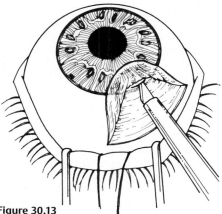

Figure 30.13

5. Enter the anterior chamber behind the insertion of the conjunctival flap (microsurgical knife) (**Fig. 30.13**).
6. Extend entry site for ~2–3 mm.

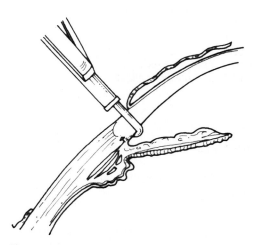

Figure 30.14

7. Perform sclerectomy ~2–3 mm long and 1–2 mm wide (Kelly Descemet punch) (**Fig. 30.14**).
    a. Hold posterior lip of the wound with 0.12 mm forceps to facilitate placing punch.
    b. The sclerectomy should be ~1–2 mm wide, its posterior extent at the level of the scleral spur.
8. Cauterize the posterior lip of the sclerectomy to expand the opening and prevent bleeding.
9. Perform broad basal iridectomy (Jeweler's forceps, Vannas scissors).
10. Reposition and secure the conjunctival flap as in Steps 22 to 30 above.
11. Inject subconjunctival Decadron (4–8 mg) 180 degrees away from filter site into the conjunctival fornix.
12. Apply topical antibiotic, steroid ointment, and 1% atropine drops.
13. Apply light dressing and shield.

Postoperative Procedure

1. Atropine 1% twice per day until eye is quiet (to prevent posterior synechiae and help maintain deep chamber).
2. Topical antibiotic drops (e.g., moxifloxacin 0.5% [Vigamox, Alcon Laboratories, Inc., Fort Worth, TX, US], gatifloxacin 0.3% [Zymar, Allergan, Inc., Irvine, CA, US]) 4 times per day for 10–14 days.
3. Topical steroid (e.g., prednisolone acetate 1%): from 4 times per day up to every hour, depending upon the degree of inflammation, for ~3 weeks.
4. *Optional*: Oral steroid (e.g., prednisone 80 mg for 4 days tapering 20 mg/day every 4 days).
5. Keep patient at moderate activity (e.g., bed rest with bathroom privileges, head of bed elevated 30 degrees).
6. Use light patch and Fox shield on first postoperative day, then Fox shield only. May discharge with instructions to wear glasses during the day and Fox shield for protection when sleeping (see Chapter 6.)
7. Avoid aqueous suppressors. Restart carbonic anhydrase inhibitors only if essential for the health of the contralateral eye (since decreased aqueous production can compromise the bleb).
8. Avoid rubbing the eye since minor trauma may precipitate shallowing of the anterior chamber.
9. Apply digital pressure as needed if anterior chamber is deep, IOP too high, and bleb not elevated.

Complications

1. Postoperative flat anterior chamber
   a. Etiology
      i. Overfiltration or choroidal effusion
      ii. Wound leak
      iii. Aqueous diversion syndrome (malignant glaucoma)
      iv. Decreased aqueous formation secondary to inflammation
      v. Pupillary block with imperforate or blocked peripheral iridectomy
   b. Treatment modalities for postoperative flat chamber secondary to overfiltration or choroidal effusion
      i. Medical treatment
         I. Vigorous cycloplegia (e.g., cyclopentolate 1% plus phenylephrine 10% every 15 minutes for 2 hours, then 4 times per day and atropine 1% 4 times per day).
         II. Keep patient at relative rest.
         III. Keep head of bed at 30 degrees or have patient sit to decrease gravitational filtration.
         IV. Oral and topical steroids if choroidal effusion appears inflammatory in origin.
      ii. Pressure patch to decrease filtration.
      iii. Tamponade filter with glaucoma shell or large soft contact lens.
      iv. If patient has Seidel-positive wound leak, one or several of the following may be used:
         I. Torpedo pressure patch.

      II. Glaucoma shell tamponade or large oversized soft contact lens.
      III. Medical treatment.
         A. Decreasing or discontinuing steroids may facilitate wound healing.
         B. β-blockers (e.g., timolol maleate 0.5%) and carbonic anhydrase inhibitors decrease aqueous flow through the wound gape and may hasten healing.
      IV. Resuture for large leaks or if other modalities are ineffective.
      v. If a flat chamber with choroidal effusions persists for 5 days, perform a choroidal tap with reformation of anterior chamber (see Chapter 34).
2. Hyphema.
3. Failure to filter.
   a. Sutures too tight. Treatment: cut sutures with laser.
   b. Encapsulated bleb. Treatment: bleb needling.
   c. Uveal tissue incarceration into sclerostomy. Treatment: laser or surgical revision.
4. Hypotony.
5. Bleb infection.
6. Cataract formation.
7. Corneal endothelial damage.

■ Combined Trabeculectomy, Extracapsular Cataract Extraction, Posterior Chamber Intraocular Lens

Indications

■ Visually significant cataract in selected patients with moderately severe glaucoma (requiring multiple medications).
■ Selected patients with cataract and glaucoma requiring filtration surgery for pressure control. If the patient has advanced glaucoma that is poorly controlled, however, a staged procedure filter followed by cataract extraction may have a better prognosis for long-term adequate filtration.
■ Visually significant cataract in a glaucoma patient in whom a transient postoperative pressure rise may be damaging to the optic disc.

Preoperative Procedure

See Chapter 3.

1. The preoperative management of IOP and changes to consider in the patient's preoperative medical regimen are described in the Trabeculectomy/Posterior Lip Sclerectomy section at the beginning of this chapter.
2. Pupil management.
   a. If IOP allows, discontinue pilocarpine 24 hours or more preoperatively.

b. Discontinue cholinesterase inhibitors 2 weeks pre-operatively (to allow increased pupil dilation and to decrease bleeding and postoperative inflammation).

c. *Optional:* If possible, consider discontinuing prosta-glandin analog medications 1 week preoperatively or switch to an α-agonist (i.e., brimonidine tartrate 0.1% [Alphagan P] Allergan, Inc.).

d. Dilate pupil.

   i. Cyclopentolate 1%, tropicamide 1%, and phenyl-ephrine 2.5% every 15 minutes starting 1 hour before surgery.

   ii. *Optional:* Topical nonsteroidal anti-inflammatory agent (e.g., flurbiprofen 0.03% [Ocufen, Allergan, Inc.],) every 30 minutes starting 2 hours before surgery to minimize intraoperative miosis.

3. The eye should be as quiet as possible preoperatively to enhance the prognosis for successful filtration.

a. *Optional:* Steroid drop 4 times per day to every hour 1 week preoperatively to decrease postoperative inflammation.

b. *Optional:* Oral steroids (e.g., prednisone 80 mg), starting 1 day preoperatively.

Instrumentation

- Lid speculum (e.g., Lieberman)
- Sutures (4–0 silk, 7–0 Vicryl, 10–0 nylon)
- Needle holder
- Elschnig forceps
- Kalt needle holder
- Smooth forceps (Chandler or Bracken)
- Westcott scissors
- Cautery (microdiathermy)
- Fine tissue forceps (e.g., 0.12 mm Castroviejo, Pierse)
- Castroviejo calipers
- Cellulose sponges
- Scarifier (e.g., Grieshaber #681.01, Beaver #57)
- Wheeler or 15 degree microsurgical knife
- 3 ml syringe with 30 gauge irrigation cannula
- Microsurgical knife (e.g., #75M Beaver, Superblade)
- Descemet membrane punch
- Jeweler's forceps
- Vannas scissors
- DeWecker scissors
- Gills-Vannas scissors
- Viscoelastic substance (e.g., Healon, Viscoat, Amvisc)
- Cystotome
- Left- and right-handed corneoscleral scissors
- Tying forceps (straight and angled McPherson)
- Lens loop
- Muscle hook
- Irrigation/aspiration unit (automated or manual)
- Capsule polisher
- Acetylcholine solution (e.g., Miochol)

Operative Procedure

Note: The following will describe the technique of combined trabeculectomy/cataract extraction using a fornix-based conjunctival flap. The procedure may be similarly performed using a limbus-based flap as described in the Trabeculectomy/Posterior Lip Sclerectomy section at the beginning of this chapter.

1. Anesthesia: Retrobulbar or peribulbar injection plus lid block. May use general anesthesia if preferred, and for younger or uncooperative patients, hearing or mentally impaired patients, those with language obstacles, or patients with ruptured globes.

2. Apply ocular massage for approximately 10 minutes to decompress the eye and orbit and minimize positive vitreous pressure.

3. Prep and drape.

a. Use povidone-iodide 5% on a cotton-tipped applicator to gently clean eyelashes and lid margins.

b. Place 1 or 2 drops of povidone-iodide in the conjunctival fornix.

4. For traction suture: Place 4–0 silk bridle suture under superior rectus tendon, taking care not to injure conjunctiva (Kalt needle holder, Elschnig forceps). Alternatively, place 7–0 Vicryl braided corneal traction suture through the peripheral cornea.

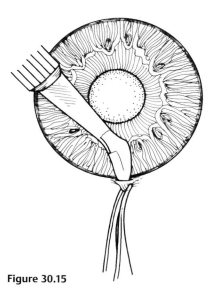

Figure 30.15

5. Prepare a fornix-based conjunctival flap.

a. Perform peritomy at the limbus from ~9:30 to 2:30.

   i. Incise conjunctiva (**Fig. 30.15**).

      I. Handle conjunctiva gently and at the edges with smooth (Bracken or Chandler) or Pierse forceps.

      II. Tent conjunctiva as close to cornea as possible and carefully incise with Westcott scissors or scarifier.

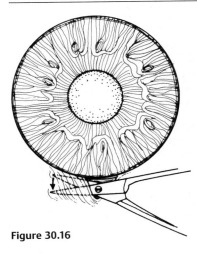

Figure 30.16

6. Always keep the conjunctival flap moist with BSS.
7. Perform meticulous hemostasis (monopolar microdiathermy).
8. Remove residual Tenon capsule from episclera (0.12 mm forceps, Westcott scissors).
9. Use calipers to measure width of scleral flap. (Flap may be rectangular or triangular with an ~3 mm base and 3 mm posterior extent.)
10. Outline edges of scleral flap with monopolar microdiathermy.

ii. Extend peritomy.
  I. Bluntly spread beneath conjunctiva with Westcott scissors parallel to the limbus (**Fig. 30.16**).
  II. Incise conjunctiva along limbus. Hug limbus to make peritomy as close to cornea as possible with minimal loss of conjunctiva from the flap.

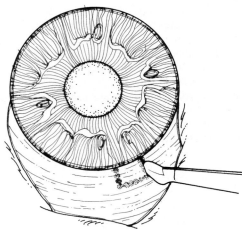

Figure 30.18

11. Make a partial-thickness (approximately one half to two thirds) scleral groove incision over the diathermy outline using scarifier (extend groove over limbus) (**Fig. 30.18**).

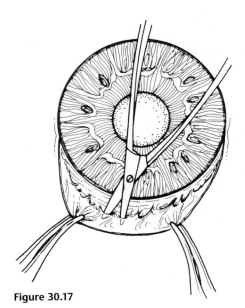

Figure 30.17

b. Fashion a thin conjunctival flap superiorly, freeing the conjunctiva from subjacent adhesions to Tenon capsule (**Fig. 30.17**).
  i. Spread Westcott scissors in conjunctiva–Tenon plane while applying counter traction to the edge of conjunctiva with smooth forceps.
  ii. With assistant elevating flap, lyse adhesions from conjunctiva to Tenon with sharp and blunt dissection.
  iii. Do not buttonhole conjunctiva.

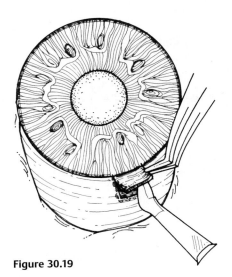

Figure 30.19

12. Perform a lamellar dissection of the scleral flap with a scarifier (**Fig. 30.19**).
  a. Flap should be ~50% deep.
  b. Apply countertraction with forceps to facilitate dissection.

c. Extend dissection anteriorly over the limbus.

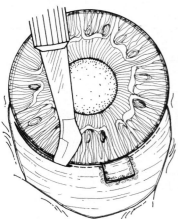

Figure 30.20

13. Make a partial-thickness (approximately one half to two thirds) scleral groove incision using scarifier or no. 57 Beaver blade. When making the scleral flap, care must be taken not to enter the anterior chamber before applying the antifibrotic agent (**Fig. 30.20**).
   a. Stop groove where it abuts trabeculectomy flap. (Do not cut over trabeculectomy bed.)
   b. Length of groove should be 11 mm in chord length.

Note: When an antifibrotic agent is used, it should be applied to the eye before the anterior chamber is entered to avoid the toxic effects of the antifibrotic agents inside of the eye.

14. *Optional but highly recommended:* An antifibrotic agent is generally used in combined trabeculectomy and cataract extraction procedures to improve the success rate of the trabeculectomy. Use an antifibrotic agent such as MMC 0.2–0.5 mg/ml (preferably 0.4 mg/ml) or 5-fluorouracil 50 mg/ml.
   a. Soak the cut end of a cellulose sponge in the solution.
   b. Place the sponge on top of the scleral flap with the conjunctival flap draped over the sponge.

Note: Do not allow the edges of the conjunctival flap to contact the antifibrotic agent.

   c. Exposure time may be titrated according to the desired effect and may vary up to 3 minutes for MMC and up to 5 minutes for 5-fluorouracil.
   d. Remove sponge and copiously irrigate area with BSS solution to remove any residual antifibrotic agent.
15. Cauterize planned entry site with monopolar diathermy.
16. Perform paracentesis through clear cornea just inside limbus in quadrant neighboring filter site with a Wheeler or similar microsurgical knife (see Chapter 7). Note the surrounding landmarks to relocate site at end of case.
17. Enter the anterior chamber under the scleral flap as anteriorly as possible and extend incision horizontally for ~2 mm (microsurgical knife).

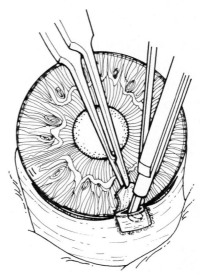

Figure 30.21

18. Perform sclerectomy with Descemet punch (**Fig. 30.21**).
   a. Hold the posterior lip of the wound with 0.12 mm forceps to facilitate placing punch.
   b. The sclerostomy should be ~2–3 mm long and 1–2 mm wide, its posterior extent at the level of the scleral spur.
   c. Alternatively, the trabeculectomy block may be removed in one piece with a knife and Vannas scissors.
19. Cauterize the posterior lip of sclerostomy to expand the opening and prevent bleeding (microdiathermy).
20. Perform broad, basal iridectomy (Jeweler's forceps, Vannas or DeWecker scissors).
21. In the case of a miotic pupil, papillary stretching, iris hooks, or inferior sphincterotomies may be helpful in achieving adequate lens exposure.
22. Irrigate viscoelastic into anterior chamber to maintain chamber depth.

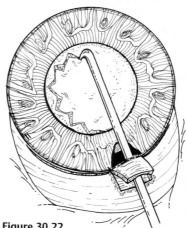

Figure 30.22

23. Perform a 360 degree, beer can–style anterior capsulectomy with a cystotome, measuring ~5 mm in diameter (**Fig. 30.22**).

24. Extend cataract wound with corneoscleral scissors to the right and left.
25. Remove anterior capsular flap (angled McPherson forceps).
26. Place 7–0 Vicryl sutures on either side of the trabeculectomy flap, separated by 7 mm and left untied.
27. Loop sutures out of wound.

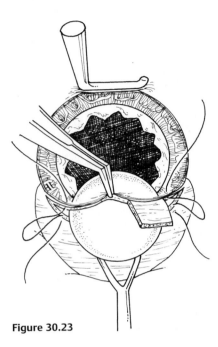

Figure 30.23

28. Express lens nucleus with lens loop and muscle hook (see Chapter 9) (**Fig. 30.23**).
29. Tie sutures.
30. Remove residual cortical material with an automated or manual irrigation/aspiration device. (Add more sutures to the cataract wound as necessary to maintain anterior chamber depth during cortical cleanup.) (See Chapter 9.)
31. *Optional:* gently polish posterior capsule.

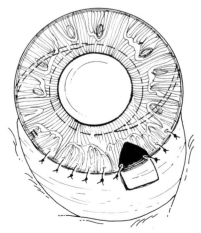

Figure 30.24

32. Irrigate viscoelastic into capsular bag.
33. Place posterior chamber intraocular lens (see Chapter 9).
34. Remove viscoelastic with the irrigation/aspiration device using minimum suction.
35. Irrigate Miochol into anterior chamber to constrict pupil.
36. Close cataract wound securely with interrupted 10–0 nylon sutures (**Fig. 30.24**).
    a. Place sutures at junction of scleral flap and cataract incision.
    b. Remove Vicryl sutures.
37. Close scleral flap with 2 interrupted 10–0 nylon sutures tied loosely at corners and bury knots. (Add more sutures; tie more tightly if less filtration is desired.)
38. Bury all sutures.
39. Remove bridle suture or corneal traction suture.
40. Reposition conjunctival flap.

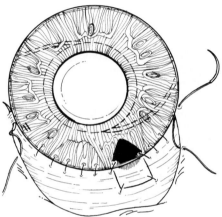

Figure 30.25

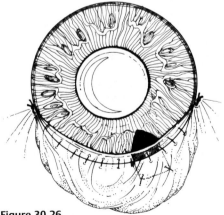

Figure 30.26

41. Secure conjunctival flap (**Figs. 30.25 and 30.26**).
    a. Overlap limbus by 0.5–1.0 mm with flap.
    b. Secure with one or two interrupted 7–0 Vicryl sutures at each corner of the flap. (Place through conjunctiva and episclera at the limbus.)
    c. Ensure that conjunctiva is stretched securely over the limbus.

42. Check patency of sclerostomy site by irrigating BSS through the previously placed paracentesis.
    a. Conjunctival bleb should elevate and anterior chamber should reform.
    b. If buttonhole is noted, close with an interrupted or mattress 10–0 nylon suture (BV needle).
    c. Paracentesis site usually does not need to be sutured.
43. Inject subconjunctival Decadron (4–8 mg) 180 degrees away from filter site into the conjunctival fornix.
44. Apply topical antibiotic and steroid ointment.
45. Apply light dressing and shield.

Postoperative Procedure

1. Topical antibiotic drops (e.g., moxifloxacin 0.5% [Vigamox, Alcon Laboratories, Inc.], gatifloxacin 0.3% [Zymar, Allergan, Inc.]) 4 times per day for the first 2–3 weeks.
2. Topical steroid (e.g., prednisolone acetate 1%): First apply at each dressing change until anterior chamber is well formed and patient stable. Then use from 4 times per day up to every hour depending upon degree of inflammation.
3. *Optional:* Oral steroid (e.g., prednisone 80 mg for 4 days, tapering 20 mg/day every 4 days).
4. Keep patient at moderate activity (e.g., bed rest with bathroom privileges, head of bed elevated 30 degrees).
5. Patient should use light patch and Fox shield on first postoperative day, then Fox shield only. May wear glasses during the day and Fox shield for protection when sleeping (see Chapter 6).
6. Avoid aqueous suppressors. Restart carbonic anhydrase inhibitors only if essential for the health of the contralateral eye, because decreased aqueous production can compromise the bleb.
7. Avoid rubbing the eye, as minor trauma may precipitate shallowing of the anterior chamber.
8. Carefully apply digital pressure as needed if anterior chamber is deep, IOP is too high, bleb is not elevated, and wound is secure.

Complications

1. Posterior capsule rupture
2. Vitreous loss (see Chapter 12)
3. Hyphema
4. Postoperative flat anterior chamber
5. Wound leak
6. Failure to filter
7. Hypotony
8. Cystoid macular edema
9. Retinal detachment
10. Bleb infection
11. Pseudophakic bullous keratopathy

■ Combined Trabeculectomy, Phacoemulsification, Posterior Chamber Intraocular Lens

Indications

■ Visually significant cataract in patients with moderately severe glaucoma and good pressure control on multiple medications
■ Patients with cataract and glaucoma requiring filtration surgery for pressure control
■ Visually significant cataract in an advanced glaucoma patient in whom a transient postoperative pressure rise may be damaging to the optic disc

Preoperative Procedure

See Chapter 3.

1. The preoperative management of IOP and changes to consider in the patient's preoperative medical regimen are described in the Combined Trabeculectomy, Extracapsular Cataract Extraction, Posterior Chamber Intraocular Lens section earlier in this chapter.
2. Pupil management:
    a. If IOP allows, discontinue pilocarpine 24 hours or more preoperatively.
    b. Discontinue cholinesterase inhibitors 2 weeks preoperatively to allow increased pupil dilation and to decrease bleeding and postoperative inflammation.
    c. Dilate pupil.
        i. Cyclopentolate 1%, tropicamide 1%, and phenylephrine 2.5% every 15 minutes starting 1 hour before surgery.
        ii. Optional: Topical nonsteroidal anti-inflammatory agent (e.g., flurbiprofen 0.03% [Ocufen, Allergan, Inc.],) every 30 minutes starting 2 hours before surgery to minimize intraoperative miosis.
3. The eye should be as quiet as possible preoperatively to enhance the prognosis for successful filtration.
    a. *Optional:* Steroid drop 4 times per day to every hour 1 week preoperatively to decrease postoperative inflammation.
    b. *Optional:* Oral steroids (e.g., prednisone 80 mg starting 1 day preoperatively).

Instrumentation

■ Lid speculum (e.g., Lieberman)
■ Sutures (6–0 silk or 6–0 Vicryl if a corneal bridle suture is used; 8–0 Vicryl; 10–0 nylon)
■ Elschnig forceps
■ Kalt needle holder
■ Smooth forceps (Chandler or Bracken)
■ Westcott scissors
■ Cautery (microdiathermy)
■ Fine tissue forceps (e.g., 0.12 mm Castroviejo, Pierse)

- Castroviejo calipers
- Cellulose sponges
- Scarifier (e.g., Grieshaber #681.01, Beaver #57)
- Wheeler or 15 degree microsurgical knife
- 3 ml syringe with 30 gauge irrigation cannula
- Microsurgical knife (e.g., #75 M Beaver, Superblade)
- Kelly Descemet membrane punch
- Jeweler's forceps
- Vannas scissors
- DeWecker scissors
- Viscoelastic substance (e.g., Healon, Viscoat, Amvisc)
- Cystotome
- Utrata forceps
- Keratome (e.g., Beaver #55)
- Tying forceps (straight and angled McPherson)
- Lens loop
- Muscle hook
- Kuglen hook
- Phacoemulsification unit
- Capsule polisher
- IOL forceps
- Sinskey hook
- Acetylcholine solution (e.g., Miochol)

Operative Procedure

Note: The following will describe the technique of combined trabeculectomy/phacoemulsification using a fornix-based conjunctival flap. The procedure may be similarly performed using a limbus-based flap as described in the Combined Trabeculectomy, Extracapsular Cataract Extraction, Posterior Chamber Intraocular Lens section earlier in this chapter.

1. Anesthesia: Retrobulbar or peribulbar injection plus lid block. May use general anesthesia if preferred, and for younger or uncooperative patients, hearing or mentally impaired patients, those with language obstacles, or patients with ruptured globes.
2. Apply ocular massage for approximately 10 minutes to decompress the eye and orbit, minimizing positive vitreous pressure
3. Prep and drape.
   a. Use povidone-iodide 5% on a cotton-tipped applicator to gently clean eyelashes and lid margins.
   b. Place one or two drops of povidone-iodide in the conjunctival fornix.
4. Place lid speculum.
5. Ensure adequate pupillary dilation (prefer pupil diameter of 7 mm or more).
6. *Optional, but usually not needed for fornix-based combined surgery:* Place 6–0 silk or 6–0 Vicryl braided corneal traction suture through the peripheral cornea.
7. Prepare a fornix-based conjunctival peritomy at the limbus measuring ~4–5 mm (Westcott scissors, smooth tissue forceps). (See combined trabeculectomy, extracapsular cataract extraction, posterior chamber intraocular lens section in this chapter for details of handling the conjunctiva when creating a fornix-based conjunctival flap.)

8. Remove residual Tenon capsule from episclera (0.12 mm forceps, Westcott scissors).
9. Perform meticulous hemostasis (monopolar microdiathermy).
10. Use calipers to measure width of scleral flap. (Flap may be rectangular or triangular with an ~3-mm base and 2 to 3 mm posterior extent.)
11. *Optional:* Outline edges of scleral flap with monopolar microdiathermy.

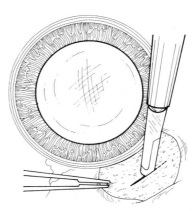

Figure 30.27

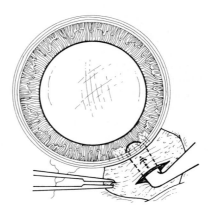

Figure 30.28

12. Make a partial-thickness (approximately one half to two thirds) scleral groove incision using scarifier or No. 57 Beaver blade). When making the scleral flap, care must be taken not to enter the anterior chamber before applying the antifibrotic agent (**Figs. 30.27 and 30.28**).

Note: When an antifibrotic agent is used, it should be applied to the eye before the anterior chamber is entered to avoid the toxic effects of the antifibrotic agents inside of the eye.

13. *Optional but highly recommended:* An antifibrotic agent is generally used in combined trabeculectomy and cataract extraction procedures to improve the success rate of the trabeculectomy. Use an antifibrotic agent such as MMC 0.2–0.5 mg/ml (preferably 0.4 mg/ml) or 5-fluorouracil 50 mg/ml.

a. Soak the cut end of a cellulose sponge in the solution.
b. Place the sponge on top of the scleral flap with the conjunctival flap draped over the sponge.

Note: Do not allow the edges of the conjunctival flap to contact the antifibrotic agent.

c. Exposure time may be titrated according to the desired effect and may vary up to 3 minutes for MMC and up to 5 minutes for 5-fluorouracil.
d. Remove sponge and copiously irrigate area with BSS solution to remove any residual antifibrotic agent.

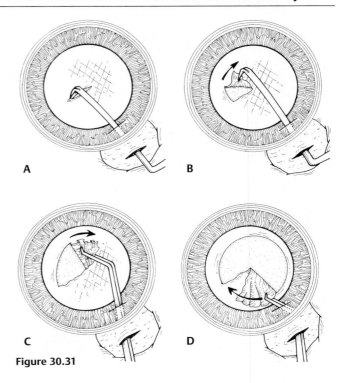

Figure 30.31

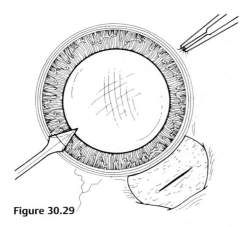

Figure 30.29

14. Perform a paracentesis through peripheral clear cornea adjacent to the limbus (see Chapter 7) (**Fig. 30.29**).
    a. Place at 10 or 2 o'clock on side of nondominant hand.
    b. Use a microsurgical knife (e.g., Beaver No. 75).
15. Irrigate viscoelastic into anterior chamber.

17. Nick the anterior capsule with cystotome and perform a 360 degree continuous curvilinear capsulorrhexis (measuring ~5–6 mm in diameter) with Utrata forceps (**Figs. 30.31A–30.31D**).
18. Remove anterior capsular flap (angled McPherson forceps).

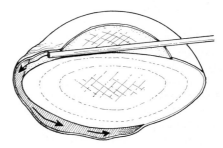

Figure 30.32

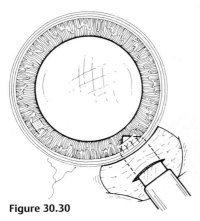

Figure 30.30

16. Enter anterior chamber with a keratome (2.8–3.2 mm) beneath the trabeculectomy flap at the posterior limbus on the side of the dominant hand with a microsurgical knife (**Fig. 30.30**).

19. Hydrodissect the lens nucleus by injecting BSS solution through a 30 gauge cannula between the anterior capsular flap and the lens nucleus. Gently rotate the nucleus using a Kuglen hook, cyclodialysis spatula, or nucleus rotator (**Fig. 30.32**).
20. Prepare phacoemulsification unit (see Chapter 8 for details).

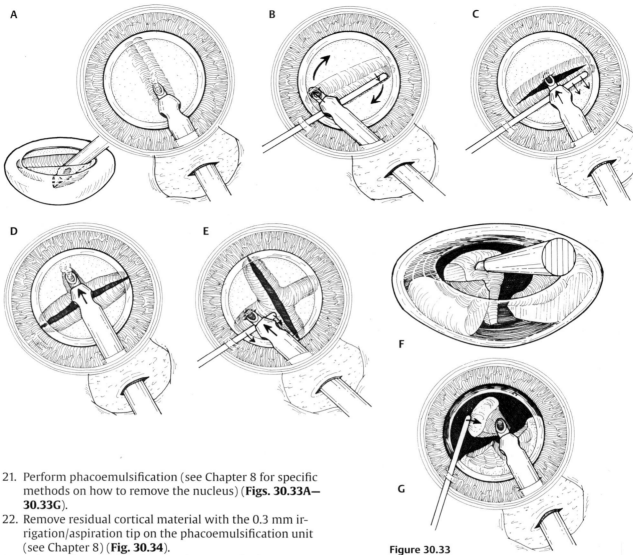

A

B

C

D

E

F

G

Figure 30.33

21. Perform phacoemulsification (see Chapter 8 for specific methods on how to remove the nucleus) (**Figs. 30.33A— 30.33G**).
22. Remove residual cortical material with the 0.3 mm irrigation/aspiration tip on the phacoemulsification unit (see Chapter 8) (**Fig. 30.34**).
23. Irrigate viscoelastic substance into capsular bag.
24. If planning a foldable IOL insertion, fold silicone or acrylic intraocular lens (IOL) into lens insertion device (see Chapter 8). If inserting a nonfoldable lens, the wound may be enlarged parallel and posterior to the limbus starting from the base of the scleral flap.
25. Place posterior chamber IOL into the capsular bag and center (Sinskey hook).
26. Remove viscoelastic with I/A instrument using minimum suction, or alternatively, remove viscoelastic after sclerectomy and peripheral iridectomy is performed (step 28, below).
27. Irrigate Miochol into anterior chamber to constrict pupil.
28. Perform sclerectomy with Descemet punch (see Combined Trabeculectomy, Extracapsular Cataract Extraction, Posterior Chamber Intraocular Lens section earlier in this chapter).
29. Perform broad, basal iridectomy (Jeweler's forceps, Vannas or DeWecker scissors).

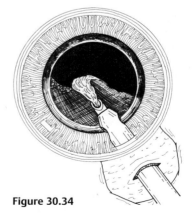

Figure 30.34

30. If needed, cauterize the edges of the sclerostomy and iridectomy to prevent bleeding (microdiathermy).
31. Close scleral flap with two interrupted 10–0 nylon sutures tied loosely at corners and bury knots (add additional sutures and/or tie more tightly if leakage or overfiltration is noted).
32. Alternatively, close scleral flap with two releasable 10–0 nylon sutures.
33. Reform the anterior chamber with BSS through a 30 gauge cannula inserted into the paracentesis to check for excess aqueous flow beneath the trabeculectomy flap and to maintain the anterior chamber depth.
34. Reposition conjunctival flap.
35. Secure conjunctival flap (see Combined Trabeculectomy, Extracapsular Cataract Extraction, Posterior Chamber Intraocular Lens section earlier in this chapter for details).
36. Check patency of sclerostomy site by irrigating BSS through the previously placed paracentesis. (See Combined Trabeculectomy, Extracapsular Cataract Extraction, Posterior Chamber Intraocular Lens section earlier in this chapter for details.)
37. If initially placed, remove corneal bridle suture.
38. Inject subconjunctival Decadron (4–8 mg) and antibiotic of choice 180 degrees away from filter site into the conjunctival fornix.
39. Apply topical antibiotic and steroid ointment.
40. Apply light dressing and Fox shield.
41. *Optional:* The phacoemulsification and trabeculectomy may be performed at two separate sites rather than at one site as just described. When performed at two separate sites, the trabeculectomy is performed superiorly and nasally at the limbus and the phacoemulsification is performed temporally at the limbus or preferably through clear cornea.

Postoperative Procedure

Basic medications for routine case:

1. Topical steroid (e.g., prednisolone acetate 1%) 4 times per day or up to every 1–2 hours while awake initially, depending upon degree of inflammation. Taper gradually over at least 3 months.

   Optional (e.g., in uveitis patients): Oral steroid (e.g., prednisone 80 mg for 4 days tapering 20 mg per day every 4 days).
2. Antibiotic eye drop (e.g., moxifloxacin 0.5% [Vigamox, Alcon Laboratories, Inc.], gatifloxacin 0.3% [Zymar, Allergan, Inc.]) 4 times per day for 3 weeks for prophylaxis. An antibiotic may be used longer in cases where a releasable suture was placed.
3. Keep patient at minimum activity (e.g., no bending, no heavy lifting, no straining, head of bed elevated 30 degrees).
4. May remove light patch and Fox shield on first postoperative day. Thereafter, use Fox shield only. Patient may wear glasses during the day and Fox shield for protection when sleeping.

5. Use aqueous suppressors or carbonic anhydrase inhibitors only if essential for the health of the contralateral eye, because decreased aqueous production can compromise the bleb.
6. Avoid rubbing the eye.
7. Carefully apply digital pressure as needed if the anterior chamber is deep, the IOP is too high, the bleb is not elevated, and the wound is secure.
8. May laser suture lyse or pull releasable 10–0 nylon scleral flap sutures if pressure becomes too high.
9. May give 5-fluorouracil postoperatively as subconjunctival injections (50 mg/ml concentration, 0.1 ml dose) 180 degrees away from the bleb as needed.
10. Bleb needling may be indicated for late fibrosis over and of the scleral flap.

Complications

1. Posterior capsule rupture
2. Vitreous loss (see Chapter 12)
3. Hyphema
4. Postoperative flat anterior chamber
5. Wound leak
6. Failure to filter (e.g., sclerostomy blockage, fibrosis, Tenon cyst)
7. Hypotony
8. Cystoid macular edema
9. Retinal detachment
10. Bleb infection
11. Pseudophakic bullous keratopathy
12. Suprachoroidal hemorrhage or choroidal effusion

■ Glaucoma Tube and Shunt Procedures

Indications

■ Glaucoma uncontrolled by maximally tolerate medical therapy, laser trabeculoplasty, and trabeculectomy with antifibrotic drugs
■ Advanced glaucomatous damage with poor visual potential
■ Neovascular or uveitic glaucoma that has failed conventional medical and filtering surgery or when filtering surgery has a poor prognosis

Preoperative Procedure

See Chapter 3.

1. Preoperative IOP should be < 30 mm Hg. If IOP is too high, intravenous or oral carbonic anhydrase inhibitors or osmotics may be used.
2. The eye should be as quiet as possible preoperatively to enhance the prognosis for successful surgery.

Instrumentation

- Lid speculum (eg., Lieberman)
- Sutures (4–0 silk, 7–0 Vicryl, 8–0, 9–0, 10–0 nylon)
- Kalt needle holder
- Elschnig forceps
- 3 mm syringe with 30 G irrigating cannula
- Smooth forceps (Chandler or Bracken)
- Cautery (polar microdiathermy)
- Westcott scissors.
- Iris spatula
- Castroviejo calipers
- Scalpel (e.g., No. 15 Bard-Parker blade or No. 69 Beaver blade)
- Cellulose sponges
- Fine tissue forceps (e.g., 0.12 mm Castroviejo, Pierse forceps)
- Microsurgical knife (e.g., Beaver No. 75 M, Superblade)
- 23 gauge needle
- Scarifier (e.g., Grieshaber No. 681.01, Beaver No. 57)
- Wheeler or 15 degree microsurgical knife
- Tying forceps
- Needle holder
- Glaucoma shunt device (e.g., Ahmed, Baerveldt, Molteno implants)
- Donor sclera, dura, pericardium, etc.

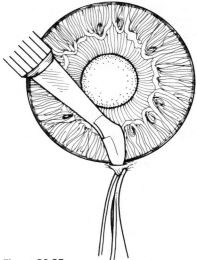

Figure 30.35

Operative Procedure

1. Anesthesia: Retrobulbar or peribulbar injection plus lid block. May use general anesthesia if preferred, and for younger or uncooperative patients, hearing or mentally impaired patients, those with language obstacles, or patients with ruptured globes.
2. Prep and drape.
   a. Use povidone-iodide 5% on a cotton tipped applicator to gently clean eyelashes and lid margins.
   b. Place one or two drops of povidone-iodide in the conjunctival fornix.
3. Select position for drainage device placement, usually in the superotemporal quadrant in the area between the rectus muscles.
4. Prepare a fornix-based conjunctival flap in the region of the limbus selected (Bracken or Chandler smooth forceps, Westcott scissors) (see Combined Trabeculectomy, Extracapsular Cataract Extraction Cataract Extraction, Posterior Chamber Intraocular Lens section earlier in this chapter) (**Figs. 30.35, 30.36, and 30.37**).
5. Episclera is exposed under Tenon capsule with meticulous cauterization of bleeding vessels.
6. Superior and lateral rectus muscles are exposed with muscle hooks and held with 4–0 silk bridle sutures.
7. The reservoir or silicone plate for collection of aqueous is placed under the conjunctiva and between the rectus muscles and sutured to the sclera using 8–0 or 9–0 nylon, with its anterior border 8–10 mm posterior to the limbus.

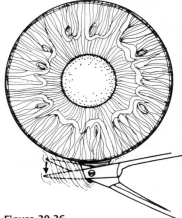

Figure 30.36

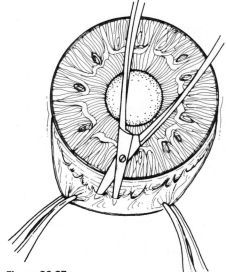

Figure 30.37

8. *Optional:* Dissection of half-scleral thickness flap up to the limbus. Alternative modification is the use of a donor scleral, dural, pericardial, or fascial patch to cover the tube and sutured to the sclera with 10–0 nylon suture.

9. The long silicone tube is trimmed, bevel up, to allow its insertion 2–3 mm into the anterior chamber.

10. A paracentesis is performed at 9 o'clock in the peripheral cornea adjacent to the limbus with a Wheeler or Beaver #75 M Superb

11. The anterior chamb   superiorly for introduction of the tub   nife or a 23 gauge
needle. Special ca   rv parallel
to the iris plane   of the
tube once insi
site wound s
leakage.

12. The tube is
ter good r
confirm

13. *Option*
Vicry
non
If th
ing t
to op
from
cluded

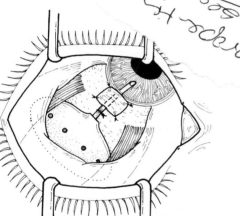

Figure 30.38

14. *Optional:* Donor sclera/pericardium may be sutured over the tube and tube insertion site with 10–0 nylon or 8–0 Vicryl suture to prevent erosion through the conjunctiva at the limbus (**Fig. 30.38**).

15. Tenon tissue and conjunctiva are repositioned and sutured at the limbus with 7–0 Vicryl suture.

16. The anterior chamber is deepened by irrigating BSS through a 30 gauge cannula that is inserted into the paracentesis site. The anterior chamber should remain deep and well formed. The paracentesis site usually does not need to be sutured.

17. Inject subconjunctival Decadron (4–8 mg) 180 degrees away from the device site into the conjunctival fornix.

18. Apply topical antibiotic, steroid ointment, and 1% atropine drops.

19. Apply light dressing and Fox shield.

Postoperative Procedure

1. Atropine 1% 2 times per day until eye is quiet to prevent posterior synechiae and help maintain deep chamber.

2. Topical fluoroquinolone (e.g., moxifloxacin 0.5% [Vigamox, Alcon Laboratories, Inc.], gatifloxacin 0.3% [Zymar, Allergan, Inc.]) four times a day for 2 weeks.

3. Topical steroid (e.g., prednisolone acetate 1%) first apply
       ach dressing change until anterior chamber is well
              nd patient stable. Then use from 4 times per day
                     r, depending on degree of inflammation.
                         (e.g., prednisone 80 mg for 4 days
                          ry 4 days).
                           bed rest with bath-
                             30 degrees and no
                               t postoperative day,
                               ear glasses during
                               ion when sleeping (see

                               start carbonic anhydrase
                             the health of the contra-
                          sed aqueous production can
                      e and cause complications.

             tive flat anterior chamber
       ology.
       i. Overfiltration/choroidal effusion
       ii. Wound leak.
       iii. Aqueous diversion syndrome (malignant glaucoma)
       iv. Decreased aqueous formation secondary to inflammation
       v. Pupillary block with imperforate or blocked peripheral iridectomy
2. Hyphema
3. Failure to filter
4. Hypotony
5. Infection
6. Cataract formation
7. Corneal endothelial damage
8. Tube contact or blockage by corneal endothelium, iris, lens, or vitreous
9. Erosion of tube through the conjunctiva
10. Retinal detachment
11. Vitreous hemorrhage
12. Phthisis bulbi

31

Peripheral Iridectomy

Indications

- Relief of pupillary block in eyes with angle closure glaucoma
- Prophylaxis in eyes with anatomy predisposing toward angle closure
- Select cases of chronic or secondary angle closure glaucoma in which at least 25% of angle is not permanently closed
- Aphakic or pseudophakic pupillary block
- Specific indications for surgical rather than laser iridectomy:
    - Patient unable to cooperate with laser treatment
    - Poor anterior segment visualization (e.g., secondary to corneal edema)
    - Flat anterior chamber

Preoperative Procedure

1. See Chapter 3.
2. Pilocarpine 2% every 6 hours on day before surgery and every 15 minutes starting 1 hour preoperatively to constrict pupil.

Instrumentation

- Lid speculum (e.g., Lieberman)
- Sutures (4–0 silk, 9–0 silk, 7–0 and 9–0 Vicryl, or 10–0 nylon)
- Wheeler or similar microsurgical knife
- Fine-toothed tissue forceps (e.g., 0.12 mm Castroviejo)
- Smooth-tipped forceps (e.g., Jeweler's forceps)
- Vannas or DeWecker scissors
- Scarifier (e.g., Beaver #64, Grieshaber #681.01)
- Microsurgical knife (e.g., Beaver #75M, Superblade)
- Keratome
- Westcott scissors
- Cautery (e.g., disposable, underwater unipolar microdiathermy)
- Muscle hook
- Iris spatula
- Acetylcholine solution (e.g., Miochol)

Operative Procedures

1. Anesthesia: Retrobulbar or peribulbar plus lid block. May use general anesthesia for younger, hearing or mentally impaired, or uncooperative patient.
2. Prep and drape eye.
3. Place lid speculum.
4. Optional: Place 4–0 silk superior rectus bridle suture (see Chapter 9).
5. Perform anterior chamber paracentesis through clear cornea at 10 or 2 o'clock with Wheeler knife (see Chapter 7).

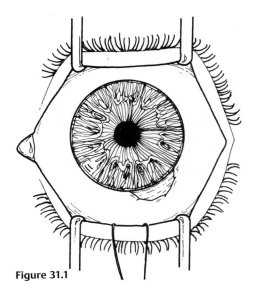

Figure 31.1

6. Fashion fornix or limbus-based peritomy in superotemporal or superonasal quadrant for 2–3 clock hours opposite the paracentesis site (Westcott scissors). Do not traumatize conjunctiva, which may be needed for later filtration surgery (**Fig. 31.1**).
7. Secure hemostasis with cautery.
8. Make a 2–3 mm groove with the scarifier approximately two thirds deep at the midanterior limbus.
   a. Place at ~10 or 2 o'clock.
   b. Groove should be perpendicular to eye.
9. *Optional:* Preplace 9–0 silk, 7–0 Vicryl, or 10–0 nylon interrupted suture through groove and loop it out of the wound.

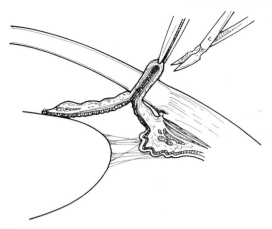

Figure 31.3

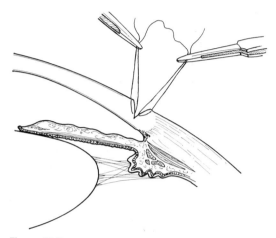

Figure 31.2

10. Have assistant gape the wound using the preplaced suture loops for traction on the wound margins (**Fig. 31.2**).
11. Enter anterior chamber with microsurgical knife at the base of the groove.
    a. Carefully scratch down at base of groove to obtain controlled entry into anterior chamber.
    b. Perform the incision perpendicular to the iris (do not shelve the incision to facilitate iris prolapse).
    c. Internal aspect of wound should be ~2 mm in length.
12. Traction on the wound margins using the preplaced suture should prolapse the iris. If not, apply gentle pressure to the posterior lip of the wound with an iris spatula.
13. If iris does not prolapse with these maneuvers, carefully use smooth-tipped forceps to grasp the iris at the wound without touching the lens or zonules.

14. After the iris prolapses, grasp it with 0.12 mm forceps and perform a basal iridectomy with Vannas or DeWecker scissors (**Fig. 31.3**).
    a. Ascertain that the iridectomy is full thickness by inspecting for iris pigment epithelium in the resected specimen and by directly observing the iridectomy.

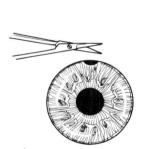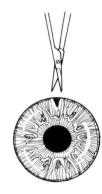

Figure 31.4

    b. Shape of iridectomy is determined by direction of the cut (**Fig. 31.4**).
       i. Holding scissors parallel to the limbus results in a broad, basal iridectomy.
       ii. Holding scissors perpendicular to the limbus results in a narrow iridectomy pointing toward the pupil.

15. Reposit the iris. The following maneuvers may be used:
    a. Irrigate the wound with balanced salt solution.
    b. With a muscle hook, gently stroke the cornea in a radial fashion, starting from the wound margin and proceeding centrally.
    c. Irrigate Miochol into the anterior chamber through the previously placed paracentesis. (Do not irrigate through the iridectomy since this may damage the lens or reprolapse the iris.)
16. Inspect to ensure that the pupil is round and that there is no iris incarceration in the wound.
17. Close the wound with the preplaced suture if present, and add suture if necessary.
18. If necessary, reform the anterior chamber through the paracentesis site with BSS.
19. If needed, close conjunctiva over limbal wound (7–0 or 9–0 Vicryl, or cauterize conjunctiva closed).
20. Apply topical antibiotic and steroid ointment.
21. Optional: Apply cycloplegic (e.g., cyclopentolate 1%).
22. Apply patch and place Fox shield.

Postoperative Procedure

1. Cycloplegia (e.g., cyclopentolate 1%) 2 times per day if eye inflamed and prone to posterior synechiae.
2. Steroid drops (e.g., prednisolone acetate 1%) 4 times per day and tapered as degree of inflammation warrants.
3. Topical antibiotic (e.g., moxifloxacin 0.5% [Vigamox, Alcon Laboratories, Inc., Fort Worth, TX, US], gatifloxacin 0.3% [Zymar, Allergan, Inc., Irvine, CA, US]) 4 times per day.
4. Monitor intraocular pressure and treat glaucoma as necessary.

Complications

1. Imperforate iridectomy
2. Hyphema
3. Lens damage
4. Malignant glaucoma

32

Cyclodestructive Procedures

■ Cyclocryotherapy

Indications

- Treatment of glaucoma that has failed multiple procedures (e.g., filtration, cyclodialysis, or tube/shunt procedures), especially in aphakic or pseudophakic eyes
- Control of increased intraocular pressure (IOP) in eyes with poor potential for good central acuity
- As a possible alternative to enucleation or evisceration of an eye that is blind and painful because of secondary glaucoma.

Preoperative Procedure

See Chapter 3.

1. Topical steroids (e.g., prednisolone acetate 1%) as indicated to decrease inflammation.
2. Cycloplegia (e.g., atropine 1% twice daily) in painful eyes.
3. Glaucoma medications are continued up to the time of the procedure to diminish postoperative rise in IOP.
4. Administer a topical nonsteroidal anti-inflammatory drug (NSAID) (e.g., flurbiprofen 0.03% [Ocufen, Allergan, Inc., Irvine, CA, US]) to inhibit postoperative prostaglandin release.

Instrumentation

- Lid speculum (e.g., Lieberman)
- Castroviejo calipers
- Cryosurgical unit with glaucoma cryoprobe (2.5 mm diameter tip)

Operative Procedure

1. Anesthesia:
   a. Peribulbar or retrobulbar with lid block if necessary.
   b. General anesthesia in uncooperative patient.

2. *Optional:* In a blind painful eye, retrobulbar alcohol may be injected for long-lasting anesthesia (see Chapter 4).
3. Prep and drape.
4. Place lid speculum.
5. Test cryosurgical unit. (The optimal treatment temperature is ~80 degrees centigrade.)
6. Plan number and position of applications.
   a. Measuring with calipers, place anterior edge of cryoprobe 1.0 to 1.5 mm from anterior border of limbus (e.g., centered directly over pars plicata).
   b. Separate spots by 1 clock hour.
   c. Titrate number of applications to desired pressure-lowering effect. A typical treatment covers 6 to 9 clock hours (180–270 degrees). This number should rarely be exceeded, as the risk of complications increases with more applications.

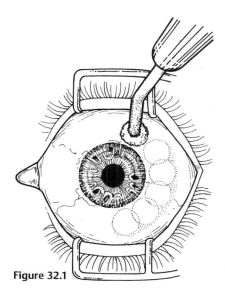

Figure 32.1

7. Apply cryoprobe and perform treatment (**Fig. 32.1**).

a. Press cryoprobe firmly over desired position, indenting sclera.
b. Activate cryo-unit.
c. Observe development of iceball and decrease in cryoprobe temperature to at least −60 degrees centigrade (−80°C is optimal).
d. Maintain freezing application for 60 seconds.
e. Iceball should extend to limbus but not too far over clear cornea.
8. Stop the freeze and irrigate the tip of the probe at the end of each application to facilitate its removal from the globe.
9. Apply topical antibiotic and steroid ointment.
10. Place patch.

Postoperative Procedure

1. Control inflammation.
   a. Topical steroids (e.g., prednisolone acetate 1%) every 1 to 2 hours and taper as inflammation warrants.
   b. Oral steroids if inflammation is severe.
   c. NSAIDs to inhibit prostaglandin release.
2. Control pain and discomfort.
   a. Cycloplegia (e.g., atropine 1% twice daily).
   b. NSAID.
   c. Narcotics as needed.
   d. Antiemetics as needed.
3. Control IOP.
   a. Continue glaucoma medications postoperatively, as hypotensive effect of cyclocryotherapy may take several days to develop.
   b. Measure IOP 4–6 hours postoperatively and daily thereafter until stable.
   c. If IOP increases, the following may be added to the medical regimen.
      i. Osmotics (e.g., mannitol 20% intravenously or oral hyperosmotics).

Note: Some surgeons routinely administer mannitol postoperatively to prevent pressure spike.

      ii. Carbonic anhydrase inhibitors (e.g., dorzolamide hydrochloride 2% [Trusopt, Merck & Co., Inc., Whitehouse Station, NJ, US]) 3 times per day or Diamox sequels 500 mg orally 2 times per day.
      iii. β-blockers (e.g., timolol maleate 0.5% 2 times a day).
      iv. α-agonists (e.g., brimonidine tartrate 0.10% [Alphagan P, Allergan, Inc.]) 2 or 3 times per day.
   d. Repeat cyclocryotherapy if IOP is not satisfactorily controlled with medication.
      i. Wait at least 1 month before repeating treatment to allow time for the full effect of initial treatment to be manifested.
      ii. When performing repeat cyclocryotherapy, may re-treat the initial sites first in an attempt to avoid overtreatment, hypotony, and consequent phthisis. Additional spots may be cautiously added if deemed necessary for adequate pressure control. However, total treatment of more than 300 degrees is rarely, if ever, indicated.

Complications

1. Severe ocular pain
2. Inflammation
3. Transient increase in IOP
4. Macular edema
5. Suprachoroidal effusion or hemorrhage
6. Hyphema (especially in eye with neovascular glaucoma)
7. Vitreous bleeding
8. Hypotony and phthisis bulbi
9. Cataract
10. Dellen and limbal scars
11. Staphyloma
12. Anterior segment necrosis

■ Laser Cyclophotocoagulation

Indications

■ Treatment of glaucoma that has failed multiple procedures (e.g., filtration, cyclodialysis, or tube/shunt procedures), especially in aphakia or pseudophakia.
■ Control of increased IOP in eyes with poor potential for good central visual acuity.
■ As a possible alternative to enucleation or evisceration of a blind and painful eye due to secondary glaucoma.

Preoperative Procedure

See Chapter 3.

1. Topical steroid (e.g., prednisolone acetate 1%) as indicated to decrease inflammation.
2. Cycloplegia (e.g., atropine 1% twice daily) in painful eyes. Glaucoma medications (e.g., β-blockers, α-agonists, or carbonic anhydrase inhibitors) are continued up to the time of the procedure to diminish postoperative rise in IOP.
3. Administer aspirin or NSAID to inhibit postoperative prostaglandin release.

Instrumentation

■ Shields contact lens and Nd:YAG laser with a slit lamp delivery system in the continuous thermal mode for noncontact laser cyclophotocoagulation.
■ Lid speculum (e.g., Lieberman)
■ Semiconductor diode laser with a contact probe (e.g., G-Probe) for contact laser cyclophotocoagulation.
■ Castroviejo calipers

Operative Procedure

1. Anesthesia:
   a. Peribulbar or retrobulbar with lid block if necessary.
   b. General anesthesia in uncooperative patient.

2. *Optional:* In a blind and painful eye, retrobulbar alcohol may be injected for long-lasting anesthesia (see Chapter 4).
3. Prep and drape.
4. Place lid speculum.
5. Test laser unit.
6. Plan number and position of applications.
   a. Measuring with calipers, Shields contact lens, or G-Probe 1.0 to 1.5 mm posterior to the limbus.
   b. Titrate number of applications to desired pressure-lowering effect. A typical treatment covers 6 to 9 clock hours (180–270 degrees). Approximately 5–8 applications can be made per quadrant.
7. For noncontact laser cyclophotocoagulation, apply the Shields contact lens with methylcellulose to the eye.

   Laser parameters:

   a. Maximum offset of nine on the Lasag Microrupter II.
   b. Power: 8.0 Joules.
   c. Duration: 20 ms.
   d. Applications: 32 spots sparing the 3 and 9 o'clock positions to avoid the long posterior ciliary arteries.
8. Contact laser cyclophotocoagulation
   a. Laser parameters.
      i. Duration: 2–4 seconds
      ii. Power: 1.2–3 W
      iii. Applications: Five to eight spots per quadrant; occasionally a popping sound may be heard with each application.
9. Inject subconjunctival steroid and apply topical cycloplegic, antibiotic, and steroid ointment.
10. Place patch over eye.

Postoperative Procedure

1. Control inflammation.
   a. Topical steroids (e.g., prednisolone acetate 1%) every 1–2 hours and taper as inflammation warrants.
   b. Aspirin or NSAID to inhibit prostaglandin release.
2. Control pain and discomfort.
   a. Cycloplegia (e.g., atropine 1% twice daily).
   b. Aspirin or NSAID.
3. Control IOP.
   a. Continue glaucoma medications postoperatively, as hypotensive effects of laser cyclophotocoagulation may take several days to develop.
   b. Measure IOP 2–6 hours postoperatively and weekly thereafter until stable.
   c. If IOP increases, the following may be added to the medical regimen.
      i. β-blockers (e.g., timolol maleate 0.5% twice daily).
      ii. α-agonists (e.g., brimonidine tartrate 0.10% [Alphagan P, Allergan, Inc.]) drops 2 or 3 times per day.
      iii. Carbonic anhydrase inhibitors (e.g., dorzolamide hydrochloride 2% [Trusopt, Merck & Co., Inc.]) 3 times a day or Diamox 500 mg sequels orally 2 times per day.

d. Repeat laser cyclophotocoagulation if IOP is not satisfactorily controlled with medication.
   i. Wait at least 1 month before repeating treatment to allow time for the full effect of initial treatment to be manifested.
   ii. When performing repeat laser cyclophotocoagulation, may re-treat the initial sites first in an attempt to avoid overtreatment, hypotony, and consequent phthisis. Additional spots may be cautiously added if deemed necessary for adequate pressure control.

Complications

1. Severe ocular pain, but less frequent than with cyclocryotherapy
2. Inflammation
3. Transient increase in IOP
4. Macular edema
5. Suprachoroidal effusion or hemorrhage
6. Hyphema (especially in an eye with neovascular glaucoma)
7. Vitreous bleeding
8. Hypotony and phthisis bulbi
9. Cataract
10. Conjunctival scarring
11. Loss of vision

■ Cyclodialysis

Indications

■ Performed infrequently, but may help select aphakic eyes that have failed filtering surgery and other glaucoma procedures.
■ With cyclodialysis, the goal is to disinsert a portion of the ciliary muscle from the scleral spur and create a cleft in the angle to provide direct communication between the anterior chamber and the suprachoroidal space.

Preoperative Procedure

See Chapter 3.

1. Apply topical steroids (e.g., prednisolone acetate 1%) as inflammation dictates. An inflamed eye has a poor chance of success.
2. Discontinue strong cycloplegics 1 week preoperatively.

Instrumentation

■ Lid speculum (e.g., Lieberman)
■ Sutures (4–0 silk, 7–0, 8–0 Vicryl)
■ Needle holder
■ Fine-toothed tissue forceps (e.g., 0.12 mm Castroviejo)
■ Westcott scissors

- Wheeler or similar microsurgical knife
- Cautery
- Castroviejo calipers
- Scarifier (e.g., Grieshaber #681.01 or Beaver #57)
- Cyclodialysis spatula
- Syringe with 30 gauge needle or cannula

Operative Procedure

1. Anesthesia:
   a. Peribulbar or retrobulbar with lid block if necessary.
   b. General anesthesia in uncooperative patient.
2. Prep and drape.
3. Place lid speculum.
4. *Optional:* Place 4–0 silk bridle sutures through insertions of superior and inferior rectus muscles.
5. Select site for cyclodialysis.
   a. Select superior site if possible to allow blood to drain away from the cleft postoperatively.
   b. Avoid the area of a previous iridectomy.
   c. Select site between rectus muscles to avoid ciliary vessels at 3, 6, 9, and 12 o'clock.
   d. In reoperations, perform cyclodialysis in area of previous cleft to avoid compromising the remaining angle.
6. Perform a fornix-based conjunctival peritomy at the anticipated cyclodialysis site (Westcott scissors, 0.12 mm forceps).
7. Secure hemostasis with cautery.
8. Perform anterior chamber paracentesis away from cyclodialysis site with Wheeler or similar microsurgical knife (see Chapter 7).
9. Verify patency of paracentesis with 30 gauge cannula on syringe.
10. Measure 4–5 mm posterior to limbus and mark cyclodialysis site with calipers or cautery.
11. Cauterize sclera over planned sclerostomy site to minimize bleeding.

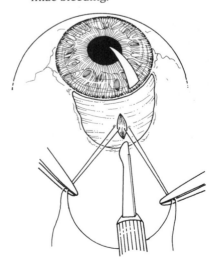

Figure 32.2

12. Carefully scratch down sclera to suprachoroidal space with scarifier (**Fig. 32.2**).

a. Make incision radial, centered 4.5 mm posterior to limbus, and ~3 mm in length.
b. Before reaching suprachoroidal space, may place 7–0 Vicryl traction suture through partial thickness (one half to two thirds) sclera. This is used to spread the lips of the sclerostomy to facilitate a controlled entry.
c. Stop as soon as uveal tissue is reached.

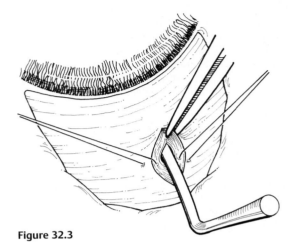

Figure 32.3

13. Enter sclerostomy with cyclodialysis spatula (**Fig. 32.3**).
    a. Have assistant spread wound with traction sutures.
    b. Carefully place cyclodialysis spatula into sclerostomy site and advance it radially toward limbus in the supraciliary space
       i. Apply countertraction on sclera with 0.12 mm forceps, grasping anterior aspect of wound and pulling up and posteriorly.

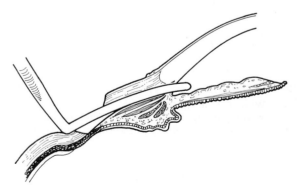

Figure 32.4

      ii. Hug sclera with cyclodialysis spatula during all movements to avoid penetrating uvea (**Fig. 32.4**).
         I. Depress heel of spatula while lifting up on tip.
         II. Visualize spatula tip lifting up on sclera.

c. Advancement should be smooth and not forced. There may, however, be some resistance when the scleral spur is ultimately reached and separated.

14. Visualize tip of cyclodialysis spatula in anterior chamber (**Fig. 32.4**).
    a. Avoid stripping Descemet membrane.
        i. Do not force spatula anteriorly.
        ii. Tilt tip of spatula down slightly once anterior chamber has been entered.
    b. Do not enter eye behind iris. If this occurs, pull back on the spatula and reenter anterior chamber more anteriorly.

15. Advance tip of spatula ~2 mm into anterior chamber.

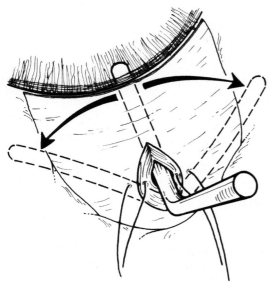

Figure 32.5

16. Slowly sweep spatula ~60 degrees in one direction (**Fig. 32.5**).
    a. Use sclerostomy site as fulcrum of sweep.
    b. Hug sclera with spatula at all times but tilt tip slightly down to avoid stripping Descemet membrane while executing the sweep.

17. Remove spatula, reenter sclerostomy site, advance spatula into anterior chamber, and sweep 60 degrees in opposite direction.

18. Remove spatula.
19. If bleeding is encountered, inject air through paracentesis site for tamponade (30 gauge cannula).
20. Irrigate balanced salt solution into anterior chamber through paracentesis to reconstitute anterior chamber and restore IOP.
21. Close sclerostomy with preplaced 7-0 Vicryl suture.
22. Remove bridle sutures.
23. Reposition conjunctiva and secure with interrupted sutures (e.g., 8-0 Vicryl).
24. Perform subconjunctival injections of antibiotic (e.g., gentamicin 20-40 mg) and steroid (e.g., Decadron 4-8 mg).
25. Remove lid speculum.
26. Apply Phospholine Iodide ¼% drops, antibiotic, and steroid ointment.
27. Place patch and Fox shield.

Postoperative Procedure

1. Position patient to allow any anterior chamber blood to settle away from cyclodialysis cleft.
2. Apply steroid drops (e.g., prednisolone acetate 1%) every 2 hours and taper as inflammation warrants.
3. Phospholine Iodide ¼% twice per day to mechanically pull cleft open.
4. Phenylephrine 2.5% every 12 hours to mechanically pull ciliary body centrally and thereby widen cleft.
5. Carbonic anhydrase inhibitor (e.g., acetazolamide 250 mg 4 times per day). If IOP is lower than 12 mm Hg during early postoperative period, the carbonic anhydrase inhibitor may be discontinued and the IOP followed closely.
6. Avoid dilating pupil, as this may compromise cleft.
7. Danger of rebleed is highest on postoperative days 3-5.

Complications

1. Hemorrhage (operative and postoperative)
2. Hypotony and phthisis
3. Cataract formation in phakic eye
4. Uveitis
5. Cleft closure with precipitant increase in IOP

33

Glaucoma Laser Procedures

■ Laser Iridotomy

Indications

- Relief of pupillary block in eyes with primary angle closure glaucoma
- Prophylaxis in eyes with anatomy predisposing toward angle closure
- Aphakic or pseudophakic pupillary block
- Pupillary seclusion with iris bombe
- Selected cases of chronic or secondary angle closure glaucoma
- Specific indications for use of laser rather than surgical iridectomy:
  - Treatment of imperforate surgical iridectomy
  - Treatment of nanophthalmic eyes that frequently develop severe choroidal effusions with invasive procedures
  - Prophylactic treatment of the fellow eye in ciliary block glaucoma

Preoperative Procedure

1. Examine anterior chamber angle with gonioscopy lens to assess degree of angle closure and anterior chamber depth.
2. Constrict pupil with pilocarpine 1% 30 minutes before procedure.
3. Place one drop of α-adrenergic agonist (e.g., brimonidine tartrate 0.10%, [Alphagan P, Allergan, Inc., Irvine, CA, US]).

Instrumentation

- Argon, Nd:YAG, or Diode laser
- Abraham iridotomy lens with peripheral 66 diopter button

Operative Procedure

Argon or Diode Laser

Technique 1: Drumhead method
1. Apply topical anesthetic (e.g., proparacaine).
2. Place Abraham lens with methylcellulose solution.
3. Select iridotomy site:
   a. Superonasal or superotemporal peripheral iris, approximately two thirds of distance from pupillary margin to limbus.
   b. Select iris crypt for easier penetration.
   c. In shallow anterior chamber, choose site where iris is most distant from cornea (to prevent endothelial trauma).
   d. Choose site as peripheral as possible but central to arcus senilus to facilitate visualization.
4. Focus at base of iris crypt, ensuring that laser is not aimed at macula or optic nerve.

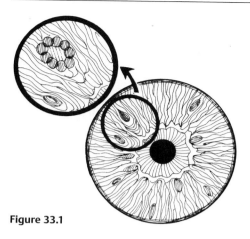

Figure 33.1

5. Apply stretch burns (**Fig. 33.1**).
   a. Approximately four to eight overlapping burns centered around planned penetration site.
   b. Laser parameters:
      i. Spot size: 200 μm.
      ii. Duration: 0.2 seconds.
      iii. Power: 100–200 mW.

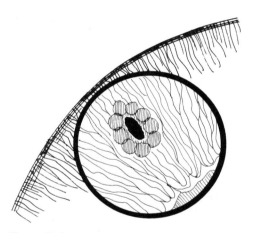

Figure 33.2

6. Apply penetrating burns (**Fig. 33.2**):

Note: there are variations in parameters, depending on iris color.

   a. Aim at center of stretch burns.
   b. Laser parameters:
      i. Spot size: 50 μm.
      ii. Duration: 0.1 sec.
      iii. Power: 500–1500 mW (adjust as iris reaction indicates).
   c. Apply burns directly over each other until penetration is achieved.
   d. Number of applications required averages ~25 but may be more than 100.

7. Verify patency by visualizing anterior lens capsule or vitreous (in aphakes) directly through iridotomy with slit beam. (A red reflex by retroillumination does not confirm patency.)
8. When iris is penetrated, enlarge iridotomy by chipping away at its edges.
   a. Laser parameters:
      i. Spot size: 50 μm.
      ii. Duration: 0.05–0.1 sec.
      iii. Power: 500 mW.
   b. Do not aim laser directly through iridotomy to avoid damaging lens.

Technique 2: Chipping away method

1. Prepare eye and select iridectomy site as described for drumhead method.
2. Focus laser at base of selected iris crypt.
3. Perform iridotomy using the following parameters:
   a. Spot size: 50 μm.
   b. Duration: 0.1 sec.
   c. Power: 500–1500 mW. (Adjust as iris reaction indicates.)
4. Apply burns directly over each other until penetration is achieved.
5. Verify patency of iridotomy with slit beam.
6. Upon achieving patency, enlarge iridotomy and remove residual pigment by chipping away at edge of opening using the following parameters.
   a. Spot size: 50 μm.
   b. Duration: 0.05–0.1 sec.
   c. Power: 500 mW.

Nd:YAG Laser

1. Apply topical anesthetic (e.g., proparacaine).
2. Place Abraham lens with methylcellulose solution.
3. Select iridotomy site as described in argon laser drumhead method (see step 3, above)
4. Focus Helium-Neon laser aiming beam at desired site.
5. *Optional:* Apply stretch/cautery burns with argon laser. (May decrease bleeding caused by subsequent YAG applications.)
   a. Apply ~4–8 overlapping burns.
   b. Laser parameters.
      i. Spot size: 200 μm.
      ii. Duration: 0.2 sec.
      iii. Power: 100–200 mW.
6. Perform YAG laser treatment.
   a. Power: ~4–8 mJoules (start at 4 mJoules).
   b. May need to wait a few minutes between applications while debris disperses away from site.
   c. Apply 1–10 applications until patency is achieved.

Note: YAG laser iridotomies have less propensity for late closure than do argon laser iridotomies.

7. If bleeding occurs at laser site, apply brief pressure to the eye with contact lens.

Postoperative Procedure

1. Reexamine angle with gonioscopy lens to assess effect of laser treatment on depth of anterior chamber.
2. Apply steroid drops (e.g., prednisolone acetate 1%) 4 times per day for 1 week, then taper to treat inflammation.
3. Place 1 drop of α-adrenergic agonist (e.g., brimonidine tartrate 0.10% [Alphagan P, Allergan, Inc.]) after laser treatment for prophylaxis against intraocular pressure spikes.
4. Continue pilocarpine 1% every 6 hours if unsure of iridotomy patency and if angle closure remains a possibility.
5. If iridotomy is patent and inflammation is severe, dilate pupil (e.g., cyclopentolate 1%) to avoid posterior synechiae.

Follow-up Schedule

1. Measure IOP 1 hour postlaser to check for pressure elevation.
2. Follow-up in 1 week to measure intraocular pressure (IOP) and examine iridotomy site.
3. Routine follow-up every 3 to 6 months thereafter.

Complications

1. Iritis
2. Hyphema (more common with YAG laser)
3. Transient elevation of intraocular pressure.
4. Closure of iridotomy (more common with argon laser)
5. Lens damage (localized)
6. Localized corneal endothelial damage: shattered glass appearance.
7. Retinal damage

■ Laser Trabeculoplasty

Indications

■ Chronic open angle glaucoma uncontrolled by maximally tolerated medical therapy.
■ Glaucoma patients who are noncompliant with medications.
■ Selected secondary open angle glaucomas uncontrolled by medical therapy, for example:
  ❑ Pseudoexfoliative glaucoma.
  ❑ Pigmentary glaucoma.
■ Laser trabeculoplasty is not useful for the angle closure or inflammatory glaucomas.

Preoperative Procedure

Examine Anterior Chamber Angle with Gonioscopy Lens

1. Identify landmarks.
2. If angle is narrow, a laser iridotomy or gonioplasty may be performed initially to facilitate laser trabeculoplasty.
3. Apply one drop of 1% pilocarpine to stretch iris.

Instrumentation

■ Argon green or blue-green or diode laser
■ Goldmann 3-mirror contact lens or similar gonioscopy lens.

Operative Procedure

1. Apply topical anesthetic (e.g., proparacaine).
2. Place contact lens (e.g., Ritch trabeculoplasty lens) with methylcellulose solution.
3. Examine the entire angle, identifying landmarks (e.g., scleral spur) before proceeding.
4. Laser parameters.
   a. Spot size: 50 μm.
   b. Duration: 0.1 sec.
   c. Power: start at ~800–1000 mW and adjust as necessary to produce desired effect (see step 5e, below).
5. Apply laser spot (**Fig. 33.3**).

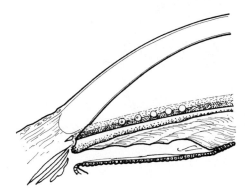

Figure 33.3

a. Apply at junction of anterior nonpigmented trabecular meshwork and posterior pigmented meshwork. (If trabecular meshwork is completely nonpigmented, aim for its center.)
b. Apply 100 evenly spaced spots over the entire 360 degrees of angle in two sessions.
   i. Apply 50 spots over 180 degrees during each session.
   ii. By convention, start treatment with nasal or inferior half (180 degrees) of angle.
   iii. Separate sessions by 3 weeks to allow for assessment of pressure response.
   iv. Alternatively, some surgeons treat 360 degrees at one session.

c. Focus aiming beam at desired location.
   i. Tilt the contact lens as necessary to produce a round, not elliptical, spot.
   ii. Rotate the lens as necessary to keep the application site centered in the mirror.

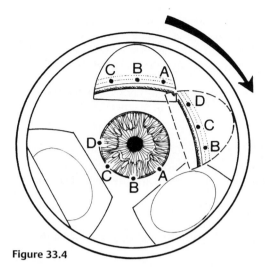

Figure 33.4

d. Start treatment at the 6 o'clock angle (contact lens mirror at 12 o'clock) and proceed superiorly (**Fig. 33.4**).
   i. Remember: Laser applications are reflected off a plano mirror. Therefore, spots placed counterclockwise through the mirror will actually be placed clockwise on the angle.
   ii. However, again because of the plano mirror effect, when the lens is rotated clockwise, a given point on the angle will likewise appear to move clockwise in the mirror. Therefore, if applications are centered in the mirror, moving the lens clockwise will result in laser bums placed clockwise in the opposite angle.
e. Titrate laser power to produce slight depigmentation and bubble formation at the application site, avoiding pigment dispersion and excessive bubble formation.

Postoperative Procedure

1. Topical steroid (e.g., prednisolone acetate 1%) 4 times per day for 1 week.
2. Continue prelaser glaucoma medications until hypotensive response is demonstrated (usually 4 to 6 weeks postoperatively) and then taper conservatively.
3. Treat any acute increase in IOP with additional α–agonists, β–blockers, or topical carbonic anhydrase inhibitors as needed. (Approximately 25% of eyes have IOP elevation during the first 3 weeks postlaser.)

Follow-up Schedule

1. Measure IOP 1–2 hours postlaser to check for early pressure elevation.
2. Recheck IOP in 1 week.
3. Follow-up in 4 weeks, and thereafter as indicated for the patient.
   i. Perform gonioscopy at each visit to check for development of peripheral anterior synechiae.
   ii. Monitor IOP at each visit (maximal pressure lowering effect of laser trabeculoplasty may not be seen for more than 1 month).

Complications

1. Hemorrhage from laser sites
2. Transient increase in IOP
3. Rare cases of persistently elevated IOP
4. Inflammation
5. Peripheral anterior synechiae
6. Localized corneal endothelial damage

■ Selective Laser Trabeculoplasty

Indications

■ Open angle glaucoma uncontrolled by maximally tolerated medical therapy
■ May also be used in patients who have failed argon laser trabeculoplasty (either 180 or 360 degrees)
■ Glaucoma patients who cannot tolerate or are noncompliant with their glaucoma medications
■ Long-term success rates in secondary open angle glaucomas are yet to be determined; however, selective laser trabeculoplasty has been shown to work well with patients with pigmentary, pseudoexfoliation, juvenile and angle recession glaucomas.

Preoperative Procedure

1. Examine anterior chamber angle by gonioscopy.
2. Identify landmarks to plan area of laser treatment.

Instrumentation

■ Coherent Selecta 7000 frequency doubled, Q-switched Nd:YAG laser emitting at 532 nm (Coherent Inc., Palo Alto, California, US).
■ Goldmann 3-mirror gonioscopy lens, 1-mirror Latina gonioscopy lens, or Ritch trabeculoplasty lens.

Operative Procedure

1. Using pilocarpine 1% may improve the view of the angle to facilitate laser treatment.
2. Apply topical α-adrenergic agent to prevent postlaser intraocular pressure elevations.
3. Apply topical anesthetic (e.g., proparacaine).
4. Place gonioscopy lens with methylcellulose solution.
5. Examine the entire angle, identifying landmarks before proceeding.
6. Laser parameters.
   a. Spot size: 400 μm.
   b. Duration: 3 nsec.
   c. Power: start at ~0.8 mJ and then energy is titrated to threshold energy (see step 7e, below).
7. Apply laser spot.
   a. Apply at the junction of the anterior nonpigmented trabecular meshwork and the posterior pigmented trabecular meshwork.

Note: The system's 400 μm spot size is large enough to irradiate the entire anteroposterior height of the trabecular meshwork.

   b. Focus aiming beam at desired location.
      i. Tilt the contact lens as necessary to produce a round, not elliptical, spot.
      ii. Rotate the lens as necessary to keep the application site centered in the mirror.
   c. Using single-burst mode, apply 50–55 contiguous, but not overlapping, laser spots along 180 degrees.

Note: The remaining 180 degrees may be treated at another session, if needed. Separate sessions by 3 to 4 weeks to allow for assessment of pressure response.

   d. According to the surgeon's view, moving the lens (e.g., clockwise) in the opposite direction of the laser spot applications (e.g., counterclockwise) will more easily allow continuous contiguous placement of the laser sports.

Note: Unlike argon laser trabeculoplasty, the visible end points of bubble formation or blanching of the trabecular meshwork are generally not seen.

   e. The threshold energy for bubble formation is determined by starting at 0.8 mJ; energy is increased by 0.1 mJ until bubble formation is noted.
   f. Once the threshold energy is identified, or if bubble formation is already noted at 0.8 mJ, laser energy is decreased by 0.1 mJ until no bubble formation is observed.

Note: This lower energy is the treatment energy.

Postoperative Procedure

1. Optimal postoperative medications are yet to be determined.
2. Topical steroids (e.g., prednisolone acetate 1%) 4 times per day for 4–7 days may be used.
3. Note: Some of the pressure-lowering effect may partly be due to migration and phagocytosis of trabecular meshwork debris by macrophages, so some have also advocated using milder topical steroids for only a few days, using topical NSAIDs, or not even using any anti-inflammatory drops postlaser.
4. Continue prelaser glaucoma medications until hypotensive response is demonstrated and then taper conservatively.

Follow-up Schedule

1. Measure eye pressure 1–2 hours postlaser to check for early pressure elevations; treat any pressure elevations as needed.
2. Recheck eye pressure after 24 hours if patient cannot tolerate pressure fluctuations.
3. Follow up in 1 week, 4 weeks, and thereafter as indicated for the patient.
4. Monitor eye pressure at each visit.

Note: Maximal pressure-lowering effect of selective laser trabeculoplasty may not be seen for 1 month or longer.

5. Consider gonioscopy if IOP is elevated.

Complications

1. Increase in IOP
2. Anterior chamber inflammation
3. Hemorrhage from laser sites
4. Peripheral anterior synechiae
5. Localized corneal endothelial damage

■ Laser Gonioplasty and Iridoplasty

Indications

Laser Gonioplasty or Peripheral Iridoplasty

- Deepening of the peripheral anterior chamber angle to facilitate visualization of the trabecular meshwork for laser trabeculoplasty
- Treatment of plateau iris syndrome
- Medically unresponsive attack of angle closure glaucoma when an iridotomy cannot be performed
- Lysis of recently formed (less than 1 year) peripheral anterior synechiae from an attack of acute angle closure glaucoma

Laser Iridoplasty or Pupilloplasty

- Medically unresponsive attack of angle closure glaucoma when an iridotomy is unable to be performed.
- Enlargement of a chronically miotic pupil.

Preoperative Procedure

1. Examine anterior chamber iris and angle with gonioscopy lens.
2. Identify landmarks.

Instrumentation

- Argon green or blue-green or diode laser
- Goldmann 3-mirror contact lens or similar gonioscopy lens for gonioplasty and peripheral iridoplasty procedure
- Pupilloplasty procedure does not require a contact lens

Operative Procedure

1. Apply topical anesthetic (e.g., proparacaine).
2. Place contact lens with methylcellulose solution onto the cornea.
3. Examine the entire anterior chamber angle and identify landmarks (e.g., scleral spur) before proceeding.
4. Laser parameters:
   a. Spot size: 500 μm.
   b. Duration: 0.2–0.5 sec.
   c. Power: start at ~200 mW and may increase (maximum is ~800 mW) and adjust as necessary to produce a visible shrinking of the iris stroma with each laser burn.
5. Apply laser spot.
   a. Gonioplasty or peripheral iridoplasty:

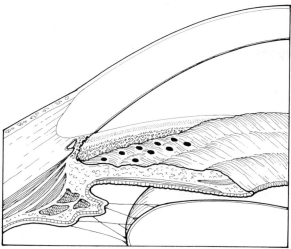

Figure 33.5

i. Apply laser burns at the peripheral roll of iris closest to the anterior chamber angle (**Fig. 33.5**).
ii. Visible shrinking of the peripheral iris should be seen and the peripheral iris stroma should flatten immediately.
iii. Two applications of the laser per clock hour are usually sufficient and retreatment is often necessary as the condition may recur.
   b. Laser pupilloplasty:

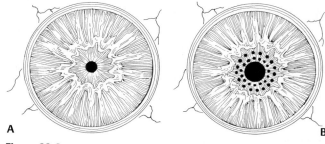

A   B

Figure 33.6

i. Apply laser burns to the region of the iris collarette (**Figs. 33.6A and 33.6B**).

Note: Burns may be applied even more centrally at pupillary border.

ii. Treatment of one section of the iris may be sufficient to cause a distortion of the pupil border and break the pupillary block.
iii. For photomydriasis, laser burns can be placed circumferentially near the pupillary border to create a slow contraction of the iris surface.

Note: Adding laser applications in a radial pattern from the pupillary border to the mid-iris area (**Fig. 33.6B**).

Postoperative Procedure

1. Topical steroid (e.g., prednisolone acetate 1%) starting at 4 times per day and taper over 1 week.
2. Continue prelaser glaucoma medications until hypotensive response is demonstrated and then taper conservatively.
3. Treat any acute increase in intraocular pressure with additional α agonists, β-blockers, or topical carbonic anhydrase inhibitors as needed.

Follow-up Schedule

1. Measure IOP 1–2 hours postlaser to check for early elevation.
2. Follow up in 1 week (sooner for severe glaucoma), 4 weeks, and thereafter as indicated for the patient.
   a. Perform gonioscopy at each visit to check for reformation of peripheral anterior synechiae.
   b. Monitor IOP at each visit.

Complications

1. Transient increase in IOP
2. Inflammation
3. Peripheral anterior synechiae
4. Distortion of the pupillary border
5. Localized corneal endothelial damage
6. Hemorrhage (from laser site)
7. Persistently elevated IOP

■ Laser Suture Lysis

Indications

Elevated IOP after trabeculectomy during the early postoperative period, caused by inadequate filtration from tight suture closure of the scleral trabeculectomy flap.

Preoperative Procedure

Carefully examine the trabeculectomy flap and conjunctiva to be sure that the trabeculectomy flap sutures are visible through the conjunctiva. Success of this procedure depends on clear visualization of the trabeculectomy flap sutures.

Instrumentation

- Argon green or blue-green or diode laser
- Hoskins or Ritch lens or a rounded corner of a Zeiss four-mirror lens.

Operative Procedure

1. Apply topical anesthetic (e.g., proparacaine).
2. Carefully examine the conjunctiva and scleral flap with the slit lamp biomicroscope and identify landmarks (e.g., dark nylon sutures) before proceeding. Place the lens over the conjunctiva to clearly visualize the sutures.
3. Laser parameters.
   a. Spot size: 50 μm.
   b. Duration: 0.05–0.1 sec.
   c. Power: Start at ~250–1000 mW and adjust as necessary to cut the suture. The more fibrosis covering the suture, the higher the energy required to cut the suture.
4. Apply laser spot.

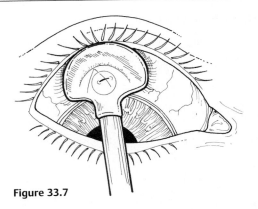

Figure 33.7

a. Carefully focus the aiming beam directly on the suture and apply energy (**Fig. 33.7**).
b. One or more sutures may be cut depending on the desired effect. The greater the number of sutures cut and the shorter the postoperative period when the sutures are cut, the greater the hypotensive effect.

Note: The tightest suture should be cut first.

c. Focal pressure on the edge of the scleral flap after the procedure may allow the flap to open and encourage aqueous outflow.

Postoperative Procedure

Continue as per trabeculectomy (see Trabeculectomy/Posterior Lip Sclerectomy section in the beginning of Chapter 30).

Complications

1. Hypotony with shallow anterior chamber
2. Conjunctival perforation
3. Subconjunctival hemorrhage
4. Conjunctival and scleral inflammation

■ Goniophotocoagulation

Indications

Neovascular glaucoma in the absence of synechial closure of the anterior chamber angles. This is a supplementation, not a replacement, for panretinal photocoagulation, which treats the underlying neovascularization process.

Preoperative Procedure

Examine the anterior chamber angle carefully with a gonioscopy lens and identify the areas where neovascularization is occurring without peripheral anterior synechial closure of the angle.

Instrumentation

- Argon green or blue-green or diode laser
- Goldmann three-mirror contact lens or similar gonioscopy lens.

Operative Procedure

1. Apply topical anesthetic (e.g., proparacaine).
2. Place contact lens with methylcellulose solution.
3. Examine the entire anterior chamber angle and identify landmarks for treatment.
4. Laser parameters.
    a. Spot size: 100–200 μm.
    b. Duration: 0.1–0.2 sec.
    c. Power: 200–400 mW and adjust as necessary to produce blanching of the treated blood vessels.
5. Apply laser spot (**Fig. 33.8**).

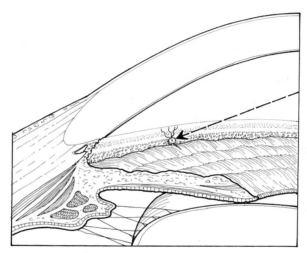

Figure 33.8

    a. Apply laser burn directly to each vessel as it crosses the scleral spur or to the vessel root in the area of the ciliary body band.
    b. The trabecular meshwork should not be treated directly to avoid peripheral anterior synechial formation and scarring.

    c. Treat the entire open angle available and avoid treatment to peripheral anterior synechiae.
    d. Multiple treatment sessions may be required for optimum effect.
    e. In most cases panretinal laser photocoagulation should be combined with goniophotocoagulation to prevent progressive neovascularization of the anterior segment.

Postoperative Procedure

1. Topical steroid (e.g., prednisolone acetate 1%) 4 times per day for 1 week, then taper to treat iritis.
2. Cycloplegic (e.g., atropine 1% drops) 2 times per day for comfort and to dilate the pupil.
3. Treat any acute increase in IOP with additional β-blockers, α-agonists, or topical carbonic anhydrase inhibitors as needed.

Follow-up Schedule

1. Measure IOP 1–2 hours postlaser to check for early elevation.
2. Follow up in 1 week and thereafter as indicated for the patient.
    a. Perform gonioscopy at each visit to check for development of peripheral anterior synechiae and regression of neovascularization.
    b. Monitor IOP at each visit.

Complications

1. Inflammation
2. Hemorrhage from laser site
3. Transient or persistent increase in IOP
4. Peripheral anterior synechiae

34

Choroidal Tap

Indications

■ Treatment of flat anterior chamber secondary to choroidal effusion after glaucoma filtration surgery.
■ Treatment of select hemorrhagic choroidal detachments.

Preoperative Procedure

See Chapter 3.

1. Indirect ophthalmoscopic examination or ultrasound to confirm presence and location of choroidal effusion.
2. Topical and oral steroids as inflammation warrants.

Instrumentation

■ Lid speculum
■ Wheeler or similar microsurgical knife
■ Castroviejo calipers
■ Fine-toothed tissue forceps (e.g., 0.12 mm Castroviejo forceps)
■ Westcott scissors
■ Cautery
■ Scarifier (e.g., Grieshaber #681.01, Beaver #57)
■ Sutures (7–0 Vicryl)
■ Needle holder
■ Cellulose sponges
■ Syringe with 30 gauge needle or cannula

Operative Procedure

1. Anesthesia:
   a. Peribulbar or retrobulbar with lid block.
   b. General anesthesia or retrobulbar plus lid block in uncooperative patient.
2. Prep and drape.
3. Place lid speculum.

4. Perform anterior chamber paracentesis with a Wheeler or similar microsurgical knife (see Chapter 7).
5. Use calipers to measure location of desired sclerostomy.
   a. Center ~5 mm from limbus.
   b. Choose area where the choroidal detachment is high.
   c. If the choroidal effusion is not localized, perform the tap inferotemporally or inferonasally.
6. Expose sclera at desired sclerostomy location.
   a. Perform conjunctival peritomy or
   b. Radial incision down to sclera over incision site (Westcott scissors).
7. Cauterize sclera over sclerostomy site to minimize bleeding.

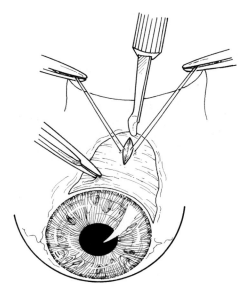

Figure 34.1

8. Carefully scratch down sclera to suprachoroidal space with scarifier (**Fig. 34.1**).

a. Make incision radial and ~3 mm in length.
b. Before reaching choroid, may place a 7–0 Vicryl traction suture through partial thickness (one half to two thirds) sclera. This is used to spread the lips of the sclerostomy to facilitate a controlled entry into the suprachoroidal space.
c. Stop as soon as choroid is reached.

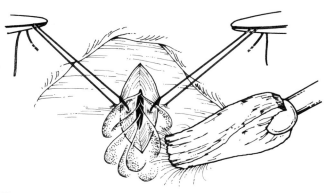

Figure 34.2

9. Upon entry into the suprachoroidal space, effusion fluid should spontaneously drain. This may be facilitated by:
   a. Pressure on the surrounding sclera with cellulose sponges (**Fig. 34.2**).
   b. Slow irrigation of balanced salt solution through the paracentesis to restore pressure within the globe and to reform the anterior chamber (syringe with 30 gauge needle or cannula).
   c. Spreading the lips of the sclerostomy with the traction suture.

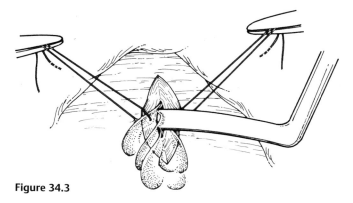

Figure 34.3

d. Careful insertion of cyclodialysis spatula into suprachoroidal space (**Fig. 34.3**).
   i. Enter parallel to limbus to avoid inadvertent cyclodialysis.
   ii. May gently elevate spatula within the suprachoroidal space to encourage egress of fluid.

10. Repeat step 9 until effusion has been satisfactorily drained. (The fundus may be examined with indirect ophthalmoscope to verify flattening of choroidals.)
11. Perform a second sclerostomy at another site if additional drainage is necessary.
12. Restore anterior chamber depth with balanced salt solution or viscoelastic irrigated through the paracentesis (leave eye with normal intraocular pressure at end of the case).
13. *Optional:* Close sclerostomy site.
    a. May leave site open to encourage continued drainage postoperatively. (Some surgeons cauterize lips of sclerostomy to gape edges.)
    b. May close with interrupted 7–0 Vicryl suture.
14. Close conjunctiva (7–0 Vicryl).
15. Optional: Inject subconjunctival Decadron (4–8 mg) away from any filtration sites into the conjunctival fornix.
16. Apply topical antibiotic, steroid ointment, and 1% atropine drops.
17. Apply light patch and Fox shield.

Postoperative Procedure

1. Steroid drops (e.g., prednisolone acetate 1%) 4 times per day up to every hour, as degree of inflammation warrants.
2. *Optional:* Oral steroid if choroidal effusion appears inflammatory in etiology.
3. Cycloplegia (e.g., atropine 1% twice per day) until the eye is quiet.
4. Topical antibiotic (e.g., moxifloxacin 0.5% [Vigamox, Alcon Laboratories, Inc., Fort Worth, TX, US], gatifloxacin 0.3% [Zymar, Allergan, Inc., Irvine, CA, US]), 4 times per day for 1 week.
5. Repeat ophthalmoscopic examination to evaluate the effect of the procedure.
6. Repeat ultrasound if suspect reformation of choroidal effusion (e.g., shallowing of anterior chamber).
7. Discharge patient when anterior chamber depth is stable.

Complications

1. Inadvertent cyclodialysis
2. Choroidal hemorrhage

VII

Pediatrics and Strabismus

35

Probe and Irrigation

Indications

- Tearing associated with a nasal lacrimal duct obstruction in a child.
- There is a lower success rate in children older than 2 years and in adults.

Preoperative Procedure

See Chapter 3.

A thorough evaluation of the nasal lacrimal duct system, including the inspection of both the upper and the lower puncta, is essential to ensure that they are not absent and to rule out seclusio punctum.

Instrumentation

- Punctal dilator
- Bowman lacrimal probes
- Nasal speculum
- Headlight
- Lacrimal cannula on a syringe
- Fluorescein strip
- Sterile saline
- Flexible nasal suction cannula
- Hemostat or Freer periosteal elevator (if infracture of the inferior turbinate will be performed)

Operative Procedure

1. Afrin nasal spray may be given ~20 minutes preoperatively into the nostril to decrease bleeding.
2. Anesthesia: General

Note: This may be performed in the office (with or without sedation) if the infant is small enough (usually younger than 6 months) to be restrained with a blanket or papoose board.

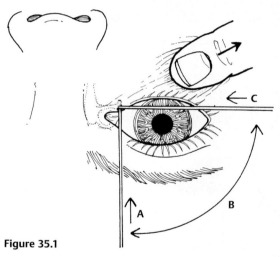

Figure 35.1

3. Dilate the lower punctum (**Fig. 35.1**).
   a. Insert the dilator vertically into the punctum for 1 mm.
   b. Rotate the dilator so it is pointing medially.
   c. Pull the lower eyelid laterally with a finger for countertraction while applying gentle medial pressure with the dilator.
4. Probe the nasal lacrimal duct.
   a. Insert a small-diameter Bowman lacrimal probe (usually a 2–0 or 1–0) vertically into the inferior punctum for 1 mm.
   b. Rotate the probe so it is pointing medially.
   c. Pull the lower eyelid laterally with a finger to provide countertraction. (This helps prevent the creation of a false passage.)

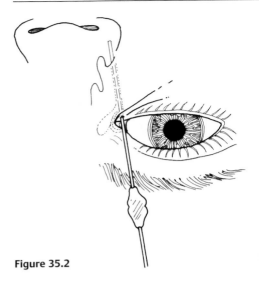

Figure 35.2

d. Push the probe medially. There should be little resistance. The end point is when a "hard stop" is felt. This indicates that the probe is pushing the lacrimal sac against the bone of the lacrimal fossa. If a soft stop is felt, there is extraneous tissue between the probe and the lacrimal sac. Pull out the probe laterally part way and try redirecting it medially (**Fig. 35.2**).

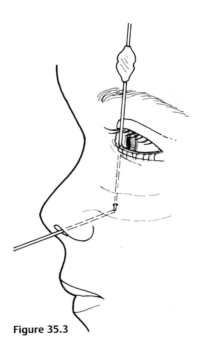

Figure 35.3

5. Rotate the probe to point inferiorly and gently guide it into the bony canal of the nasal lacrimal duct. The probe should point slightly medially and posteriorly. A pop may be felt when the probe perforates the membrane within the bony canal or overlying the exit of the duct. This ends the procedure if the child is not under general anesthesia (**Fig. 35.3**).

6. Check the probe in the nose. (These following steps are usually not performed if the child is not under general anesthesia.)
   a. Stand next to the head on the opposite side of the eye being probed.
   b. Insert the nasal speculum into the nasal ala.
   c. With the aid of the headlight, look under the inferior turbinate to visualize the tip of the probe. Look in the same direction as the patient's shoulder opposite to you. Make sure the probe tip is clearly visualized without any overlying membrane.
7. An alternative method to direct visualization of the probe tip is to insert one of the larger probes (usually a size 3 or 4) under the inferior turbinate and feel for metal on metal contact with the probe tip. This is less precise, as a thin membrane over the probe tip cannot be ruled out.
8. Remove the original probe and probe the system with progressively larger probes (e.g., 1–0, 0, and 1).
9. Infracture of the inferior turbinate can be optionally performed at this time using a Freer elevator or a hemostat.
   a. The Freer elevator is placed under the inferior turbinate and then pushed medially to rotate the inferior turbinate medially.
   b. Alternatively, a hemostat can be used to grasp the inferior turbinate and then used to rotate the inferior turbinate medially.
10. Irrigate the nasal lacrimal duct system.
   a. Place the fluorescein strip into a small cup of sterile saline and draw up the mixture into a syringe with a lacrimal cannula.
   b. Place the nasal suction cannula into the nose underneath the inferior turbinate.
   c. Insert the lacrimal cannula into the inferior punctum and medially into the lacrimal sac.
   d. Inject a small amount of fluid and recover it from the nose with the suction. (The fluorescein dye helps identify the irrigant.)
11. Instill a drop of antibiotic/steroid combination.

Postoperative Procedure

1. Discharge the patient when stable.
2. Instill a drop of antibiotic/steroid combination 4 times per day for 1 week.
3. Advise the parents that drops of blood from the nose and pink tears from the eye for a couple of days are normal.

Complications

1. Recurrence of the nasal lacrimal duct obstruction. Consideration may be given for a repeat probing, silicone tube intubation, or balloon dacryoplasty.
2. Creation of a false passageway

36

Forced Duction Testing

Indications

- Determination of restrictive component of limited ductions.
- Performed in the operating room before strabismus surgery or in the office with a cooperative adult.

Preoperative Procedure

None.

Instrumentation

- Lid speculum (e.g., Lancaster, Barraquer)
- Toothed forceps (e.g., Bishop-Harmon, 0.5 mm Castroviejo)

Operative Procedure

1. Anesthesia: General anesthesia or topical (e.g., proparacaine or tetracaine). If topical, augment the anesthesia by holding a cotton pledget soaked with anesthetic in the area to be grasped.
2. Place lid speculum if patient is under general anesthesia.
3. Perform forced ductions on the recti muscles (**Fig. 36.1**).
   a. If the patient is awake, ask him to look in the direction of intended forced duction testing (e.g., medially if testing adduction).
   b. Grasp the conjunctiva with toothed forceps at the limbus opposite the direction of intended rotation (e.g., at the lateral limbus if testing adduction).
   c. Proptose the globe by gently pulling it anteriorly.
   d. Rotate the globe in the desired direction and note any resistance. It is helpful to compare the resistance of the opposite eye to note any differences.

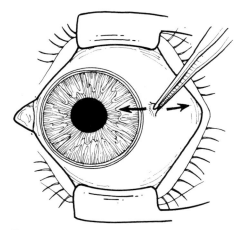

Figure 36.1

   e. Remove the eyelid speculum when testing supraduction and infraduction so the speculum will not get in the way.
4. Perform forced ductions on the superior oblique muscle. This is usually performed under general anesthesia (**Fig. 36.2**).
   a. Grasp the conjunctiva with toothed forceps at the limbus at 3 o'clock and 9 o'clock.
   b. Retropulse the globe by gently pushing it posteriorly.
   c. Excyclotort the globe and move it superonasally.
   d. Rock the inferior forceps temporally to feel the tendon.
5. Perform forced ductions on the interior oblique muscle. This is usually performed under general anesthesia.
   a. Grasp the conjunctiva with toothed forceps at the limbus at 3 o'clock and 9 o'clock.
   b. Retropulse the globe by gently pushing it posteriorly.
   c. Incyclotort the globe and move it inferonasally.
   d. Rock the superior forceps temporally to feel the tendon.

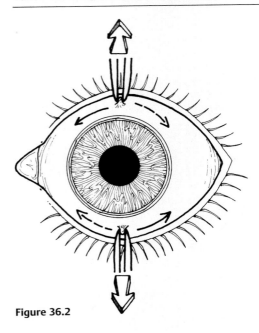

Figure 36.2

Postoperative Procedure

As per strabismus surgery protocol if performed in conjunction with eye muscle surgery.

Complications

1. Corneal abrasion
2. Subconjunctival hemorrhage

37

Horizontal Rectus Recession

Indications

Extraocular muscle imbalance requiring muscle weakening for correction (e.g., medial rectus recession in esotropia).

Preoperative Procedure

See Chapter 3.

A complete strabismus evaluation with determination of the detailed surgical plan is necessary.

Instrumentation

- Lid speculum (e.g., Lancaster, Barraquer)
- Needle holder
- Sutures (6–0 silk with spatula needle, double-armed 6–0 Vicryl with spatula needle (S29 or S14 needle), 7–0 Vicryl suture)
- Toothed forceps (e.g., Bishop-Harmon, 0.5 mm Castroviejo)
- Two locking 0.5 mm toothed forceps
- Westcott scissors (rounded tips)
- Cautery (bipolar forceps)
- Muscle hooks (e.g., Green, Jameson)
- Stevens tenotomy hooks
- Castroviejo caliper

Operative Procedure

Note: Figures are drawn from the surgeon's viewpoint with the surgeon standing at the head of the patient.

Limbal Approach

1. Anesthesia: General anesthesia or retrobulbar/peribulbar injection plus eyelid block.
2. Place a drop of neosynephrine 2.5% into the eye to constrict the blood vessels and decrease bleeding. Prep and drape.
3. Place lid speculum.

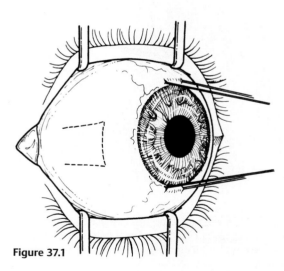

Figure 37.1

4. Place a 6–0 silk episcleral stay suture at the limbus at 6 and 12 o'clock (**Fig. 37.1**).

   Optional: Use locking Castroviejo forceps instead of stay suture.

5. Secure the globe with stay sutures to expose surgical field.

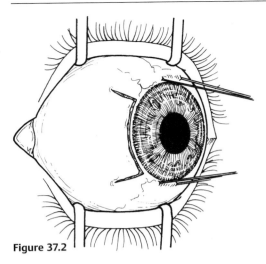

Figure 37.2

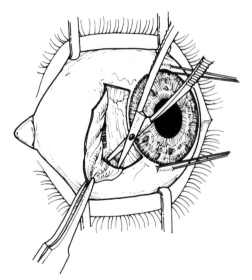

Figure 37.3

6. Prepare a fornix-based, winged limbal peritomy down to bare sclera with Westcott scissors (**Fig. 37.2**).

7. Buttonhole Tenon capsule and intermuscular septum with sharp and blunt dissection with Westcott scissors to reach bare sclera on either side of the muscle insertion (**Fig. 37.3**).
   a. Aim 45 degrees between the horizontal and vertical recti to avoid injuring the muscles.
   b. Bluntly spread the incision with Westcott scissors.
   c. Repeat on the opposite side of the muscle insertion.
8. Isolate the muscle (**Fig. 37.4**).
   a. First, sweep the Stevens tenotomy hook through the fascial buttonhole and under the muscle. Hold the hook parallel to and flush with bare sclera to facilitate passage.
   b. Follow with a Green muscle hook perpendicular to the sclera and just posterior to the Stevens hook. Keep the tip of the Green hook pressed against the sclera.
   c. Remove the Stevens tenotomy hook.

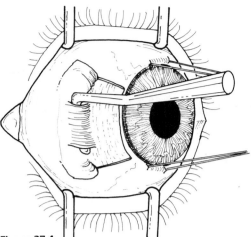

Figure 37.4

   d. Follow with a second Green muscle hook perpendicular to the sclera and just posterior to the first Green hook. Once again, keep the tip of the Green hook pressed against the sclera.
   e. Remove the first Green hook.
   f. The tip of the muscle hook can be visualized on the other side of the muscle. If not, repeat steps 8d–e.

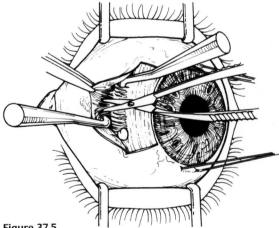

Figure 37.5

9. Tent the overlying conjunctiva with two Stevens tenotomy hooks and use Westcott scissors to minimally cut the check ligaments to the muscle sheath. Take care not to cut the muscle sheath or muscle or bleeding may occur. If bleeding occurs, apply direct pressure with a dental roll until it stops (**Fig. 37.5**).

Note: Be sure to dissect the lateral rectus intermuscular septal attachments to the inferior oblique to avoid the "J Syndrome."

10. Incise the intermuscular septum superior and inferior to the muscle minimally if necessary to obtain adequate muscle exposure. Be careful not to cut the inferior oblique muscle if incising along the inferior border of the lateral rectus.

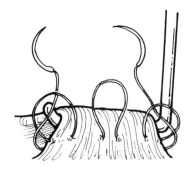

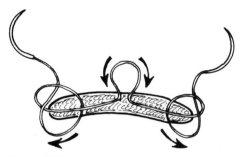

Figure 37.6

11. Suture the muscle 1 mm from its insertion with the double-armed 6–0 Vicryl with spatula needles (**Fig. 37.6**).
    a. Elevate muscle with the muscle hook.
    b. First throw is through half-thickness muscle from the center to one edge of the muscle, 1 mm from the insertion. Second throw is through full-thickness muscle, posterior to anterior, 1 mm from the edge of the muscle. Lock the second throw.
    c. Perform superiorly and inferiorly.
    d. Do not cut off the needles.

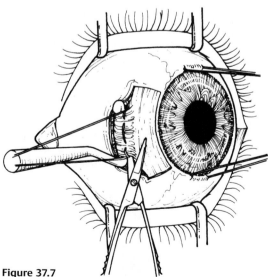

Figure 37.7

12. Detach the muscle at its insertion with Westcott scissors (**Fig. 37.7**).

a. Hold the muscle hook and sutures up to avoid cutting the sutures.
b. Cut the muscle flush with the sclera.
c. Inspect the muscle to ensure that it is properly sutured and not split, and that the lock bites are in place and adequate.

13. Gently cauterize (as needed) or apply direct pressure with a dental roll on the insertion site to achieve hemostasis.
14. Measure the length of recession from the original insertion site with calipers. Mark with the caliper tips the superior and inferior suture sites, keeping the original width of the muscle.

Note: Always recheck the accuracy of the calipers before using.

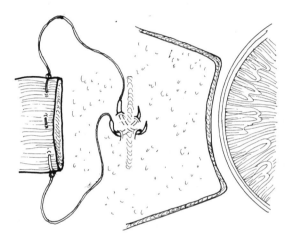

Figure 37.8

15. Reattach the muscle to sclera at the new position using the two ends of the previously placed 6–0 Vicryl suture (**Fig. 37.8**).
    a. Secure globe with toothed forceps.
    b. Enter the sclera at the previously marked location. Keep the needle parallel to the sclera to decrease the chance of penetration.
    c. Bring the needle partial thickness through the sclera almost parallel to the original insertion site.
    d. The needles should exit very close to each other in a crossed-swords fashion.
    e. Always visualize the needle tip through sclera to avoid penetrating the globe. Burrow through for partial thickness.
16. Securely tie muscle to sclera.
    a. Gently pull the muscle to its new insertion site. Retract the Tenon capsule and intermuscular septum to avoid dragging it with the suture into the scleral tunnel.
    b. Tie a 2–1–1 surgeon's knot.
    c. The assistant may hold the first throw down with a needle holder or tying forceps to prevent slippage.
    d. Inspect the muscle to ensure that it is in its proper position and no soft tissue is dragged into the suture tracts.

17. Reposition the conjunctiva. Wetting the eye may help differentiate conjunctiva (pink) from Tenon capsule (white).

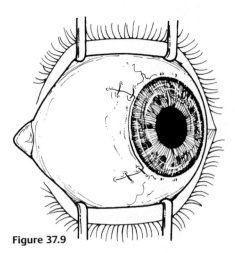

Figure 37.9

18. Suture the conjunctiva into position with interrupted 7–0 Vicryl sutures in a buried fashion (**Fig. 37.9**).
19. Remove stay sutures.
20. Apply antibiotic and steroid ointment.

Fornix Approach

The figures shown will be for a right medial rectus recession. This technique requires a knowledgeable assistant.

1. Anesthesia: General anesthesia or retrobulbar/peribulbar injection plus lid block.
2. Place a drop of neosynephrine 2.5% into the eye to constrict the blood vessels and decrease bleeding. Prep and drape.
3. Place lid speculum.

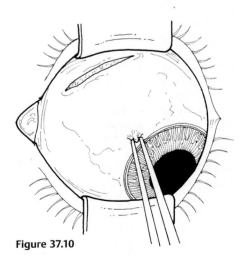

Figure 37.10

4. Create a fornix conjunctival incision (**Fig. 37.10**).

a. The assistant grasps the globe at the limbus at either the 4:30 position (for access to the right medial or left lateral rectus) or the 7:30 position (for access to the right lateral or left medial rectus).
b. The assistant then exposes the inferior fornix by elevating and abducting the globe (for access to the medial rectus) or elevating and adducting the globe (for access to the lateral rectus).
c. Create an 8 mm incision parallel to the fornix and 1 mm from the fornix on the bulbar conjunctiva with Westcott scissors.

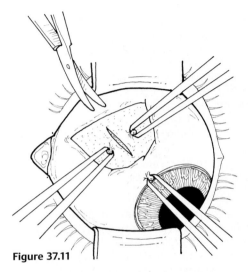

Figure 37.11

5. Create a radial incision through the Tenon capsule to expose the sclera (**Fig. 37.11**).
   a. The assistant and surgeon grasp the Tenon capsule less than 10 mm from the limbus.
   b. Cut the Tenon capsule between the forceps and radially toward the limbus.
   c. The incision should reach bare sclera. If layers of Tenon remain, repeat steps a–b.
   d. The incision should not extend more than 10 mm from the limbus or orbital fat may be exposed and adherence syndrome may occur.

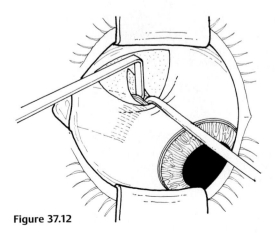

Figure 37.12

6. Isolate the rectus muscle with a Stevens hook (**Fig. 37.12**).
   a. First sweep the Stevens tenotomy hook through the fornix incision and under the muscle. (Hold the hook parallel to and flush with bare sclera to facilitate passage.)
   b. The assistant releases the forceps fixating the globe.
7. Isolate the muscle with the Green hook.
   a. Sweep a Green muscle hook perpendicular to the sclera and just posterior to the Stevens hook. Keep the tip of the Green hook pressed against the sclera.
   b. Remove the Stevens tenotomy hook.
   c. Follow with a second Green muscle hook perpendicular to the sclera and just posterior to the first Green hook. Once again, keep the tip of the Green hook pressed against the sclera.
   d. Remove the first Green hook.

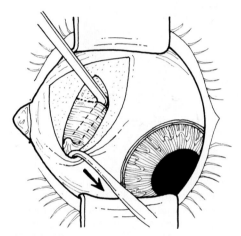

Figure 37.13

8. Expose the muscle insertion by using a Stevens hook to retract the Tenon capsule and conjunctiva over the tip of the Green hook (**Fig. 37.13**).

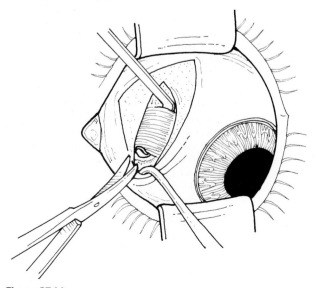

Figure 37.14

9. Incise the intermuscular septum at the tip of the Green hook with Westcott scissors (**Fig. 37.14**).

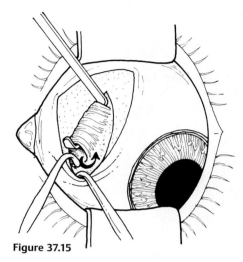

Figure 37.15

10. Check to ensure that the entire muscle is hooked (**Fig. 37.15**).
    a. The assistant exposes the superior pole of the muscle insertion with a Stevens hook.
    b. Sweep a Stevens hook from posterior to the insertion, around the superior pole and then anterior to the insertion in an arc. There should be no significant resistance felt.
    c. If there is significant resistance and it appears that the muscle is split, repeat steps 9c–d and 12a–b.
11. Incise the intermuscular septum anterior to the muscle to expose the muscle insertion.

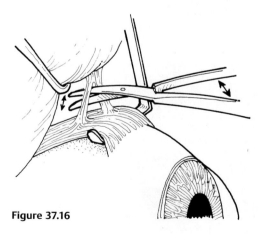

Figure 37.16

12. Tent the overlying conjunctiva with a Stevens tenotomy hook and use Westcott scissors to minimally cut the check ligaments to the muscle sheath (**Fig. 37.16**). Take care not to cut the muscle sheath or muscle as bleeding may occur. If bleeding occurs, apply direct pressure with a dental roll until it stops.

13. Incise the intermuscular septum superior and inferior to the muscle if necessary to obtain adequate muscle exposure. Be careful not to cut the inferior oblique muscle if incising along the inferior border of the lateral rectus.

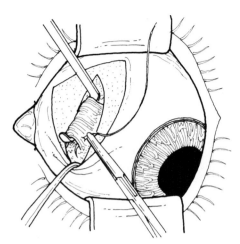

Figure 37.17

14. Suture the muscle 1 mm from its insertion with the double-armed 6–0 Vicryl with spatula needles (**Fig. 37.17**).
    a. Elevate the muscle with the muscle hook.
    b. First throw is through half-thickness muscle from the center to one edge of the muscle, 1 mm from the insertion. Second throw is through full-thickness muscle, posterior to anterior, 1 mm from the edge of the muscle. Lock the second throw.

Note: locking bite should be ~1 mm of muscle edge.

    c. Perform superiorly and inferiorly.
    d. Do not cut off the needles.

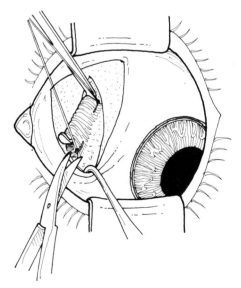

Figure 37.18

15. Detach the muscle at its insertion with Westcott scissors (**Fig. 37.18**).
    a. Hold the muscle hook and sutures up to avoid cutting the sutures.
    b. Cut the muscle flush with the sclera.
    c. Inspect the muscle to ensure it is properly sutured and not split.
16. Gently cauterize or apply direct pressure with a dental roll on the insertion site to achieve hemostasis.

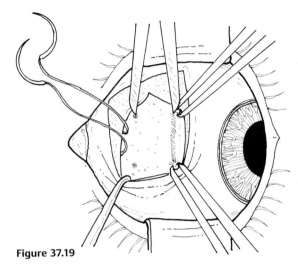

Figure 37.19

17. Mark the length of recession (**Fig. 37.19**).
    a. Fixate the globe with a locking 0.5 Castroviejo forceps at the superior and inferior pole of the original muscle insertion site. The assistant will rotate the globe either superiorly or inferiorly to help expose the surgical field.
    b. Retract the conjunctiva and Tenon capsule with a Stevens hook.
    c. Measure the length of recession from the original insertion site with calipers. Mark with the caliper tips the superior and inferior suture sites (keeping the original width of the muscle).

Note: Always recheck the accuracy of the calipers prior to using.

18. Reattach the muscle to sclera at the new position using the two ends of the previously placed 6–0 Vicryl suture (**Fig. 37.20**).
    a. Enter the sclera at the previously marked location. Keep the needle parallel to the sclera to decrease the chance of penetration.
    b. Bring the needle partial thickness through the sclera aiming almost parallel to the original insertion site.
    c. The needles should exit very close to each other in a crossed-swords fashion.
    d. Always visualize the needle tip through sclera to avoid penetrating the globe.

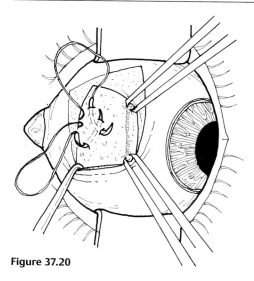

Figure 37.20

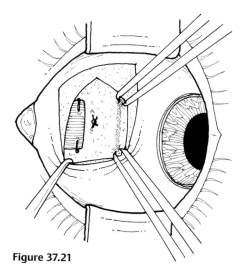

Figure 37.21

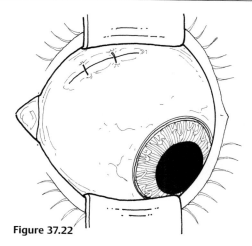

Figure 37.22

20. Reposition the conjunctival incision into the fornix (**Fig. 37.22**).
   a. If the incision site is gaping, suture the conjunctiva closed with interrupted 7–0 Vicryl sutures in a buried fashion.
   b. Wetting the eye may help differentiate conjunctiva (pink) from the Tenon capsule (white).
21. Apply antibiotic and steroid ointment.

Postoperative Procedure

1. Discharge patient when stable.
2. Apply antibiotic or antibiotic/steroid ointment 4 times a day for 5–14 days (e.g., erythromycin, TobraDex, Maxitrol).
3. The patient should avoid dirty water (e.g., swimming pool) or dusty conditions (e.g., sandbox, basement) for 2 weeks. It is fine to start taking a shower the next day.

Follow-up Schedule

1. One or two visits at postoperative days 1 through 10.
2. Another visit 6–12 weeks postoperatively, and then as necessary.
3. Advise patient to report severe pain or decreased vision immediately.

Complications

1. Perforation of sclera with suture needle
2. Retinal detachment
3. Cellulitis
4. Endophthalmitis
5. Dellen formation in limbal incisions
6. Muscle slippage back from its sutured position
7. Conjunctival inclusion cyst
8. Conjunctival scarring
9. Foreign body granuloma
10. Anterior segment ischemia secondary to concurrent surgery on multiple muscles

19. Securely tie muscle to sclera (**Fig. 37.21**).
   a. Gently pull the muscle to its new insertion site. Retract the Tenon capsule and intermuscular septum to avoid dragging it with the suture into the scleral tunnel.
   b. Tie a 2-1-1 surgeon's knot.
   c. The assistant may hold the first throw down with a needle holder or tying forceps to prevent slippage.
   d. Inspect the muscle to ensure that it is in its proper position and no soft tissue is dragged into the suture tracts.

38

Horizontal Rectus Resection

Indications

Extraocular muscle imbalance requiring muscle strengthening for correction (e.g., lateral rectus resection in esotropia).

Preoperative Procedure

See Chapter 3.
A complete strabismus evaluation with the determination of the detailed surgical plan is necessary.

Instrumentation

- Lid speculum (e.g., Lancaster, Barraquer)
- Needle holder
- Sutures (6–0 silk with spatula needle, double-armed 6–0 Vicryl with spatula needle (S29 or S14), 7–0 Vicryl suture)
- Toothed forceps (e.g., Bishop-Harmon, 0.5 mm Castroviejo)
- Two locking 0.5 mm toothed forceps
- Westcott scissors (rounded tips)
- Cautery (bipolar forceps)
- Muscle hooks (e.g., Green, Jameson)
- Stevens tenotomy hooks
- Castroviejo caliper
- Muscle clamp (e.g., Apt or Jameson) or Hartman mosquito hemostat
- Scalpel with #15 blade

Operative Procedure

Note: Figures are drawn from the surgeon's viewpoint with the surgeon standing at the head of the patient.

Limbal Approach

1. Anesthesia: General anesthesia or retrobulbar/peribulbar injection plus lid block.
2. Place a drop of neosynephrine 2.5% into the eye to constrict the blood vessels and decrease bleeding. Prep and drape.
3. Place lid speculum.
4. Place a 6–0 silk episcleral stay suture at the limbus at 6 and 12 o'clock.

Optional: May use locking Castroviejo forceps instead of stay sutures.

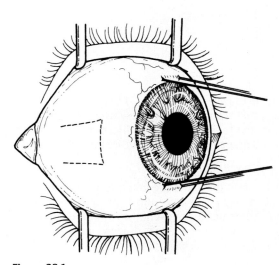

Figure 38.1

5. Secure globe with stay sutures to expose surgical field (see **Fig. 38.1**).

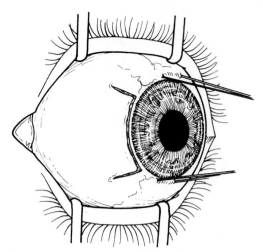

Figure 38.2

6. Prepare a fornix-based winged limbal peritomy down to bare sclera with Westcott scissors (see **Fig. 38.2**).

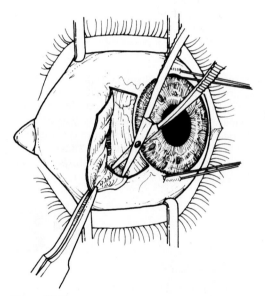

Figure 38.3

7. Buttonhole the Tenon capsule and intermuscular septum with sharp and blunt dissection with Westcott scissors to reach bare sclera on either side of the muscle insertion (see **Fig. 38.3**).
   a. Aim 45 degrees between the horizontal and vertical recti to avoid injuring the muscles.
   b. Bluntly spread the incision with Westcott scissors.
   c. Repeat on the opposite side of muscle insertion.
8. Isolate the muscle (see **Fig. 38.4**).
   a. First sweep the Stevens tenotomy hook through the fascial buttonhole and under the muscle. Hold hook parallel to and flush with bare sclera to facilitate passage.

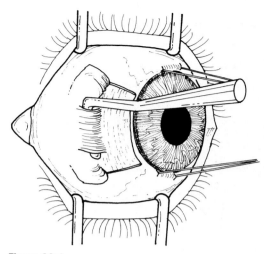

Figure 38.4

   b. Follow with a Green muscle hook perpendicular to the sclera and just posterior to the Stevens hook. Keep the tip of the Green hook pressed against the sclera.
   c. Remove the Stevens tenotomy hook.
   d. Follow with a second Green muscle hook perpendicular to the sclera and just posterior to the first Green hook. Once again, keep the tip of the Green hook pressed against the sclera.
   e. Remove the first Green hook.
   f. The tip of the muscle hook can be visualized on the other side of the muscle. If not, repeat steps 8d–e.

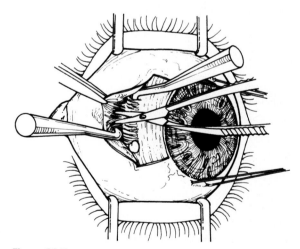

Figure 38.5

9. Tent the overlying conjunctiva with Stevens tenotomy hook and use Westcott scissors to carefully cut the check ligaments to the muscle sheath. Take care not to cut the muscle sheath or the muscle as bleeding may occur. If bleeding occurs, apply direct pressure with a dental roll or cellulose sponge until it stops (see **Fig. 38.5**).

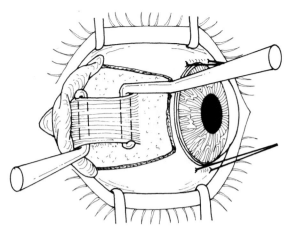

Figure 38.6

10. Incise the intermuscular septum superior and inferior to the muscle to obtain adequate muscle exposure. Be careful not to cut the inferior oblique muscle if incising along the inferior border of the lateral rectus.
11. Place the second Green hook under the muscle and expose the muscle (**Fig. 38.6**).

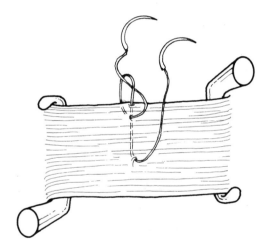

Figure 38.7

12. Suture the muscle with two double-armed 6–0 Vicryl sutures (**Fig. 38.7**).
    a. Measure the length of resection with the calipers. Do not stretch the muscle while measuring.
    b. The first throw of the first suture is placed at the measured site from the center of the muscle to the superior edge through half-thickness muscle. The second throw is through full-thickness muscle starting from underneath the muscle, 2 mm from the edge of the muscle. Lock the second throw.
    c. Tape the free ends of the sutures to the drape. Do not cut off the needles.

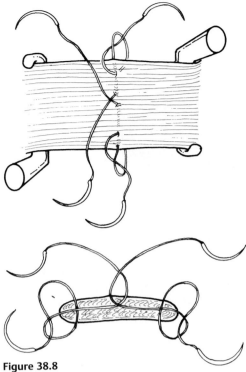

Figure 38.8

d. The first throw of the second suture is placed at the measured site from the center of the muscle to the inferior edge through half-thickness muscle. The second throw is through full-thickness muscle starting from underneath the muscle, 2 mm from the edge of the muscle. Lock the second throw (**Fig. 38.8**).
e. Tape the free ends of the sutures to the drape. Do not cut off the needles.

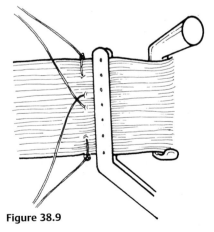

Figure 38.9

13. Clamp the muscle (with a muscle clamp or Hartman hemostat) just anterior to the suture (**Fig. 38.9**).
14. Detach the muscle's insertion from the globe with Westcott scissors. Cut flush with the sclera.

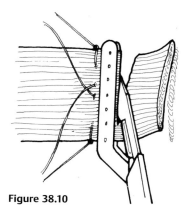

Figure 38.10

15. Gently cauterize or apply direct pressure with a dental roll or cellulose sponge on the insertion site to achieve hemostasis.
16. Cut the muscle flush with the clamp using the scalpel (**Fig. 38.10**).
17. Cauterize the muscle stump, if needed, along the muscle clamp/hemostat.

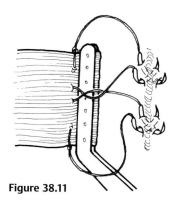

Figure 38.11

18. Suture the muscle to the insertion site (**Fig. 38.11**).
    a. Untape the superior most suture and pass the needles in a crossed-swords fashion partial thickness through the superior half of the insertion site.
    b. Untape the inferior suture and pass the needles in a crossed-swords fashion partial thickness through the inferior half of the insertion site.
    c. Make sure that the needle passes through the sclera in addition to the stump of the muscle tendon.
19. Remove the muscle clamp/hemostat.
20. Release the tension on the stay sutures.

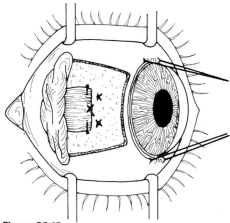

Figure 38.12

21. Tie the sutures (**Fig. 38.12**).
    a. First gently pull the sutures parallel to the globe to bring the muscle up to the insertion site.
    b. Tie the superior suture and then the inferior suture securely using a 2–1-1 surgeon's knot.
22. Reposition the conjunctiva. Wetting the eye may help differentiate conjunctiva (pink) from the Tenon capsule (white).

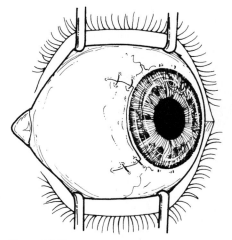

Figure 38.13

23. Suture the conjunctiva into position with interrupted 7–0 Vicryl sutures in a buried fashion (see **Fig. 38.13**).
24. Remove stay sutures.
25. Apply antibiotic and steroid ointment.

Fornix Approach

The figures shown will be for a right medial rectus resection. This technique requires a knowledgeable assistant.

1. Anesthesia: General anesthesia or retrobulbar/peribulbar injection plus lid block.

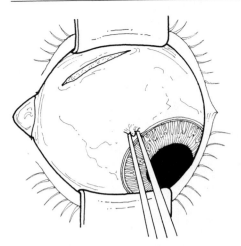

Figure 38.14

2. Place a drop of neosynephrine 2.5% into the eye to constrict the blood vessels and decrease bleeding. Prep and drape.
3. Place lid speculum.
4. Create a fornix-based conjunctival incision (see **Fig. 38.14**).
   a. The assistant grasps the globe at the limbus at either the 4:30 position (for access to the right medial or left lateral rectus) or the 7:30 position (for access to the right lateral or left medial rectus).
   b. The assistant then exposes the inferior fornix by elevating and abducting the globe (for access to the medial rectus) or elevating and adducting the globe (for access to the lateral rectus).
   c. Create an 8 mm incision parallel to the fornix and 1 mm from the fornix on the bulbar conjunctiva with Westcott scissors.

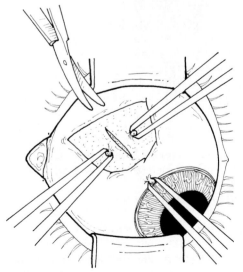

Figure 38.15

5. Create a radial incision through the Tenon capsule to expose the sclera (see **Fig. 38.15**).

a. The assistant and surgeon grasp the Tenon capsule less than 10 mm from the limbus.
b. Cut the Tenon capsule between the forceps and radially toward the limbus.
c. The incision should reach bare sclera. If layers of Tenon remain, repeat steps 5a–b.
d. The incision should not extend more than 10 mm from the limbus or orbital fat may be exposed and adherence syndrome may occur.

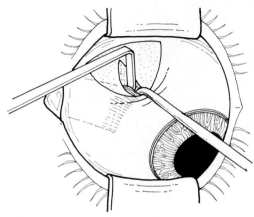

Figure 38.16

6. Isolate the rectus muscle with a Stevens hook (see **Fig. 38.16**).
   a. First sweep the Stevens tenotomy hook through the fornix incision and under the muscle. Hold the hook parallel to and flush with bare sclera to facilitate passage.
   b. The assistant releases the forceps fixating the globe.
7. Isolate the muscle with the Green hook.
   a. Sweep a Green muscle hook perpendicular to the sclera and just posterior to the Stevens hook. Keep the tip of the Green hook pressed against the sclera.
   b. Remove the Stevens tenotomy hook.
   c. Follow with a second Green muscle hook perpendicular to the sclera and just posterior to the first Green hook. Once again, keep the tip of the Green hook pressed against the sclera.
   d. Remove the first Green hook.

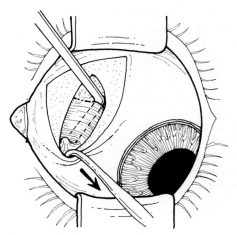

Figure 38.17

8. Expose the muscle insertion by using a Stevens hook to retract the Tenon capsule and conjunctiva over the tip of the Green hook (see **Fig. 38.17**).

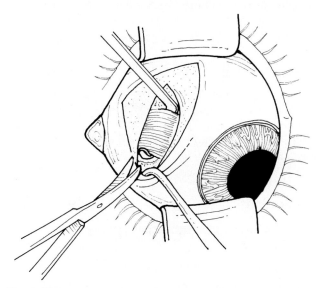

Figure 38.18

9. Incise the intermuscular septum at the tip of the Green hook with Westcott scissors (see **Fig. 38.18**).

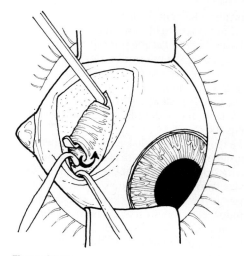

Figure 38.19

10. Check to ensure the entire muscle is hooked (see **Fig. 38.19**).
    a. The assistant exposes the superior pole of the muscle insertion with a Stevens hook.
    b. Sweep a Stevens hook from posterior to the insertion, around the superior pole and then anterior to the insertion in an arc. There should be no significant resistance felt.
    c. If there is significant resistance and it appears that the muscle is split, repeat steps 7c–d and 10a–b.
11. Incise the intermuscular septum anterior to the muscle to expose the muscle insertion.

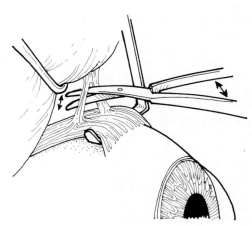

Figure 38.20

12. Tent the overlying conjunctiva with a Stevens tenotomy hook and use Westcott scissors to carefully cut the check ligaments to the muscle sheath. Take care not to cut the muscle sheath or muscle or bleeding may occur. If bleeding occurs, apply direct pressure with a dental roll until it stops (see **Fig. 38.20**).

13. Incise the intermuscular septum superior and inferior to the muscle if necessary to obtain adequate muscle exposure. Be careful not to cut the inferior oblique muscle if incising along the inferior border of the lateral rectus.
14. Place the second Green hook under the muscle and expose the muscle (see **Fig. 38.6**).
15. Suture the muscle with two double-armed 6–0 Vicryl sutures (see **Fig. 38.7**).
    a. Measure the length of resection with the calipers.
    b. The first throw of the first suture is placed at the measured site from the center of the muscle to the superior edge through half-thickness muscle. The second throw is through full-thickness muscle starting from underneath the muscle, 2 mm from the edge of the muscle. Lock the second throw.
    c. Tape the free ends of the sutures to the drape. Do not cut off the needles.
    d. The first throw of the second suture is placed at the measured site from the center of the muscle to the inferior edge through half-thickness muscle. The second throw is through full-thickness muscle starting from under the muscle, 2 mm from the edge of the muscle. Lock the second throw (see **Fig. 38.8**).
    e. Tape the free ends of the sutures to the drape. Do not cut off the needles.
16. Clamp the muscle (with a muscle clamp or Hartman hemostat) just anterior to the suture (see **Fig. 38.9**).
17. Detach the muscle's insertion from the globe with Westcott scissors. Cut flush with the sclera.
18. Gently cauterize or apply direct pressure with a dental roll on the insertion site to achieve hemostasis.
19. Cut the muscle flush with the clamp using the scalpel (see **Fig. 38.10**).
20. Cauterize the muscle stump, if needed, along the muscle clamp/hemostat.
21. Fixate the globe by grasping the sclera with two locking 0.5 mm Castroviejo forceps, one 2 mm anterior and 2 mm superior to the superior pole of the muscle insertion and one 2 mm anterior and 2 mm inferior to the inferior pole of the muscle insertion.
22. Suture the muscle to the insertion site (see **Fig. 38.11**).
    a. Untape the superiormost suture and pass the needles in a crossed-swords fashion partial thickness through the superior half of the insertion site.
    b. Untape the inferior suture and pass the needles in a crossed-swords fashion partial thickness through the inferior half of the insertion site.
    c. Make sure the needle passes through the sclera in addition to the stump of the muscle tendon.
23. Remove the muscle clamp/hemostat.
24. Tie the sutures (see **Fig. 38.12**).
    a. First gently pull the sutures parallel to the globe to bring the muscle up to the insertion site.
    b. Tie the superior suture and then the inferior suture securely using a 2-1-1 surgeon's knot.
25. Reposition the conjunctival incision into the fornix (see **Fig. 37.22**, p. 203).
    a. If the incision site is gaping, suture the conjunctiva closed with interrupted 7–0 Vicryl sutures in a buried fashion.
    b. Wetting the eye may help differentiate conjunctiva (pink) from the Tenon capsule (white).
26. Apply antibiotic and steroid ointment.

Postoperative Procedure

1. Discharge patient when stable.
2. Apply antibiotic or antibiotic/steroid ointment four times a day for 5–14 days (e.g., erythromycin, TobraDex, Maxitrol).
3. The patient should avoid dirty water (e.g., swimming pool) or dusty conditions (e.g., sandbox, basement) for 2 weeks. It is fine to start taking a bath the next day.
4. Avoid pets.

Follow-up Schedule

1. One or two visits at postoperative days 1 through 10.
2. Another visit 6–12 weeks postoperatively, and then as necessary.

Advise patient to report severe pain or decreased vision immediately.

Complications

1. Perforation of sclera with suture needle
2. Retinal detachment
3. Cellulitis
4. Endophthalmitis
5. Dellen formation in limbal incisions
6. Muscle slippage back from its sutured position
7. Conjunctival inclusion cyst
8. Conjunctival scarring
9. Foreign body granuloma
10. Anterior segment ischemia secondary to concurrent surgery on multiple muscles

39

Inferior Oblique Recession/ Anterior Transposition

Indications

Inferior oblique muscle overaction requiring muscle weakening for correction, or concomitant dissociated vertical deviation requiring anterior transposition of the inferior oblique.

Preoperative Procedure

See Chapter 3.

A complete strabismus evaluation with determination of the detailed surgical plan is necessary.

Instrumentation

- Lid speculum (e.g., Lancaster, Barraquer)
- Needle holder
- Sutures (4–0 silk suture, double-armed 6–0 Vicryl with spatula needle, 7–0 Vicryl suture)
- Toothed forceps (e.g., Bishop-Harmon, 0.5 mm Castroviejo)
- Westcott scissors (rounded tips)
- Cautery (bipolar forceps)
- Muscle hook (e.g., Green, Jameson)
- Gass muscle hook
- Stevens tenotomy hooks
- Iris spatula
- Hartman mosquito hemostat
- Desmarres retractor
- Castroviejo caliper
- Headlight

Operative Procedure

Note: Figures are drawn from the surgeon's viewpoint with the surgeon standing at the head of the patient.

Note: Illumination of the surgical field is best obtained with a headlight.

1. Anesthesia: General anesthesia or retrobulbar/peribulbar injection plus eyelid block.
2. Place a drop of neosynephrine 2.5% into the eye to constrict the blood vessels and decrease bleeding. Prep and drape.
3. Place lid speculum.

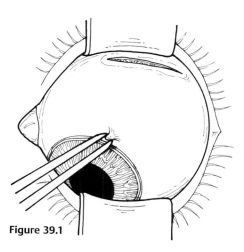

Figure 39.1

4. Create conjunctival incision in the inferotemporal fornix (**Fig. 39.1**).
   a. The assistant grasps the globe at the limbus at the inferotemporal limbus.
   b. The assistant then exposes the inferior fornix by elevating and adducting the globe.
   c. Create an 8 mm incision parallel to the fornix and 1 mm from the fornix on the bulbar conjunctiva with Westcott scissors.

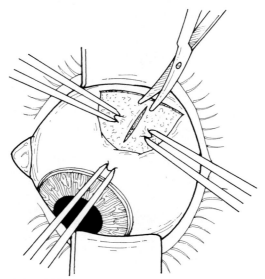

Figure 39.2

5. Create a radial incision through the Tenon capsule to expose the sclera (**Fig. 39.2**).
   a. The assistant and surgeon grasp the Tenon capsule less than 10 mm from the limbus.
   b. Cut the Tenon capsule between the forceps and radially toward the limbus.
   c. The incision should reach bare sclera. If layers of Tenon capsule remain, repeat steps 5a-b.
   d. The incision should not extend more than 10 mm from the limbus or else orbital fat may be exposed and adherence syndrome may occur.
6. Isolate the lateral rectus with a Stevens hook.
   a. First sweep the Stevens tenotomy hook through the fornix incision and under the muscle. Hold the hook parallel to and flush with bare sclera to facilitate passage.
   b. The assistant releases the forceps fixating the globe.
7. Isolate the lateral rectus with the 4–0 silk stay suture.
   a. Sweep a Gass muscle hook perpendicular to the sclera and just posterior to the Stevens hook. Keep the tip of the Gass hook pressed against the sclera.

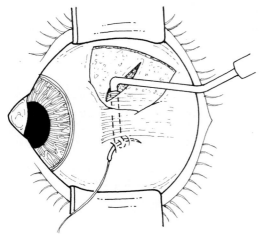

Figure 39.3

b. Remove the Stevens tenotomy hook.
c. Pass the needle of the 4–0 silk suture completely through the eyelet of the Gass hook (**Fig. 39.3**).
d. Remove the Gass hook while continuing to grasp the needle, thus pulling the free end of the 4–0 silk suture underneath the lateral rectus muscle.

Optional: Use a Green hook to hold the lateral rectus muscle in place.

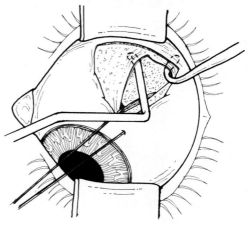

Figure 39.4

8. Elevate and adduct the globe with the 4–0 silk stay suture and attach to the drape (**Fig. 39.4**).
9. Retract the incision inferiorly with a Gass hook and temporally with a Stevens hook (**Fig. 39.4**).

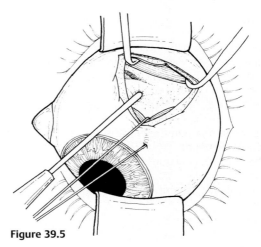

Figure 39.5

10. Depress the sclera with the iris spatula to visualize the vortex vein and the posterior border of the inferior oblique muscle. The use of a headlight will help with visualization (**Fig. 39.5**).

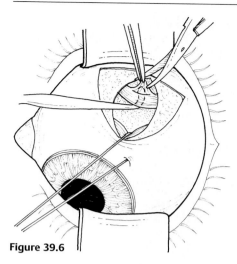

Figure 39.6

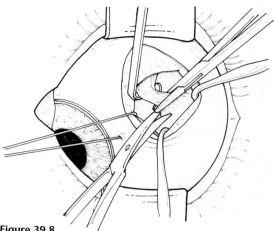

Figure 39.8

11. Hook the entire inferior oblique muscle with a Stevens hook, being careful not to split the muscle (**Fig. 39.6**).

16. Carefully cut the inferior oblique muscle close to the sclera with Westcott scissors, taking care not the cut the sclera. Remember that the muscle insertion site is approximately in the region of the macula (**Fig. 39.8**).
17. Gently cauterize the stump of the muscle on the hemostat with bipolar cautery.

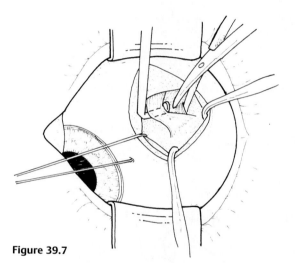

Figure 39.7

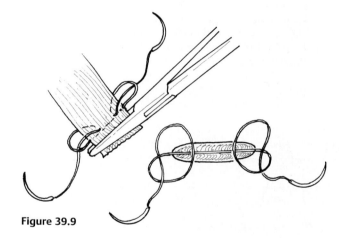

Figure 39.9

12. Pull excess Tenon capsule off the tip of the Stevens hook and snip an opening in the Tenon capsule with Westcott scissors to expose the hook tip (**Fig. 39.7**).
13. Replace the Stevens hook with a Green muscle hook.
14. Expose the intermuscular septum with Stevens hook and dissect it to the insertion of the inferior oblique with Westcott scissors.
15. Clamp the inferior oblique muscle near its insertion with the Hartman mosquito hemostat. Leave a small gap between the hemostat and insertion site to allow easier disinsertion (**Fig. 39.8**).

18. Suture the muscle stump with the double-armed 6–0 Vicryl with spatula needles (**Fig. 39.9**).
    a. First throw is through partial thickness through the muscle just proximal to the clamp.
    b. Second throw is through full-thickness muscle, 1 mm from the edge of the muscle. Lock the second throw.
    c. Third throw is through full-thickness muscle, 1 mm from the other edge of the muscle. Lock the third throw.
    d. Do not cut off the needles.
    e. Remove the Hartman hemostat.
    f. Inspect the muscle to ensure it is securely sutured. Keep the sutures organized so as not to twist the muscle.

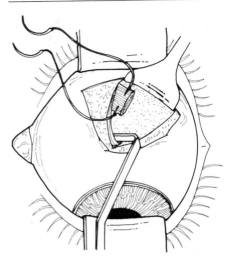

Figure 39.10

19. Hook the inferior rectus and elevate the globe (**Fig. 39.10**).
    a. Remove the 4–0 silk stay suture.
    b. Sweep a Stevens tenotomy hook through the incision site and hook the inferior rectus.
    c. Sweep a Green muscle hook perpendicular to the sclera and just posterior to the Stevens hook. Keep the tip of the Green hook pressed against the sclera.
    d. Remove the Stevens tenotomy hook.
    e. Elevate the globe.
    f. Use a Desmarres retractor to expose the surgical field.
20. Suture the inferior oblique muscle to the sclera.

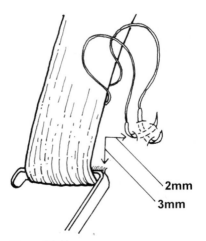

Figure 39.11

a. For a 10 mm recession (**Fig. 39.11**):
   i. Suture the anterior border of the inferior oblique muscle 3 mm posterior and 2 mm lateral to the lateral insertion edge of the inferior rectus.

ii. Suture the posterior border of the inferior oblique muscle posterolaterally by the width of the inferior oblique.

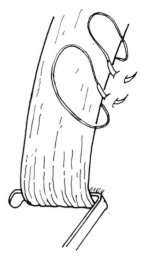

Figure 39.12

b. For a 14 mm recession (**Fig. 39.12**):
   i. Suture the anterior border of the inferior oblique muscle anterior to the inferotemporal vortex vein.
   ii. Suture the posterior border of the inferior oblique muscle posterior to the inferotemporal vortex vein.

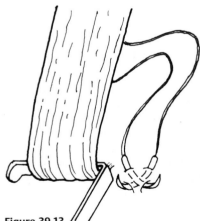

Figure 39.13

c. For anterior transposition (**Fig. 39.13**):
   i. Suture the anterior border of the inferior oblique muscle at the lateral pole of the inferior rectus insertion.
   ii. Suture the posterior border of the inferior oblique muscle lateral to the first suture at one muscle width distance.

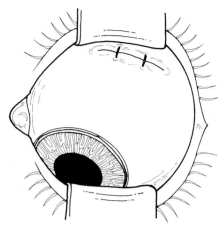

Figure 39.14

21. Reposition the conjunctival incision into the fornix (**Fig. 39.14**).
    a. If the incision site is gaping, suture the conjunctiva closed with interrupted 7–0 Vicryl sutures in a buried fashion.
    b. Wetting the eye may help differentiate conjunctiva (pink) from the Tenon capsule (white).
22. Apply antibiotic and steroid ointment.

Postoperative Procedure

1. Discharge patient when stable.
2. Apply antibiotic or antibiotic/steroid ointment 4 times per day for 5–14 days (e.g., erythromycin, TobraDex, Maxitrol).

3. The patient should avoid dirty water (e.g., swimming pool) or dusty conditions (e.g., sandbox, basement) for 2 weeks. It is fine to start taking a bath the next day.

Follow-up Schedule

1. One or two visits at postoperative days 1 through 10.
2. Another visit 6–12 weeks postoperatively, and then as necessary.
3. Advise patient to report severe pain or decreased vision immediately.

Complications

1. Missing posterior fibers of the inferior oblique producing undercorrection
2. Perforation of sclera with suture needle
3. Retinal detachment
4. Cellulitis
5. Endophthalmitis
6. Conjunctival inclusion cyst
7. Conjunctival scarring
9. Foreign body granuloma

40

Rectus Recession with Adjustable Suture Technique

Indications

Extraocular muscle imbalance requiring muscle weakening for correction (e.g., medial rectus in esotropia) in a patient who is cooperative for postoperative adjustment.

Preoperative Procedure

Test the patient's cooperativeness to postoperative adjustment. Anesthetize the eye with topical anesthetic and place an eyelid speculum in the eye. Then touch and maneuver the conjunctiva with a moistened cotton tip. A patient who does not tolerate this procedure well is a poor candidate for adjustable suture.

See Chapter 3.

A complete strabismus evaluation with determination of the detailed surgical plan is necessary.

Instrumentation

- Lid speculum (e.g., Lancaster, Barraquer)
- Needle holder
- Sutures (6–0 silk with spatula needle, double-armed 6–0 Vicryl with spatula needle (S29 or S14), 7–0 Vicryl suture, 5–0 Mersilene on a spatula needle)
- Toothed forceps (e.g., Bishop-Harmon, 0.5 mm Castroviejo)
- Two locking 0.5 mm toothed forceps
- Westcott scissors (rounded tips)
- Cautery (bipolar forceps)
- Muscle hooks (e.g., Green, Jameson)
- Stevens tenotomy hooks
- Castroviejo caliper
- Tying forceps

Operative Procedure

Note: Figures are drawn from the surgeon's viewpoint with the surgeon standing at the head of the patient.

1. Anesthesia: General anesthesia. Retrobulbar anesthesia is possible, but you will not be able to adjust the sutures until the next day when the retrobulbar block wears off completely.
2. Place a drop of neosynephrine 2.5% into the eye to constrict the blood vessels and decrease bleeding. Prep and drape.
3. Place lid speculum.

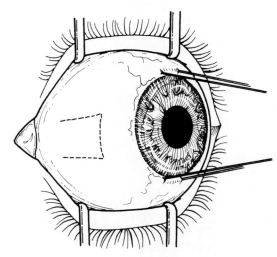

Figure 40.1

4. Place a 6–0 silk episcleral stay suture at the limbus at 6 and 12 o'clock (see **Fig. 40.1**).

   Optional: Use locking Castroviejo forceps instead of stay suture.

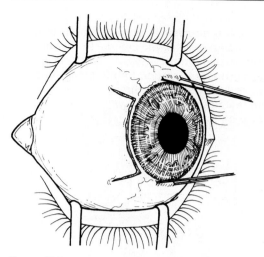

Figure 40.2

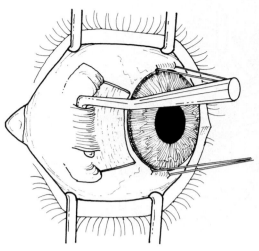

Figure 40.4

5. Secure the globe with stay sutures to expose the surgical field.
6. Prepare a fornix-based, winged limbal peritomy down to bare sclera with Westcott scissors (see **Fig. 40.2**).

8. Isolate the muscle (see **Fig. 40.4**).
    a. First sweep the Stevens tenotomy hook through the fascial buttonhole and under the muscle. Hold the hook parallel to and flush with bare sclera to facilitate passage.
    b. Follow with a Green muscle hook perpendicular to the sclera and just posterior to the Stevens hook. Keep the tip of the Green hook pressed against the sclera.
    c. Remove the Stevens tenotomy hook.
    d. Follow with a second Green muscle hook perpendicular to the sclera and just posterior to the first Green hook. Once again, keep the tip of the Green hook pressed against the sclera.
    e. Remove the first Green hook.
    f. The tip of the muscle hook can be visualized on the other side of the muscle. If not, repeat steps 8d–e.

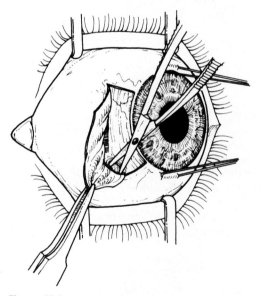

Figure 40.3

7. Buttonhole the Tenon capsule and intermuscular septum with sharp and blunt dissection with Westcott scissors to reach bare sclera on either side of the muscle insertion (see **Fig. 40.3**).
    a. Aim 45 degrees between the horizontal and vertical recti to avoid injuring the muscles.
    b. Bluntly spread the incision with Westcott scissors.
    c. Repeat on the opposite side of the muscle insertion.

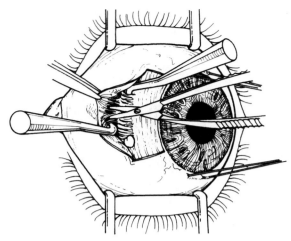

Figure 40.5

9. Tent the overlying conjunctiva with Stevens tenotomy hook and use Westcott scissors to minimally cut the check ligaments to the muscle sheath. Take care not to cut the muscle sheath or muscle, as bleeding may occur. If bleeding occurs, apply direct pressure with a dental roll until it stops (**Fig. 40.5**).

10. Incise the intermuscular septum superior and inferior to the muscle minimally if necessary to obtain adequate muscle exposure. Be careful not to cut the inferior oblique muscle if incising along the inferior border of the lateral rectus.

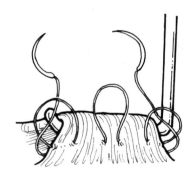

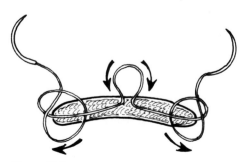

Figure 40.6

11. Suture the muscle 1 mm from its insertion with the double-armed 6–0 Vicryl with spatula needles (see **Fig. 40.6**).

a. Elevate muscle with the muscle hook.
b. First throw is through half-thickness muscle from the center to one edge of the muscle, 1 mm from the insertion. Second throw is through full-thickness muscle, posterior to anterior, 1 mm from the edge of the muscle. Lock the second throw.
c. Perform superiorly and inferiorly.
d. Do not cut off the needles.

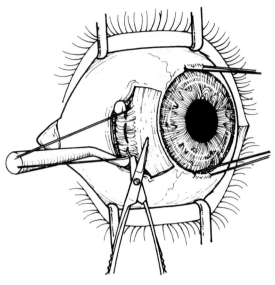

Figure 40.7

12. Detach the muscle at its insertion with Westcott scissors (**Fig. 40.7**).
a. Hold the muscle hook *and* sutures up to avoid cutting the sutures.
b. Cut the muscle flush with the sclera.
c. Inspect the muscle to ensure it is properly sutured and not split, and that the lock bites are in place and adequate.

13. Gently cauterize (as needed) or apply direct pressure with a dental roll on the insertion site to achieve hemostasis.

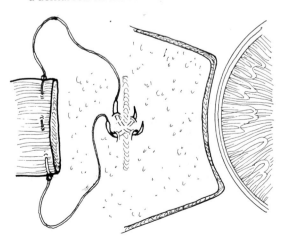

Figure 40.8

14. Reattach the muscle to the sclera at the original insertion site using the two ends of the previously placed 6–0 Vicryl suture (see **Fig. 40.8**).
    a. Secure the globe with toothed forceps.
    b. Pass the needles through the original insertion site, aiming 45 degrees toward the center of the insertion site and exiting close to each other.
    c. Make sure the needle passes through the sclera in addition to the stump of the muscle tendon.
    d. Keep the needle parallel to the sclera to decrease the chance of penetration.

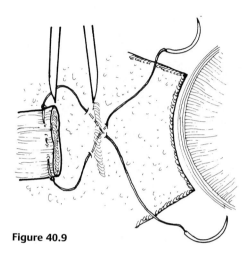

Figure 40.9

15. Hang-back the muscle (**Fig. 40.9**).
    a. Use the Castroviejo calipers to measure the amount of recession desired from the insertion site to the muscle edge.
    b. Ensure the recession is equal for both the superior and the inferior suture.

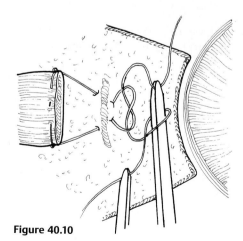

Figure 40.10

16. Tie suture with an overhand throw and then a slip knot (**Fig. 40.10**).

a. Trim the suture so the end to pull to loosen the slip knot is longer (to make it easier to identify during the adjustment).
b. Leave enough suture length to allow for easy adjustment.

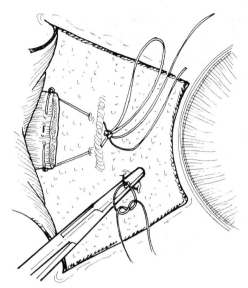

Figure 40.11

17. Place a bucket handle suture close to the limbus (**Fig. 40.11**).
    a. Suture the 5–0 Mersilene on a spatula needle partial thickness through the sclera.
    b. Tie over the closed ends of Westcott scissors to form a loop.

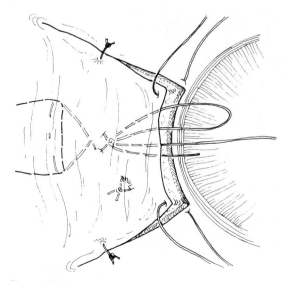

Figure 40.12

18. Close the conjunctiva with 7–0 Vicryl sutures (**Fig. 40.12**).

a. Suture permanently the radial portion of the conjunctival flap posterior to the muscle insertion.
b. Suture the two corners of the conjunctival flap to the sclera anterior to the muscle insertion with long loops of 7–0 Vicryl suture.

19. Tuck the suture ends into the fornix.
20. Remove stay sutures.
21. Apply antibiotic and steroid drops (ointment will blur the patient's vision and make the adjustment harder).
22. Bandage the eye with a pressure patch to keep it from blinking (for the patient's comfort).

Suture Adjustment

The suture adjustment may be performed later the same day (once the patient is awake and cooperative from the general anesthesia) or the next day (especially if retrobulbar anesthesia was given).

1. Remove the eye patch.
2. Anesthesia: Apply drops of proparacaine into the eye over several minutes. Warn the patient that he will still feel pressure sensations. Aggressive adjustments may cause nausea and vomiting or lightheadedness.
3. Perform strabismus test to determine if any deviations are present.
4. Place lid speculum.
5. If the desired end point is reached, go to step 7.

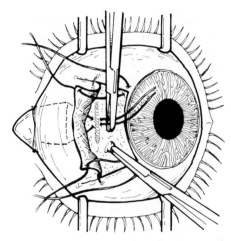

Figure 40.13

6. If an undesired amount of deviation is present, either tighten or loosen the muscle as necessary.
   a. To tighten the muscle (**Fig. 40.13**):
      i. Untie the bow of the slip knot but not the overhand throw by pulling the longer end of the suture.
      ii. Grasp each suture end with a tying forceps or needle holder.
      iii. Have the assistant grasp the bucket handle suture to stabilize the globe.

iv. Gently pull the suture (and muscle) forward parallel with the suture tracks. Do not pull too hard or the sutures may pull out from the suture tracks.
v. Once the desired amount of tightening is achieved, tighten the overhand knot and retie the slip knot. The assistant may grasp the overhand knot with tying forceps to keep it from slipping.
vi. Go back to step 3.
   b. To loosen the muscle:
      i. Untie the slip knot by pulling the longer end of the suture and loosen the overhand throw.
      ii. Grasp the suture at the approximate length to be recessed.
      iii. Grasp the bucket handle suture to stabilize the globe.
      iv. Have the patient slowly look in the direction of the muscle being adjusted and then relax.
      v. Retie the overhand and slip knot.
      vi. Go back to step 3.

7. Once the desired amount of adjustment (if any) is reached, tie the muscle suture permanently.
   a. Cut the bow of the slip knot and pull out the loose suture.
   b. Tie the suture with two more overhand throws and trim.

Note: Check rotations to be sure ductions have not been compromised.

8. Cut and remove the bucket handle suture.

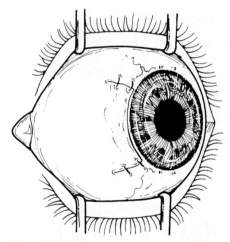

Figure 40.14

9. Close the conjunctiva using the preplaced 7–0 Vicryl sutures (see **Fig. 40.14**).
   a. Cut off the knot.
   b. Tie the sutures permanently.

Postoperative Procedure

1. Discharge patient when stable.
2. Apply antibiotic or antibiotic/steroid ointment 4 times per day for 5–14 days (e.g., erythromycin, TobraDex, Maxitrol).
3. The patient should avoid dirty water (e.g., swimming pool) or dusty conditions (e.g., sandbox, basement) for 2 weeks. It is fine to start taking a bath the next day.

Follow-up Schedule

1. Postoperative day 0–1 if adjustment will be performed in the office.
2. A visit within the next 2 weeks.
3. Another visit 6–12 weeks postoperatively, and then as necessary.
4. Advise patient to report severe pain or decreased vision immediately.

Complications

1. Perforation of sclera with suture needle
2. Retinal detachment
3. Cellulitis
4. Over- and undercorrection
5. Muscle slippage back from its sutured position
6. Conjunctival inclusion cyst
7. Conjunctival scarring
8. Endophthalmitis
9. Dellen formation in limbal incisions
10. Foreign body granuloma
11. Anterior segment ischemia secondary to concurrent surgery on multiple muscles

41

Posterior Fixation Faden Suture

Indications

Extraocular muscle imbalance that requires muscle weakening in the field of gaze of the muscle but not in primary gaze.

Preoperative Procedure

See Chapter 3.

A complete strabismus evaluation with determination of detailed surgical plan is necessary.

Instrumentation

- Lid speculum (e.g., Lancaster, Barraquer)
- Needle holder
- Sutures (6–0 silk with spatula needle, double-armed 6–0 Vicryl with spatula needle (S29 or S14), 7–0 Vicryl suture, 5–0 Mersilene with S28 or S29 needles)
- Toothed forceps (e.g., Bishop-Harmon, 0.5 mm Castroviejo)
- Two locking 0.5 mm toothed forceps
- Westcott scissors (rounded tips)
- Cautery (bipolar forceps)
- Muscle hooks (e.g., Green, Jameson)
- Stevens tenotomy hooks
- Castroviejo caliper

Operative Procedure

Note: Figures are drawn from the surgeon's viewpoint with the surgeon standing at the head of the patient.

1. Proceed with the primary strabismus surgery (usually a rectus muscle recession via limbus or fornix approach) until after the muscle reinsertion back onto the globe (or until the exposure of the muscle sheath if no recession is to be performed). Figure 41.1 is superior view of right medial rectus.

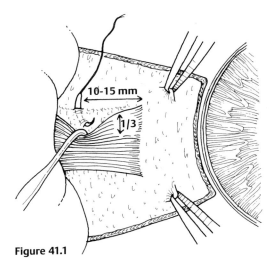

Figure 41.1

2. Retract the globe with locking Castroviejo forceps, or a Green muscle hook if the rectus muscle was not recessed (**Fig. 41.1**).
3. Suture the inferior third of the muscle with 5–0 Mersilene on a spatula needle (**Fig. 41.1**).
   a. Mark the position of the posterior fixation suture on the sclera along the inferior border of the rectus muscle using calipers (usually 10–15 mm behind the original insertion site)
   b. Retract the inferior border of the muscle with Stevens hook.
   c. Suture the 5–0 Mersilene through partial thickness sclera at the marked site.
   d. Suture through the inferior third of the muscle.

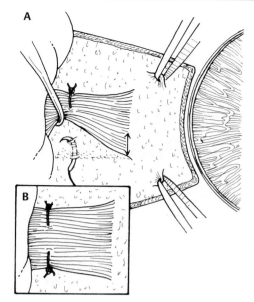

Figure 41.2

e. Tie with a 2–1–1 surgeon's knot (**Fig. 41.2A**).
4. Suture the superior third of the muscle with 5–0 Mersilene on a spatula needle.
   a. Mark the position of the posterior fixation suture on the sclera along the superior border of the rectus muscle using calipers.
   b. Retract the superior border of the muscle with Stevens hook.
   c. Suture the 5–0 Mersilene through partial thickness sclera at the marked site (**Fig. 41.2A**).
   e. Suture through the superior third of the muscle (**Fig. 41.2B**).
   f. Tie with a 2–1–1 surgeon's knot.
5. Continue with the rest of the strabismus surgery.

Postoperative Procedure

1. Discharge patient when stable.
2. Apply antibiotic or antibiotic/steroid ointment 4 times a day for 5–14 days (e.g., erythromycin, TobraDex, or Maxitrol).

The patient should avoid dirty water (e.g., swimming pool) or dusty conditions (e.g., sandbox, basement) for 2 weeks. It is fine to start taking a bath the next day.

Follow-up Schedule

1. One or two visits at postoperative days 1 through 10.
2. Another visit 6–12 weeks postoperatively, and then as necessary.
3. Advise patient to report severe pain or decreased vision immediately.

Complications

1. Perforation of sclera with suture needle
2. Retinal detachment
3. Cellulitis
4. Endophthalmitis
5. Dellen formation in limbal incisions
6. Over- and undercorrection
7. Muscle slippage back from its sutured position
8. Conjunctival inclusion cyst
9. Conjunctival scarring
10. Foreign body granuloma
11. Anterior segment ischemia secondary to concurrent surgery on multiple muscles

42

Supraplacement and Infraplacement of Horizontal Muscles for "A" or "V" Patterns

Indications

Horizontal extraocular muscle imbalance with an "A" or "V" pattern that requires muscle weakening or strengthening for correction.

Preoperative Procedure

See Chapter 3.

A complete strabismus evaluation with determination of detailed surgical plan is necessary.

Instrumentation

Same as for the primary strabismus surgery.

Operative Procedure

Note: Figures are drawn from the surgeon's viewpoint with the surgeon standing at the head of the patient.

1. Proceed with the primary horizontal strabismus surgery (rectus recession or resection via limbus or fornix approach).
2. Supra- or infraplace the muscle as planned when suturing the muscle back onto the sclera.

Note: A mnemonic to remember is "MALE" (Medial Apex—Lateral Empty). The medial rectus (MR) is shifted toward the apex or tip of the letter "A" or "V" (i.e., supraplace for "A" pattern or infraplace for "V" pattern). The lateral rectus (LR) is shifted toward the "empty" or open part of the letter "A" or "V" (i.e., infraplaced for "A" pattern or supraplaced for "V" pattern).

  a. For an "A" pattern medial rectus surgery, supraplace the muscle tendon half tendon width (or more) as planned (**Fig. 42.1A**).

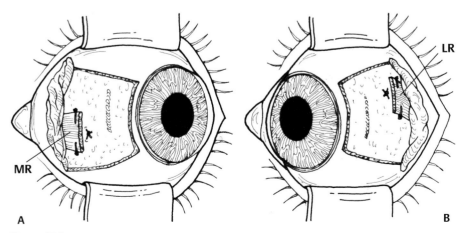

Figure 42.1

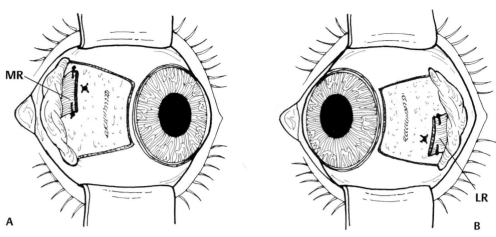

Figure 42.2

b. For an "A" pattern LR surgery, infraplace the muscle tendon half tendon width (or more) as planned (**Fig. 42.1B**).

c. For a "V" pattern MR surgery, infraplace the muscle tendon half tendon width (or more) as planned (**Fig. 42.2A**).

d. For a "V" pattern LR surgery, supraplace the muscle tendon half tendon width (or more) as planned (**Fig. 42.2B**).

3. Finish the strabismus surgery as previously described.

Postoperative Procedure

Same as for the primary strabismus surgery.

Complications

Same as for the primary strabismus surgery.

43

Pediatric Cataract Extraction

Indications

In pediatric patients, the indications for the removal of the lens include:
1. A lens opacity or cataract that causes a loss of best corrected visual acuity.
2. Lens subluxation or dislocation causing an uncorrectable decrease in visual acuity.

Surgical Management in the Pediatric Patient

Following are general recommendations for the surgical approach to cataract surgery in the pediatric patient. Specific guidelines depend on multiple factors such as the surgeon's experience with limbal versus pars plana surgery.

- Age younger than 18–24 months:
  - ❏ Lensectomy
  - ❏ Primary posterior capsulotomy
  - ❏ Anterior vitrectomy
- Age 2–6 years:
  - ❏ Phacoemulsification/irrigation and aspiration
  - ❏ Optional but recommended: Primary intraocular lens (IOL) implantation
  - ❏ Optional but recommended: Primary posterior capsulotomy and anterior vitrectomy
- Age older than ~6 years (depending if the child is able to sit for a YAG capsulotomy):
  - ❏ Phacoemulsification
  - ❏ Primary IOL implantation

Irrigation/aspiration is the preferred method for cataract extraction in children younger than 2 years.

Children 18 months to 2 years may need phacoemulsification, depending on the density of the lens.

Advantages of Phacoemulsification over Standard Extracapsular Surgery

- Smaller wound speeds recovery and minimizes astigmatism and wound-related postoperative complications.
- Surgery accomplished within a relatively closed system.

Disadvantages of Phacoemulsification Compared with Extracapsular Surgery

- Possible increased corneal endothelial damage.
- Possible increased risk of iris damage with smaller pupils.

Recommended Surgical Incision in Pediatric Patient

A scleral tunnel incision may be preferable to a clear cornea incision, as self-sealing clear cornea wounds are unreliable in a child. Perform a limbal incision, slightly anterior, within the scleral tunnel to avoid iris prolapse.

Intraocular Lens Placement

1. IOL implantation is generally recommended for children 2 years or older. Surgeons have implanted lenses in younger patients, but the long-term safety is still being investigated.
2. Polymethyl methacrylate (PMMA) lenses are recommended because of their long-term safety. Foldable acrylic lenses are suitable lens material as many studies have shown them to be well tolerated. (Silicone lenses have not been well studied in children.)
3. Multifocal lenses have been used in pediatric patients. The safety of multifocal lenses in pediatric patients has not yet been established.
4. If no IOL is used during the surgery, a contact lens must be used to achieve the best corrected vision. A secondary sulcus fixated lens or sutured lens may be planned for the future. The safety of sutured IOLs has not yet been established.

Posterior Capsular Opacification

1. A primary posterior capsulotomy and anterior vitrectomy should be performed in children younger than 4 years, as posterior capsular opacification will develop postoperatively. An anterior vitrectomy must be preformed along with a posterior capsulotomy because the anterior vitreous face can act as a scaffold for fibrous proliferation, which can occlude the visual axis.
2. Primary posterior capsulotomies may compromise capsule integrity.
3. After the age of 4, a YAG may be possible in compliant pediatric patients.
4. The surgical procedure is only part of the visual rehabilitation of the pediatric patient. Optical rehabilitation with contact lens fitting, patching, and further amblyopic care is essential.
   a. Patching of the other eye should be started, in most cases the first day after surgery according to the schedule recommended by the surgeon.
   b. If an IOL is not used, the appropriate contact lens or glasses prescriptions should be used as early as 1 week after surgery.
   c. Follow-up evaluations of posterior capsular opacification, late-onset glaucoma, and retinal detachment are also required.

Preoperative Procedure

1. Maximum dilation may be difficult to achieve because of iris hypoplasia.
2. Recommendations for dilation in the pediatric patient include the following:
   a. One drop of 2.5% neosynephrine, 1% tropicamide, and 1% cyclopentolate; alternatively use collyrium 3 and 38¼ ophthalmic solution (this contains cyclopentolate 1%, phenylephrine 2.5%, tropicamide 0.25%).
   b. Repeat above once if necessary.
   c. If refractory to adequate dilations, atropine 0.5% 1 per day for 1 week before surgery.
   d. Intraoperatively, 0.5 ml of 1:10,000 nonpreserved epinephrine added to a 500 ml bottle of balanced salt solution (BSS) may be used if approved by anesthesiology.
   e. Iris hooks (e.g., Grieshaber) may be needed intraoperatively in an otherwise unresponsive pupil.
3. Additionally, see Chapter 3.

   In children, it is essential to obtained informed consent regarding general anesthesia and IOL placement if considered.

4. Clearance for general anesthesia must be given by the pediatrician before surgery.

Calculate Intraocular Lens Power

Numerous formulas for the calculation of IOL power have been derived based on theoretical optics and empirical data. The Sanders-Retzlaff-Kraff (SRK) formula is one of the most widely used.

SRK Formula: Power of IOL = $A - 2.5(AL) - 0.9(K)$ where

1. A = constant is determined by the manufacturer of a specific lens. A typical value is A = 118.7.
2. K = average keratometry measurement in diopters.
3. AL = axial length of eye in millimeters measured with A-scan ultrasonography.

Recommended: Use nonsilicone lenses (e.g., PMMA, Acrysoft) in pediatric patients. The long-term stability of foldable acrylic lenses is still being studied.

Instrumentation

- Honan balloon (optional)
- Lid speculum
- Fine-toothed forceps (e.g., 0. 12 mm straight Castroviejo and/or Colibri)
- Elschnig forceps
- Westcott scissors
- Cautery (underwater eraser or disposable)
- Scarifier (Beaver #64 or Grieshaber #68)
- Microsurgical knife (e.g., Beaver #75M, Superblade)
- 20 gauge microvitreoretinal (MVR) blade (e.g., Beaver or Sharpoint).
- Viscoelastic substance (e.g., Healon, Amvisc, Viscoat)
- Keratome (e.g., Beaver #55, diamond or steel, 2.9 mm to 3.2 mm)
- Cystotome
- Utrata forceps
- Phacoemulsification and vitrectomy unit
- Kuglen hook
- Straight and angled McPherson tying forceps
- IOL forceps
- Sinskey hook
- Vannas scissors
- Fine needle holder
- Sutures: 10–0 nylon, 10–0 Vicryl
- Acetylcholine solution (e.g., Miochol)
- Cellulose sponges

Operative Procedure

1. Anesthesia: General.
2. *Optional:* Apply Honan balloon for ~5 minutes to decompress eye and orbit, minimizing positive vitreous pressure.
3. Prep and drape.
4. Place lid speculum.
5. Ensure adequate pupillary dilation.
6. For infants younger than ~18 months and where no IOL will be placed:
   a. Use an MVR blade to make two incisions slightly anterior to the anterior limbal vessels at 11 and 2 o'clock.
   b. Inject viscoelastic into the anterior chamber.
   c. Perform a capsulotomy: This can be performed in two ways:

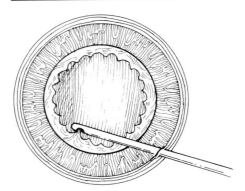

Figure 43.1

i. Use an octome vitrector to cut out a 4 mm capsulotomy (**Fig. 43.1**).
ii. Perform a continuous curvilinear capsulorrhexis with a cystotome and Utrata capsulorrhexis forceps ~4 mm in diameter. Be aware of the elasticity of the capsule in pediatric patients, as the rhexis can easily be lost under the pupil. Use a controlled technique of keeping the capsule folded on itself while performing the capsulorrhexis (**Figs. 43.2A and 43.2B**).

Note: Indocyaninegreen (ICG) has been used in children to assist in the visualization of the anterior capsule. The long-term safety for children has not yet been established.

d. Use the irrigation/aspiration system to carefully and meticulously remove all lens material (see Chapter 8). A split irrigation/aspiration system is particularly helpful in removing all cortex and epithelial cells within the capsular bag (**Figs. 43.3A and 43.3B**).

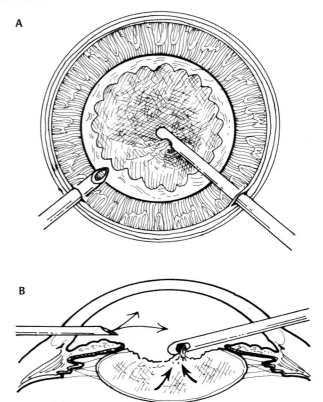

Figure 43.3

e. Use the octome vitrector to perform a posterior capsulectomy (**Fig. 43.4**). Alternatively, a primary posterior continuous curvilinear capsulorrhexis may be performed in experienced hands.
f. Perform an anterior vitrectomy (see Chapter 12).
g. A separate butterfly irrigation cannula may be placed through the paracentesis.
h. Keep the tip of the vitrectomy behind the level of the posterior capsule in attempt to remove the anterior hyaloid face.

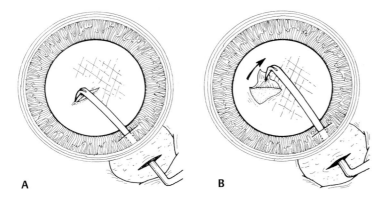

A   B   **Figure 43.2**

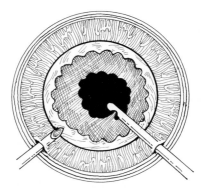

Figure 43.4

  i. Alternatively, a single-port pars plana vitrectomy may be performed (see Chapter 63).
  j. Close the MVR wounds with a 10–0 nylon suture, and bury the knot.
7. For 18 months and older.
 a. Prepare a fornix-based conjunctival peritomy at the limbus (Westcott scissors, tissue forceps) ~7 mm for one-piece lens; 4 mm if a foldable lens or if no IOL is planned. Center peritomy at approximately 10 or 2 o'clock on the side of the surgeon's dominant hand.
 b. Secure hemostasis with cautery.
 c. Create a short scleral tunnel:
  i. Use #64 Beaver blade and 0.12 mm forceps to make an initial partial-thickness, curvilinear incision perpendicular to sclera 2 mm from limbus.
  ii. Extend partial-thickness groove incision 3–3.5 mm if a foldable lens is planned and 6.0 mm if a PMMA lens is planned.
  iii. Use flat end and heel of #64 Beaver blade to construct a short scleral tunnel (~2 mm in length) of the same depth to clear cornea.
  iv. Continue tunnel construction just past the anterior limbal vessels.
 d. Perform a paracentesis through clear cornea adjacent to limbus (see Chapter 7).
  i. Place at 9 or 3 o'clock on side of nondominant hand.
  ii. Use a microsurgical knife (e.g., Beaver #75M).
 e. Inject viscoelastic into anterior chamber before or after making the clear cornea wound.
 f. Use a diamond or steel keratome (2.9 mm to 3.2 mm) to enter anterior chamber at the anterior edge of the tunnel on the side of the dominant hand (e.g., anywhere along the 10 to 2 o'clock position) in effort to avoid iris prolapse.
  i. Perform a capsulotomy. See 6c.
  ii. Perform hydrodissection with BSS if necessary:
  iii. Place tip of BSS cannula under anterior edge of capsulorrhexis. Position cannula toward equator of lens and gently inject BSS.
  iv. Usually this results in the hydration of the cortex and its subsequent elevation into the anterior chamber.

 g. Prepare phacoemulsification unit. Foot pedal functions.
  Position I = irrigation only.
  Position 2 = irrigation/aspiration
  Position 3 = irrigation/aspiration/phacoemulsification
 h. Perform phacoemulsification:
  i. In children, the lens is usually very soft and only the central nucleus rarely needs phacoemulsification. The whole lens material is often easily aspirated.
  ii. Set initial power of phacoemulsification unit to its low range and adjust up or down to achieve desired cutting effect.
  iii. Perform short linear grooves (see Chapter 8). Usually little ultrasound energy is required to remove the central nucleus in pediatric cases.
 i. Carefully and meticulously remove all cortical material with the 0.3 mm irrigation/aspiration tip on the phacoemulsification unit (see Chapter 8). A split irrigation/aspiration system is particularly helpful in removing all cortex and epithelial cells within the capsular bag.
8. For patients receiving an IOL

Note: The surgical technique depends on the decision to a nonfoldable PMMA lens or a foldable acrylic lens.

 a. If a PMMA lens is planned:
  i. Create a small scleral tunnel:
   I. Prepare a fornix-based conjunctival peritomy at the limbus (Westcott scissors, tissue forceps) ~7 mm for one-piece lens. Center peritomy at approximately 10 or 2 o'clock on the side of the surgeon's dominant hand.
   II. Secure hemostasis with cautery.
   III. Create a short scleral tunnel:
    A. Use #64 Beaver blade and 0.12 mm forceps to make an initial partial-thickness, linear incision perpendicular to sclera 2 mm from limbus.
    B. Extend partial-thickness groove incision ~6.0 mm in width.
    C. Use flat end and heel of #64 Beaver blade to construct a short scleral tunnel (~2 mm long) of the same depth to clear cornea just past the anterior limbal vessels.
  ii. Proceed with cataract removal as described in 7d–i.
  iii. A posterior capsulotomy and anterior vitrectomy should be performed if the patient will be unable to sit for a YAG capsulotomy in the near postoperative period. If the child is able to sit for a slit lamp exam and an A-scan, a YAG capsulotomy will likely be possible.
  iv. Inject viscoelastic into the capsular bag.
  v. Enlarge the wound to 6 mm with the keratome or crescent blade.
  vi. Insert the PMMA lens into capsular bag (see Chapter 8).

vii. Insert the trailing haptic with the Kelman McPherson forceps.

viii. Center IOL and spin to horizontal position with Sinskey hook. Proceed to #9.

b. If a foldable acrylic lens is planned:

i. Create a small scleral tunnel:

I. Prepare a fornix-based conjunctival peritomy at the limbus (Westcott scissors, tissue forceps) ~4 mm. Center peritomy approximately at 10 or 2 o'clock on the side of the surgeon's dominant hand.

II. Secure hemostasis with cautery.

III. Create a short scleral tunnel:

IV. Use #64 Beaver blade and 0.12 mm forceps to make an initial partial-thickness, linear incision perpendicular to sclera 2 mm from limbus.

V. Extend partial thickness groove incision 3–3.5 mm.

VI. Use flat end and heel of #64 Beaver blade to construct a short scleral tunnel (~2 mm in length) of the same depth to clear cornea.

VII. Continue tunnel construction just past the anterior limbal vessels.

ii. Proceed with the cataract extraction as noted above in 7d–k.

iii. Enlarge the wound with the keratome if needed.

iv. Insert IOL manually or with an injector (see Chapter 8).

v. Use a Kuglen or Y hook if necessary to insert trailing haptic.

vi. Center IOL and spin to horizontal position with Sinskey hook. Proceed to #9.

9. For all patients after cataract and cortex has been removed and IOL, if used, is in position.

a. Remove viscoelastic with irrigation/aspiration instrument using minimum suction.

b. Irrigate Miochol or Miostat into anterior chamber to constrict pupil.

c. Close wound with interrupted 10–0 nylon sutures.

d. Check for wound leak by applying gentle point pressure at the wound (cellulose sponges).

e. Reposition conjunctiva and secure with sutures (e.g., 7–0 Vicryl or silk) or cautery.

f. Optional: Give subconjunctival injections of cefazolin (100 mg) and Decadron (4–8 mg).

g. *Optional:* Position premeasured contact lens on eye if indicated.

h. Remove lid speculum.

i. Apply topical antibiotic and steroid ointment if no contact lens is used.

j. Apply patch and place Fox shield.

Postoperative Procedure

1. Postoperative orders may include:

a. Intravenous fluids until adequate oral intake

b. Activity may be ad lib with parents

c. Tylenol (5–10 mg/kg/dose; tablets: 80 mg, 160 mg, 325 mg, 500 mg) oral or rectal

d. Zofran (0.1 mg/kg; up to 4 mg every 4 hours);

e. A sedative as needed at night (may use chloral hydrate 25–50 mg/kg, 500 mg/5 ml syrup, maximum dose 1 g) if patient stays overnight;

f. Fox shield; no eye rubbing.

2. The parents should be instructed to keep the baby from crying if possible to minimize Valsalva.

3. Remove the shield on postoperative day 1. Patient should continue to use previously prescribed polycarbonate glasses during the postoperative period.

4. Patient should use Fox shield when sleeping for first week.

5. Steroid drops (e.g., Pred Forte 1%) every hour for first 24–48 hours, then every 2 hours for 4–7 days, then slowly tapered over ~6–8 weeks as inflammation warrants.

6. Atropine every day or every other day as long as inflammation is present and steroids are used.

7. Topical antibiotics (e.g., Ciloxan, Tobrex, Ocuflox) 4 times per day for 10–14 days.

8. Start patching nonoperated eye after surgery according to the recommendations of the surgeon.

9. Fit the patient for a contact lens in the operative eye according to the recommendations of the surgeon, ideally as soon as possible.

Follow-up Schedule

1. Postoperative day 1

2. Postoperative day 4 or 5 (highest incidence of endophthalmitis onset at this time)

3. Follow weekly postoperatively as necessary

Suture Removal

Induced astigmatism postoperatively may decrease significantly over the following weeks after surgery, and the surgeon may choose to observe. If suture removal is needed in the pediatric patient, it must be done under sedation or general anesthesia.

Complications

1. Loss of nuclear fragments into vitreous cavity

2. Transient increase in intraocular pressure

3. Hyphema

4. Corneal endothelial damage and consequent bullous keratopathy

5. Suprachoroidal effusion or hemorrhage

6. Posterior capsule opacification

7. Endophthalmitis

8. Retinal detachment

9. Cystoid macular edema

10. Amblyopia

11. Glaucoma (13–24% of postoperative pediatric cataract patients develop glaucoma and need to be followed)

44

Goniotomy and Trabeculotomy

■ Goniotomy

Indications

- Primary congenital glaucoma
- Other primary developmental glaucomas
- Pediatric secondary glaucomas
- Prevention of glaucoma secondary to aniridia

Preoperative Procedure

See Chapter 3.

1. Treatment of primary congenital glaucoma is usually surgical. Medical therapy is usually a temporizing measure before surgery.
2. Educate the parents about the possibility of multiple operations and frequent follow-up visits.
3. Perform a thorough preoperative examination of the patient in the office. Intraocular pressure (IOP) should be accurately determined in the office, as many drugs used during an examination under anesthesia alter the IOP.
4. Rule out nasolacrimal duct obstruction as a cause of epiphora.
5. Clear as much corneal edema as possible with medical treatment to lower the eye pressure. Use oral acetazolamide if needed. Goniotomy can be done with greater accuracy through a clearer cornea.
6. Apply a topical antibiotic ointment to both eyes the evening before surgery.
7. As long as an accurate eye pressure has already been obtained, a drop of 1% pilocarpine 30 minutes prior to surgery will protect the lens from the goniotomy knife.

Instrumentation

- Pilocarpine 1% (optional)
- Antibiotic ointment
- Proparacaine hydrochloride
- Alcohol containing red dye
- Handheld tonometer (e.g., Perkins)
- Calipers
- Koeppe gonioscopy lens
- Handheld microscope
- Barkan handheld light
- Direct ophthalmoscope
- No. 15 Bard-Parker blade
- Binocular loupes
- Headlight or operating microscope
- Lid speculum
- Elschnig-O'Connor locking fixation forceps
- Castroviejo 0.3 mm forceps
- Muscle hook
- Barkan operating gonioscopy lens, small and large

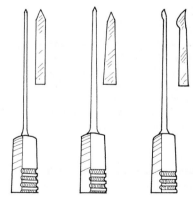

Figure 44.1

- Goniotomy knife (nontapered Swan, tapered Swan, or Barkan) (**Fig. 44.1**). (Note that the figure shows these knives in this order, from left to right.)

■ Balanced salt solution (BSS)
■ 10–0 Vicryl
■ Needle holder
■ Tying forceps
■ Vannas scissors or fine suture scissors
■ Weck-Cel sponges
■ Pediatric eye shield

Operative Procedure

1. Anesthesia: General anesthesia. If an accurate IOP was not obtained in the office, it is imperative to obtain a pressure as soon as possible after induction of anesthesia. Many barbiturates and inhalational anesthetics decrease the eye pressure, and ketamine can increase the pressure.
2. Once pressure is obtained, the patient is intubated.
3. Perform an examination under anesthesia. Measure the corneal diameters and perform gonioscopy. Examination of the optic nerve can be done through an undilated pupil with a direct ophthalmoscope through the Koeppe lens.
4. Select the area where the goniotomy will be performed.

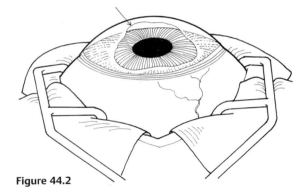

Figure 44.2

5. If the cornea is cloudy, a drop of proparacaine is place on the eye. A small amount of alcohol is painted over approximately one fourth of the cornea, 180 degrees away from the side of the angle to undergo goniotomy. After 10 seconds, the alcohol is irrigated away, and the epithelium is scraped away with a #15 Bard-Parker blade (**Fig. 44.2**). Care should be taken to preserve the limbal epithelial cells.
6. Prep and drape.
7. The surgeon is positioned to face the angle where the surgery will be performed.
8. The assistant will be opposite the surgeon.
9. Place the lid speculum.
10. Fixation of the eye:

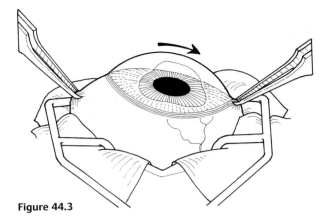

Figure 44.3

a. Castroviejo forceps are used to grab the conjunctiva near the limbus at 6 o'clock, and the eye is infraducted (**Fig. 44.3**). A muscle hook can alternatively be used to infraduct the eye.
b. Elschnig-O'Connor locking fixation forceps are used to lock the superior rectus.
c. The eye is then supraducted.
d. The other Elschnig-O'Connor locking fixation forceps are used to lock the inferior rectus.
e. The lid speculum is removed.
f. The two locking fixation forceps are handed to the assistant to position the globe.
11. Positioning of the head:

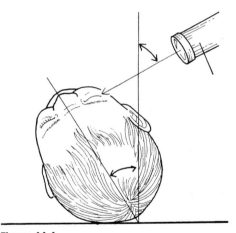

Figure 44.4

a. The patient's head is tilted 30 degrees away from the surgeon (**Fig. 44.4**). This facilitates the surgery and more easily allows removal of any air bubbles under the lens.

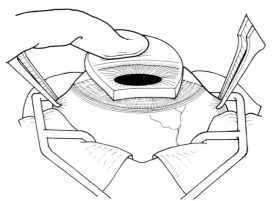

Figure 44.5

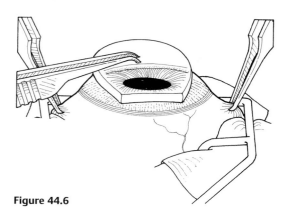

Figure 44.6

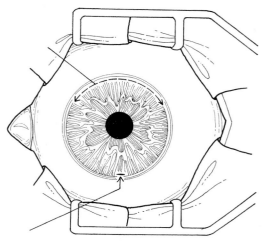

Figure 44.7

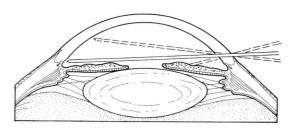

Figure 44.8

b. Barkan gonioscopy lens is placed on the cornea (**Figs. 44.5 and 44.6**). BSS is placed under the lens.

   Optional: Use Goniosol with lens.

12. Entry of the goniotomy knife into the anterior chamber.
    a. The assistant may need to provide a slow and almost imperceptible movement of the eye toward the knife as it enters the eye to provide some counterresistance as the entered knife may push the eye away from the surgeon.
    b. The knife starts to enter the anterior chamber through the cornea ~1 mm from the limbus. The entry site is 180 degrees away from the center of the area of angle to have surgery (**Fig. 44.7**).
    c. As the knife passes through the cornea, the surgeon should shift his or her view through the Barkan operating lens. The knife should be seen entering the anterior chamber.

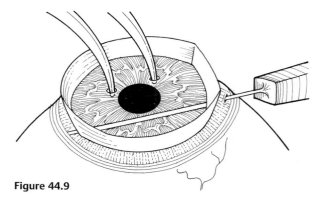

Figure 44.9

d. The knife is guided parallel to the iris (**Fig. 44.8**) and not over the pupil or the native lens (**Fig. 44.9**).

Note: (optional) If a nonirrigating knife is used, place a small amount of viscoelastic into the anterior chamber via a separate paracentesis and aspirate at conclusion of case with an air cannula.

13. Making the goniotomy incision.

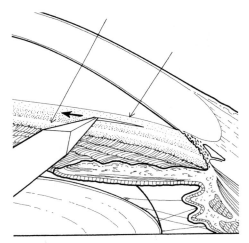

Figure 44.10

   a. The knife is directed just anterior to or at mid-trabecular meshwork (**Fig. 44.10**). When planning to operate on approximately one third of the angle, one sixth or more of the angle is incised with the knife moving clockwise. When the knife is returned to the beginning of the original incision, another sixth or more of the angle is treated with the knife moving counterclockwise. The knife is relatively superficial without incising the underlying sclera. If there is a sensation of tissue being cut, the surgeon may be too deep and into the sclera. When done correctly, a white line may be seen where the incision is made.

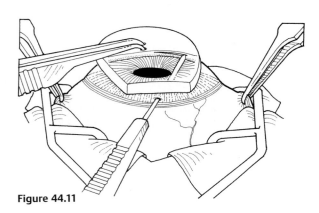

Figure 44.11

   b. After careful communication with the assistant, more clock hours of the angle can be treated if the assistant rotates the eye in the direction opposite (e.g., counterclockwise) that the surgeon intends to move the knife tip (e.g., clockwise) (**Fig. 44.11**).

14. Removing the knife.
   a. The surgeon should communicate to the assistant when this is to take place.
   b. When the knife is withdrawn, the assistant may almost imperceptibly move the eye away from the knife to provide countertraction as the withdrawing knife may pull the eye toward the surgeon.
   c. As the knife is being removed, care should be made to remove the knife over the iris and not over the pupil or native lens. The Barkan lens may be moved over the entry site to prevent egress of fluid and flattening of the anterior chamber.

15. Remove the Elschnig-O'Connor forceps and replace the lid speculum.

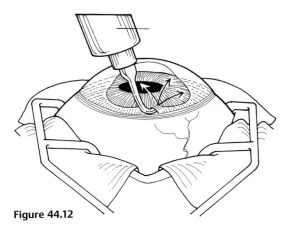

Figure 44.12

16. Immediately reform the anterior chamber with the BSS if necessary (**Fig. 44.12**).

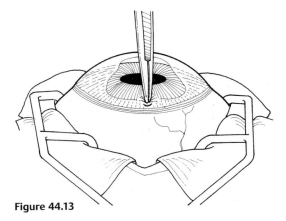

Figure 44.13

17. The wound is kept closed by the assistant with the closed ends of a blunt forceps pushing gently on the anterior lip of the wound (**Fig. 44.13**).
18. Close the wound with a 10–0 Vicryl suture. A Weck-Cel may be used to ensure a watertight wound closure.
19. Apply an antibiotic ointment and a protective eye shield to the eye.

20. If goniotomy needs to be performed on the opposite eye, the surgeon should rescrub, change gowns, and the patient should be reprepped.

Postoperative Procedure

1. Postoperative orders may include:
   a. Intravenous fluids until adequate oral intake
   b. Activity may be ad lib with parents
   c. Head of bed elevated 15 degrees
   d. Tylenol (5–10 mg/kg/dose; tablets: 80 mg, 160 mg, 325 mg, 500 mg) oral or rectal
   e. Zofran (0.1 mg/kg; up to 4 mg every 4 hours)
   f. A sedative prn qhs (may use chloral hydrate 25–50 mg/kg, 500 mg/5 ml syrup, maximum dose 1 g)
   g. Fox shield; no eye rubbing
2. Apply topical antibiotic/steroid ointment once daily for at least 5 days postoperatively. If a suture was used to close the corneal wound, the antibiotic should be continued until the suture is removed or reabsorbed.
3. The parents can be instructed to keep the baby from crying if possible to minimize Valsalva.
4. The shield can be removed on the first postoperative day.
5. Patients can be discharged from the hospital on the first or second postoperative day.
6. The intraocular pressure (IOP) may not be comfortably measured for several days.
7. If the pressure is uncertain, glaucoma medications can be continued postoperatively and gradually tapered until a reliable pressure is obtained.
8. An examination under anesthesia may be needed at 1 month if a complete office exam is not possible. Refraction should be noted.

Complications

1. Hyphema (most common)
2. Iridodialysis
3. Cyclodialysis
4. Peripheral anterior synechiae
5. Retinal detachment
6. Cataract
7. Endophthalmitis

■ Trabeculotomy

Indications

- Eyes with corneal haze that precludes a good view of the angle
- Eyes that have failed two or more goniotomies.

Preoperative Procedure

See Chapter 3.

1. Treatment of primary congenital glaucoma is usually surgical. Medical therapy is usually a temporizing measure before surgery.
2. Educate the parents about the possibility of multiple operations and frequent follow-up visits.
3. Perform a thorough preoperative examination of the patient in the office. IOP should be accurately determined in the office as many drugs used during an examination under anesthesia alter the IOP.
4. Rule out nasolacrimal duct obstruction as a cause of epiphora.
5. Clear as much corneal edema as possible with medical treatment to lower the eye pressure. Use oral acetazolamide if needed (15 mg/kg per day in four divided doses). If the cornea clears, it is usually preferable to do a goniotomy.
6. A topical antibiotic ointment applied to both eyes the evening before surgery.
7. As long as an accurate eye pressure has already been obtained and if the patient's medical condition permits, a drop of 2% pilocarpine 30 minutes before surgery.

Instrumentation

- Pilocarpine 1% (optional)
- Antibiotic ointment
- Handheld tonometer (e.g., Perkins)
- Calipers
- Koeppe gonioscopy lens
- Handheld microscope
- Barkan handheld light
- Direct ophthalmoscope
- Super sharp blade (Wheeler knife)
- Lid speculum
- Westcott scissors (blunt-tipped)
- Chandler forceps
- Hoskins forceps
- Monopolar underwater diathermy
- No. 57 Beaver blade
- Vannas scissors
- Zeiss four-mirror gonioscopy lens
- McPherson or Harms left- and right-handed trabeculotomes
- 4–0 silk superior rectus bridle suture or 6–0 silk inferior corneal bridle suture
- 6–0 Prolene suture
- 10–0 nylon suture
- 8–0 Vicryl suture
- BSS
- Needle holder
- Tying forceps
- Weck-Cel sponges
- Pediatric eye shield

Operative Procedure

1. Anesthesia: General anesthesia. If an accurate IOP was not obtained in the office, it is imperative to obtain a pressure as soon as possible after induction of anesthesia. Many barbiturates and inhalational anesthetics decrease the eye pressure, and ketamine can increase the pressure.
2. Once the pressure is obtained, the patient is intubated.
3. Perform an examination under anesthesia. Measure the corneal diameters and perform gonioscopy. Examination of the optic nerve can be done through an undilated pupil with a direct ophthalmoscope through the Koeppe lens.
4. Prep and drape.
5. Place the lid speculum.
6. Placement of bridle suture.
   a. A 4–0 silk superior rectus bridle suture may be placed to expose the superior conjunctiva.
   b. Alternatively, a 6–0 silk inferior corneal/limbal bridle suture may be placed to minimize trauma to the conjunctiva. This suture, whose ends are tied together into a closed loop, should be tucked under the inferior half of the lid speculum and clamped to the inferior drape to expose the superior conjunctiva.

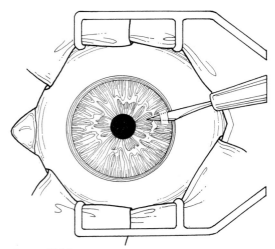

Figure 44.14

7. Make a paracentesis site through clear cornea temporally (**Fig. 44.14**).
8. Make a limbus-based conjunctival flap superotemporally or superonasally with the blunt Westcott scissors and either Chandler or Hoskins forceps (**Fig. 44.15**).
9. Use a monopolar underwater diathermy for hemostasis, minimizing trauma and inflammation. This is particularly important over the site of the future scleral flap.
10. Making the scleral flap.

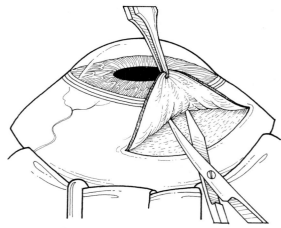

Figure 44.15

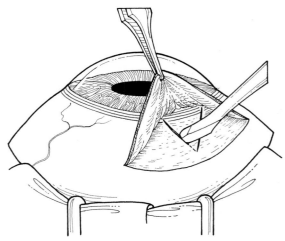

Figure 44.16

   a. Make a partial thickness scleral incision to mark out a 3–4 mm triangular or rectangular flap (**Fig. 44.16**).

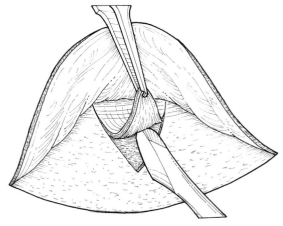

Figure 44.17

b. Pick up the flap at the edge with a Hoskins forceps (**Fig. 44.17**). Dissect the flap anteriorly toward the limbus with the # 57 blade. Care must be taken, as the sclera may be thinner in buphthalmic eyes. A thicker flap may, however, facilitate easier identification of the underlying anatomy.

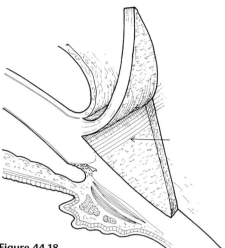

Figure 44.18

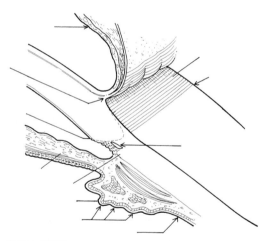

Figure 44.19

c. Continue the scleral flap dissection to ~1 mm anterior to the sclerolimbal junction (**Figs. 44.18 and 44.19**). The sclerolimbal junction is also called the surgical or posterior limbus and is the junction of the opaque white sclera and the translucent, bluish-gray limbus. The limbus is the junction of the transparent cornea and the opaque sclera. The posterior aspect of the bluish-gray limbus is the scleral spur, which has circumferentially running fibers. The Schlemm canal is the darker space at the anterior edge of this scleral spur.

11. Entering Schlemm's canal.

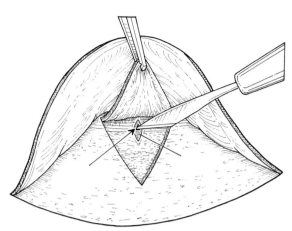

Figure 44.20

a. Make a radial scratch incision across the sclerolimbal junction to cut into the Schlemm canal and yet avoid entering the anterior chamber (**Fig. 44.20**). The Schlemm canal is right behind the trabecular meshwork.

b. Gradually deepen the radial incision until a drop of aqueous or blood is seen in the lateral wall.

c. Irrigate the incision.

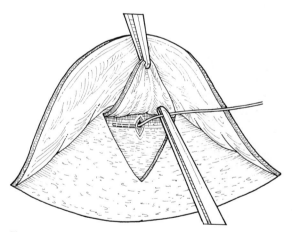

Figure 44.21

d. When entering the Schlemm canal with the 6–0 Prolene suture, there should be little resistance (**Fig. 44.21**). If placement into the Schlemm canal is uncertain, gonioscopy with the Zeiss lens will help verify the position of the Prolene suture.

12. Entering the anterior chamber with the trabeculotome.

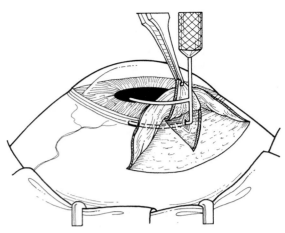

Figure 44.22

a. Once the 6–0 Prolene is removed, the internal arm of the trabeculotome is introduced into the canal (**Fig. 44.22**). There should be relatively minimal resistance. If positioning is uncertain, gonioscopy can again be performed. The right-handed surgeon may find the trabeculotome insertion to the right more difficult, so this can be done first when the view of the anterior chamber is clearer. Bleeding and shallowing of the anterior chamber may occur during the second sweep of the trabeculotome.

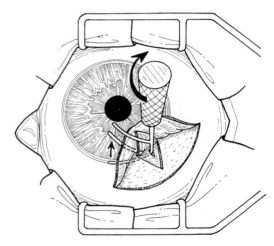

Figure 44.23

b. Once the trabeculotome is entirely in the canal, the arm is maintained parallel to the iris and rotated into the anterior chamber (**Fig. 44.23**). Care is taken to avoid the pupil and the lens.

c. If the anterior chamber shallows after removal of the trabeculotome, inject BSS into the chamber through the paracentesis.

d. Insert the other trabeculotome into the other side of the radial incision and rotate into the anterior chamber.

13. Leave the radial incision unsutured after the withdrawal of the trabeculotome.

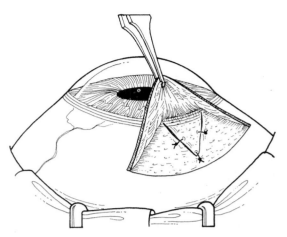

Figure 44.24

14. Close the scleral flap with three 10–0 nylon sutures (**Fig. 44.24**).
15. Close the conjunctiva and Tenon with a running suture of 8–0 Vicryl.
16. Reform the anterior chamber if necessary.
17. Place a drop of pilocarpine 1% and steroid/antibiotic drops or ointment on the eye.
18. Place a protective eye shield over the eye.
19. If a trabeculotomy needs to be performed on the opposite eye, the surgeon should rescrub, change gowns, and the patient should be reprepped.

Postoperative Procedure

1. Postoperative orders may include:
   a. Intravenous fluids until adequate oral intake
   b. Activity may be ad lib with parents
   c. Head of bed elevated 15 degrees
   d. Tylenol (5–10 mg/kg/dose; tablets: 80 mg, 160 mg, 325 mg, 500 mg) oral or rectal;
   e. Zofran (0.1 mg/kg; up to 4 mg q 4 hours);
   f. A sedative prn qhs (may use chloral hydrate 25–50 mg/kg, 500 mg/5 ml syrup, maximum dose 1 g)
   g. Fox shield; no eye rubbing.
2. Remove the shield on postoperative day 1.
3. If the anterior chamber is formed and without significant hyphema, the patient is discharged.
4. A steroid/antibiotic combination may be used 4 times per day for 2 or 3 weeks.
5. Miotics may help to keep the opening in the trabecular meshwork patent.
6. The parents can be instructed to keep the baby from crying if possible to minimize Valsalva.

7. The patient can be seen weekly in the office and attempts can be made to measure an accurate pressure.
8. If it is not possible to do a complete eye exam in the office, an examination under anesthesia may be done a month after the surgery. If possible, the IOP should be measured before intubation. Refraction should be noted. Koeppe gonioscopy should be attempted.

Complications

1. Hyphema
2. Peripheral anterior synechiae
3. Inadvertent filtering bleb
4. Choroidal detachment
5. Lens opacity
6. Infection
7. Subconjunctival iris prolapse
8. Stripping of the Descemet membrane
9. Iris trauma
10. Creation of false passage into the anterior chamber
11. Inadvertent cyclodialysis cleft

VIII

Oculoplastics

45

Chalazion Incision and Drainage

Indications

Drainage of chalazion that has not responded satisfactorily to medical management.

Preoperative Procedure

1. Treat underlying cause of chalazion formation (e.g., staphylococcal or rosacea blepharitis) with daily warm compresses, lid hygiene, diluted baby shampoo scrubs, or doxycycline as needed.
2. If skin incision is expected, advise patient of possible residual cutaneous scar.
3. **Note:** Select cases respond to intralesional corticosteroid injection.

Instrumentation

- Scleral shell (optional)
- Tissue marking pen (optional)
- Chalazion clamp
- Chalazion curette
- Scalpel (e.g., #11 or #15 Bard-Parker blade)
- Toothed forceps
- Scissors (e.g., Westcott).

Operative Procedure

1. Apply topical anesthetic.
2. *Optional:* Make fine mark with pen on skin over chalazion to prevent loss of external landmarks after infiltration with anesthetics.
3. Subconjunctival infiltration with lidocaine 2% plus epinephrine 1:100,000.
   a. Inject subconjunctivally near planned incision site, avoiding direct injection into chalazion.

4. Prep and drape.
5. *Optional:* Place scleral shell.
6. Apply chalazion clamp.

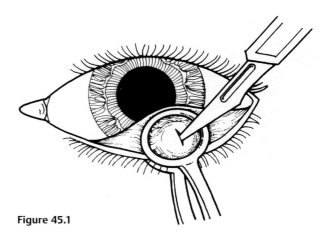

Figure 45.1

7. Incise chalazion vertically through conjunctiva and into tarsus with a scalpel (**Fig. 45.1**). *Optional:* Perform cruciate incision into tarsus with scalpel.
   a. Length of incision should be ~3 mm.
   b. Orient incision parallel to meibomian glands (to avoid excessive damage to glands).
   c. Do not place incision closer than 2.5 mm to the lid margin to prevent postoperative lid notch.

Note: Lesions that are prominent on the anterior lid surface and do not show a visible component when viewed from the conjunctival surface may be best approached with a skin incision.

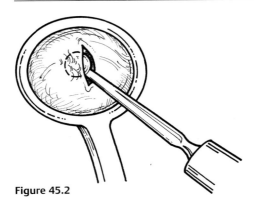

Figure 45.2

8. Remove lipogranulomatous material by curettage (chalazion curette) (**Fig. 45.2**).

Note: Send tissue from an atypical lesion for histopathology.

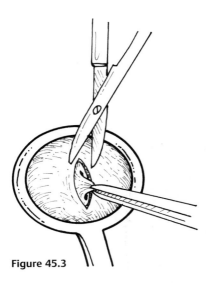

Figure 45.3

9. *Optional:* Excise capsule of chalazion if present with forceps and scissors (**Fig. 45.3**).

10. Remove chalazion clamp.
11. Remove scleral shell.
12. Apply antibiotic ointment
13. Place light patch.

Postoperative Procedure

1. Remove patch 6–24 hours after drainage has stopped.
2. Apply antibiotic ointment 3 times per day for 3 days.
3. Continue to treat underlying causes of chalazion formation.
4. Follow up results of pathology specimen if ordered.

Complications

1. Recurrence of chalazion
2. Formation of pyogenic granuloma at the operative site
3. Focal skin depigmentation and atrophy in some patients injected with steroid
4. Residual scar formation on anterior lid margin
5. Failure to diagnose malignancy in recurrent lesions not sent for histopathologic evaluation

46

Eyelid Lacerations/Eye Defects/Biopsies

■ Repair of Full-Thickness Lid Margin Lacerations and Defects

Indications

The following chapter discusses the general repair of a lid margin defect, whether of surgical or traumatic etiology. Situations in which this technique is used include:

- Full-thickness marginal lid biopsy and excision of lid margin lesions.
- Treatment of focal trichiasis.
- Repair of full-thickness lacerations involving the lid margin.
- Treatment of eyelid ectropion or entropion where full-thickness resection of eyelid is desired.

Preoperative Procedure

See Chapter 3.
For traumatic lid lacerations:

1. Rule out injury to the eye.
2. Carefully inspect injury site.
   a. Rule out involvement of canaliculus and lacrimal system. (If lacerated, see Canalicular Repair with Intubation section later in this chapter).
   b. Assess levator function to rule out injury to the levator aponeurosis. See Ptosis Repair by External Levator Aponeurosis Advancement section in Chapter 54, p. 279.
3. Administer tetanus prophylaxis as indicated.
4. Administer prophylactic intravenous or oral antibiotics.

Instrumentation

- Scleral shield
- Toothed forceps
- Scalpel with #15 Bard-Parker blade
- Scissors
- Cautery
- Needle holder
- Sutures (6–0 Vicryl on spatulated needle, 6–0 silk)

Operative Procedure

1. Apply topical anesthetic.
2. Subcutaneous infiltration with a 50:50 mixture of lidocaine 2% plus 1:100,000 epinephrine and 0.75% bupivacaine.
   a. Infiltrate area to be manipulated via cutaneous or conjunctival route.
3. Prepare and drape in the usual sterile manner.
4. Place scleral shield.

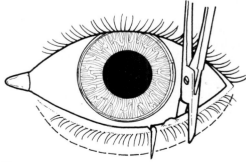

Figure 46.1

5. Incise lid margin perpendicularly at one side of area to be excised (**Fig. 46.1**).

a. Secure lid with forceps or traction suture.
b. Use #15 Bard-Parker blade scalpel or scissors to perform incision.
c. Extend incision just below edge of tarsus.
d. Excise additional several mm if excising neoplasm.
6. Similarly, perform a second vertical incision at other side of lesion, completely encompassing the area of interest (**Fig. 46.1**).

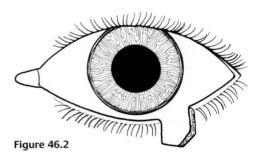

Figure 46.2

7. Excise the lid segment as a pentagon, completing the incisions inferior to the tarsus (scalpel or scissors) (**Fig. 46.2**).

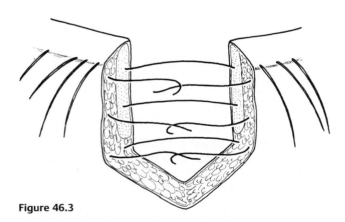

Figure 46.3

8. Approximate tarsus with three interrupted, partial thickness absorbable sutures (e.g., 6–0 Vicryl) (**Fig. 46.3**).
a. Make certain that suture does not protrude posteriorly through conjunctiva.
b. Sutures may be left untied until lid margin is approximated.

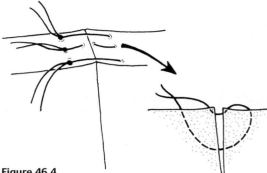

Figure 46.4

9. Approximate lid margin (**Fig. 46.4**).
a. Use nonabsorbable suture (e.g., 6–0 silk).
b. Sutures should be ~1–2 mm on each side of wound and 1–2 mm deep.
c. Suture 1: Use a vertical mattress suture through the gray line (create wound eversion to prevent lid notching) or use simple interrupted sutures.
d. Suture 2: Use an interrupted suture at lash line.
e. Suture 3 (optional): Use an interrupted suture through the posterior lid margin.

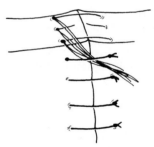

Figure 46.5

f. Keep suture ends long to subsequently secure them under the topmost skin suture to avoid contact with the cornea (**Fig. 46.5**).
10. Close skin with interrupted sutures (e.g., 6–0 silk).
11. Remove scleral shield.
12. Apply antibiotic ointment to eye and suture line.
13. Apply dressing or chilled eye pad.

Horizontal Lid Shortening

1. Prepare eye for surgery as described in steps 1–4.
2. Incise lid margin perpendicularly near area of most severe lid malposition (**Fig. 46.1**).
a. Secure lid with forceps.
b. Use scalpel (#15 Bard-Parker blade) or scissors.
c. Extend incision just inferior to tarsal margin.
3. Overlap the cut edges of the lid to assess amount of required lid shortening (may cut or crush lid margin to mark distance).

4. Perform a second vertical incision at the marked location.
5. Remove the lid segment by completing the pentagon inferior to the tarsus with scalpel or scissors (**Fig. 46.2**).
6. Close the lid defect and complete procedure as described in steps 10–14.

Repair of Full-Thickness Lid Margin Lacerations

1. Prepare eye for surgery as described above.
2. Avoid excess debridement of wound. If necessary, may clean and reshape the wound edges as needed to properly close the wound (e.g., fashion a pentagonal defect as previously described).
3. Close the lid defect and complete procedure as described in steps 8 to 13.

Postoperative Procedures

1. Administer broad-spectrum oval or intravenous antibiotics as indicated.
2. Use ice packs to decrease swelling.
3. Apply antibiotic ointment twice daily to suture line.

Suture Removal

1. Remove skin sutures after 5 days, except for the suture that directs the eyelid marginal sutures away from the cornea.
2. Remove eyelid marginal sutures and remaining skin suture in 10–14 days.

Complications

1. Infection
2. Hematoma
3. Lid notching
4. Lid malposition

■ Canalicular Repair with Intubation

Indications

■ Laceration of canaliculus from trauma
■ Laceration of canaliculus from surgery (e.g., eyelid tumor excision)

Preoperative Procedure

See Chapter 3.

1. Document medical indications for surgery. For eyelid procedures, obtain preoperative photographs.
2. If possible, discontinue aspirin and nonsteroidal anti-inflammatory agents for 10 days before surgery. Discontinue warfarin preoperatively, if medically possible.

3. Query patient about bleeding tendencies. A useful screening question is asking if the patient had unusual bleeding after dental extraction. Obtain hematological evaluation if bleeding tendency suspected.

Instrumentation

■ Scleral shield
■ Needle holder
■ Toothed forceps
■ Punctum dilators
■ Bowman lacrimal probes 0–00 and 5–6
■ Double skin hooks
■ Cautery
■ Bayonette forceps
■ Nasal speculum
■ Headlight for surgeon
■ Silastic lacrimal tubing on lacrimal probes (Quickert-Dryden, Jackson, Crawford or similar lacrimal intubation systems)
■ Retinal sponge
■ Periosteal elevator
■ Straight hemostat
■ 7–0 Vicryl, 6–0 Vicryl, 6–0 silk.

Operative Procedure

1. Use local or general anesthesia.
2. General anesthetic is preferred, because swollen tissues (after trauma) may be difficult to anesthetize and patient may be uncooperative.
3. Manipulation of tubes into the nose may be uncomfortable to some patients.
4. Apply topical anesthetic.
5. Inject local infiltrative anesthetic solution. Inject subcutaneously and subconjunctivally into medial aspects of lower and upper eyelids and at medial canthus.
   a. May use 50:50 mixture of lidocaine 2% plus 1:100,000 epinephrine and 0.75% bupivacaine.
6. Pack inferior and middle meatus of nose with 1 × 3 inch neurologic cottonoids soaked with 4% cocaine solution.
   a. This gives anesthesia and shrinks nasal mucosa, allowing for visualization of the structures within the nose.
   b. Fiber optic headlight will facilitate visualization during the procedure.
   Optional: May use oxymetazoline instead of cocaine.
7. Remove cocaine-soaked cottonoids and inject lateral wall of nose, middle meatus, and inferior meatus with anesthetic solution. Replace cocaine-soaked cottonoids in middle and inferior meatuses.
8. Prep and drape in the usual sterile manner.
9. Keep both eyes exposed for comparison during procedure.
10. Place scleral shield.
11. Dilate punctum of lacerated eyelid.

12. Introduce 0 Bowman probe though punctum of lacerated eyelid. If probe is visualized, laceration is confirmed. Withdraw probe.

13. Using magnification with operating loupes or microscope, inspect the lacerated eyelid and canthal tissues. Identify the lumen of the cut proximal end of canaliculus.
    a. Use skin hooks to retract medial canthal tissues.
    b. In the event of difficulties, the noninvolved punctum may be dilated and saline, fluorescein, or fluorescein-stained Healon may be injected to help identify the cut canaliculus.
    c. Confirm that cut end is found by inserting Bowman 0 probe into lumen to level of lacrimal sac. Probe should pass easily.

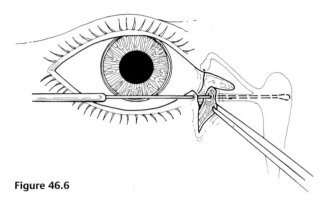

Figure 46.6

14. Again, dilate punctum with lacerated canaliculus. Advance lacrimal probe with silicone tube attached through punctum and into proximal lacerated canaliculus (**Fig. 46.6**).

15. Advance medially until hard stop of medial wall of lacrimal sac is palpated.

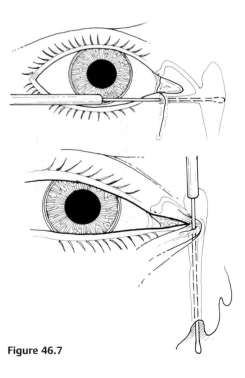

Figure 46.7

16. Remove cocaine packing from nose. Advance lacrimal probe with silicone tube attached inferiorly where it is recovered beneath inferior turbinate (**Fig. 46.7**).
    a. Use nasal speculum to visualize turbinate. The probe is often visualized directly. A Freer periosteal elevator may be used to retract turbinate medially to aid in visualization.
    b. Alternatively, insert 5–6 Bowman probe beneath inferior turbinate. Feel lacrimal probe metal on metal beneath inferior turbinate.

17. Grasp probe in nose with hemostat. Engage and withdraw from nose.

18. Dilate punctum of normal canaliculus. Insert unused probe attached to lacrimal tube through punctum to medial wall of lacrimal sac and then inferiorly. Recover tube in nose. Pull silicone tube snug through nose.

Note: Inspect as the gap in lacerated canaliculus reduces.

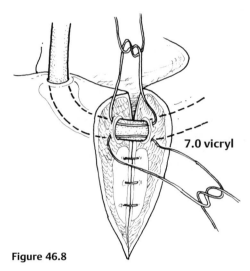

7.0 vicryl

Figure 46.8

19. Suture canaliculus with 7–0 Vicryl. Place one or two 7–0 Vicryl through two cut ends of canaliculus anterior to silicone tube and tie (**Fig. 46.8**).

Note: Make sure silicone tube is not incarcerated by moving it back and forth.

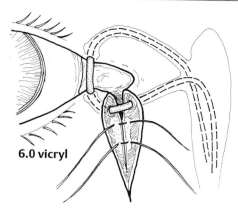

6.0 vicryl

Figure 46.9

20. Repair eyelid laceration using buried 6–0 Vicryl sutures into deep canthal tissue (**Fig. 46.9**). Use 6–0 silk to close skin.

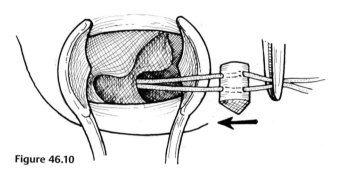

Figure 46.10

21. Cut retinal sponge to ¼ inch length and grasp with two hemostats. Use #18 needle to make two punctures in the sponge. Advance the end of Bowman probe through these holes and advance sponge into inferior meatus (**Fig. 46.10**).

22. Tie 6–8 square knots. Place muscle hook in medial canthus and advance silicone sleeve until satisfactory tension is obtained.
23. Remove scleral shell.
24. Apply to suture line.

Postoperative Procedure

1. Place ice packs to decrease swelling.
2. Elevate bed to 30 degrees to decrease swelling.
3. Apply antibiotic ointment twice daily to suture line.
4. Remove skin sutures in 5–7 days.
5. Remove tube in 6–12 weeks. Visualize bolster in nose. Cut tube in medial canthus and withdraw through the nose.

Complications

1. Nasal bleeding
2. Erosion of canaliculus from tube
3. Canalicular scarring with epiphora

47

Temporal Artery Biopsy

Indications

- Suspicion of temporal arteritis.
- If steroids have been started empirically, temporal artery biopsy should be done within 10 days.

Preoperative Procedure

See Chapter 3.

1. Obtain complete medical history, focusing on signs and symptoms of temporal arteritis.
2. Measure erythrocyte sedimentation rate and C-reactive protein.
3. If possible, discontinue aspirin and nonsteroidal anti-inflammatory agents for 10 days before surgery. Discontinue warfarin 2–3 days preoperatively, if medically possible.
4. Query patient on bleeding tendencies. A useful screening question is asking if the patient had unusual bleeding after dental extraction. Obtain hematological evaluation if bleeding tendency is suspected.

Instrumentation

- Doppler (available)
- Tissue marking pen
- Scalpel (e.g., #15 Bard-Parker blade)
- Small hemostat
- Scissors
- Sutures (4–0 and 6–0 silk, 6–0 Vicryl, 6–0 Prolene)
- Cautery

Operative Procedure

1. Identify temporal artery by palpation.

Note: May need Doppler in difficult cases.

2. Mark skin over artery (marking pen).
3. Infiltrate operative site with 2% lidocaine plus 1:100,000 epinephrine. Avoid injecting directly over artery.
4. Incise skin over artery down to subcutaneous tissue using a scalpel.

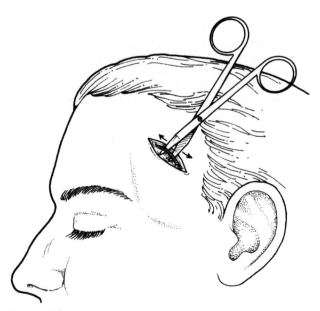

Figure 47.1

5. Expose and isolate ~3–5 cm of temporal artery using blunt dissection (scissors, hemostat) (**Fig. 47.1**).

6. Tie off accessory vessels (6–0 silk).
7. Tie off temporal artery with four sutures (4–0 silk).
   a. Biopsy specimen should be as long as possible (~2–4 cm) because, histopathologically, skip (normal) regions may be present.

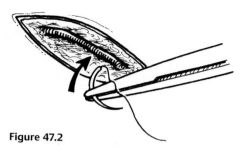

Figure 47.2

   b. Technique: Lead with the hub of needle when placing suture to avoid puncturing the vessel (**Fig. 47.2**).

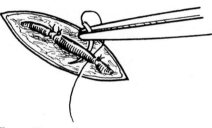

Figure 47.3

   c. Place two sutures at each end of the specimen to ensure subsequent hemostasis (**Fig. 47.3**).
8. Remove specimen with scissors, cutting artery inside of double sutures.
9. Secure hemostasis with cautery.
10. Close wound with deep absorbable sutures (e.g., 6–0 Vicryl).
11. Close skin with interrupted or running sutures (e.g., 6–0 Prolene).
12. Dress wound.

Postoperative Procedure

1. Remove skin sutures in approximately 1 week.
2. Treat medically if necessary.

Complications

1. Excessive bleeding
2. Infection
3. Facial nerve injury

48

Lateral Tarsorrhaphy

Indications

- Corneal exposure problems (e.g., facial nerve palsy, lid myopathies, thyroid ophthalmopathy).
- Neurotrophic keratitis (e.g., diabetic patient, status post-herpetic infection).
- Severe dry eye (e.g., keratoconjunctivitis sicca, ocular cicatricial pemphigoid, Stevens Johnson syndrome).
- Sterile corneal ulceration.
- Used in conjunction with amniotic membrane transplant for in ocular reconstructive procedures.

Preoperative Procedure

1. Attempt nonsurgical treatments tailored to the etiology of patient's problem (e.g., lubricants, lid taping, bandage soft contact lens, punctal occlusion).

See Chapter 3.

2. For oculoplastic procedures, discontinue aspirin and nonsteroidal anti-inflammatory agents 10 days before surgery. Discontinue warfarin 2–3 days preoperatively, if medically possible.
3. Query patient about bleeding tendencies. A useful screening question is asking if the patient had unusual bleeding after dental extraction. Obtain hematological evaluation if bleeding tendency is suspected.

Instrumentation

- Scleral shell
- Tissue marking pen
- Needle holder
- Toothed forceps
- Scalpel (e.g., #11 or #15 Bard-Parker blade)
- Scissors (e.g., Westcott)
- Sutures (6–0 Vicryl on spatulated needle, double-armed 6–0 silk [optional])

Operative Procedure

Technique 1: Lid Shaving Technique (performed less frequently than Technique 2)

1. Advantages:
   a. Quick to perform. May be performed at bedside.
   b. May be opened easily.
2. Anesthetize area with local infiltration of lidocaine 2% plus epinephrine 1:100,000.
3. Prep and drape in usual sterile manner.
4. Place scleral shell.
5. Mark upper and lower lid margins (e.g., forceps crush mark, marking pen, or scalpel nick) to delineate medial extent of desired tarsorrhaphy (usually 8–10 mm from lateral canthus).

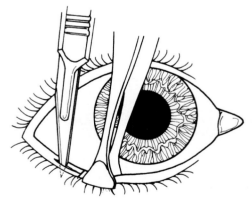

Figure 48.1

6. Shave a thin strip of lid margin tissue along gray line with scalpel or scissors from lateral commissure to medial extent of desired tarsorrhaphy (**Fig. 48.1**).
   a. Avoid shaving cilia.

b. Shaved margins of upper and lower lid should meet at lateral canthal angle.

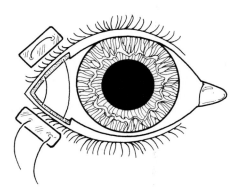

Figure 48.2

7. Place horizontal mattress sutures through upper and lower lids to secure tarsorrhaphy (**Fig. 48.2**).
   a. Use double-armed 4–0 silk sutures.
   b. Place and tie sutures through bolsters (may use piece of silicone retinal buckling band).
   c. Use one or two mattress sutures depending upon length of tarsorrhaphy.
   d. Each suture end should be placed through skin of upper lid ~5 mm above lash line, traverse the upper tarsal plate, exit through raw surface of upper lid margin, enter through raw surface of lower lid margin, traverse the lower tarsal plated, and exit through skin of lower lid ~5 mm from lash line.
   e. Remove scleral shell before tying sutures
   f. Tie over bolster.
8. *Optional:* Reinforce closure with interrupted 6–0 Vicryl sutures through lid margin.
9. Apply antibiotic ointment to wound margin.
10. Apply dressing or chilled eye pad

Technique 2: Permanent Lateral Tarsorrhaphy (performed more commonly)

1. Mark upper and lower margin to delineate medial extent of desired tarsorrhaphy (usually 8–10 mm from lateral commissure).
2. Anesthetize area with local infiltration of lidocaine 2% plus epinephrine 1:100,000.
3. Prep and drape in usual sterile manner.
4. Incise along gray line with scalpel from lateral commissure to medial extent of desired tarsorrhaphy.
   a. Avoid shaving cilia.
   b. Incision separates tarsus from orbicularis and is 4 mm in vertical height. Use scalpel to begin incision followed by scissors to deepen it.
5. Shave superficial lid margin tissue from posterior lamella of lower eyelid (scissors or scalpel) (**Fig. 48.3**).
   a. Create strip of raw surface for long-lasting adhesion to opposite eyelid.

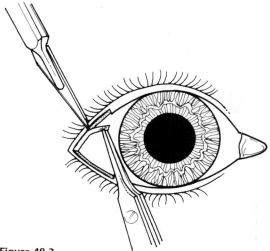

Figure 48.3

b. Do not remove tissue from anterior lamella. This avoids lash loss and undesired appearance if tarsorrhaphy is ever reversed.

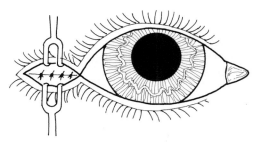

Figure 48.4

6. Suture tarsus with 3–4 partial thickness interrupted suture of 6–0 Vicryl. Tie knot anteriorly to avoid corneal abrasion (**Fig. 48.4**).
7. *Optional*: 6–0 silk sutures may be placed across anterior lamella to give added support during first 10 days of healing.
8. Apply antibiotic ointment to wound margin.
9. Apply dressing or chilled eye pad

Postoperative Procedure

1. Place ice packs to decrease swelling.
2. Elevate head of bed 30 degrees to decrease swelling.
3. Apply antibiotic ointment to tarsorrhaphy site twice per day.
4. Remove silk skin sutures in 1 week.

Complications

1. Over- and undercorrection of palpebral fissure.
2. Disruption of lash line.
3. Spontaneous breakdown of the tarsorrhaphy.

49

Gold Weight Placement

Indications

Paresis of upper eyelid orbicularis with lagophthalmos.

Preoperative Proceedure

See Chapter 3.

1. If possible, discontinue aspirin and nonsteroidal anti-inflammatory agents for 10 days before surgery. Discontinue warfarin 2–3 days preoperatively, if medically possible.
2. Query patient about bleeding tendencies. A useful screening question is asking if the patient had unusual bleeding after dental extraction. Obtain hematological evaluation if bleeding tendency is suspected.

Instrumentation

- Scleral shell
- Needle holder
- Sutures (6–0 polypropylene)
- Toothed forceps
- Scissors (e.g., Westcott)
- Cautery
- Scalpel (e.g., 15 degree blade)
- Gold weight of selected size
- Skin retractor (e.g., Blair).

Operative Procedure

1. To determine the size of the weight to be used, examine the patient in an upright position.
   a. Apply Mastisol or benzoin to pretarsal upper eyelid.
   b. Apply a gold weight or sizer weight (standard production sizes are 0.6 to 1.6 g).

Note: A 1.2 g weight is the most commonly used size.

2. Look at the position of the eyelid in primary gaze (symmetric with fellow eye desirable).
3. Look at the position with the patient asked to close gently (complete closure desired). Mark eyelid crease.
4. Apply topical anesthetic.
5. Subcutaneous infiltration with a 50:50 mixture of lidocaine 2% plus 1:100,000 epinephrine and 0.75% bupivacaine.
6. Prep and drape. Keep both eyes exposed for comparison during procedure.
7. Place scleral shield.

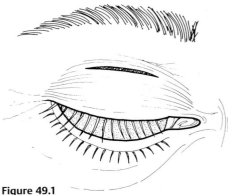

Figure 49.1

8. Make lid crease incision across upper eyelid with scalpel (**Fig. 49.1**).
9. Tent skin edges upward with forceps and button hole orbicularis muscle with Westcott scissors.

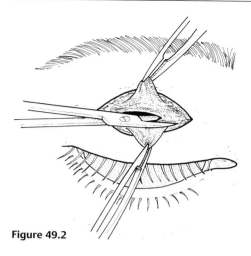

Figure 49.2

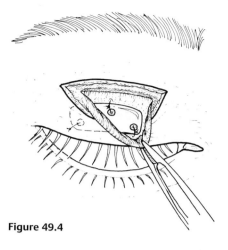

Figure 49.4

10. Use scissors to open the orbicularis muscle horizontally slightly wider than the width of the gold weight (**Fig. 49.2**).

Note: The orbital septum may or may not be open, depending on the specific anatomy of the patient.

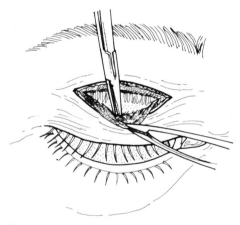

Figure 49.3

11. Dissect inferiorly and beneath the orbicularis onto the surface of the tarsal plate (**Fig. 49.3**).
    a. Dissect until lash follicles are first seen.
    b. Do not dissect any more medially or laterally than required to minimize risk of ptosis.
12. Place weight centrally onto tarsal plate. Orient the gold weight horizontally, and place rounded end of the weight inferiorly (toward lashes).

13. Place three 6–0 polypropylene sutures through partial-thickness tarsus and into the holes in the gold weight (**Fig. 49.4**).
    a. Evert lid to be certain bites are not full thickness and abrading cornea.
    b. Inferior edge of weight should rest 4 mm above lid margin.
14. Close orbicularis with buried 6–0 Vicryl suture.
15. Close skin with 6–0 Prolene or 6–0 fast-absorbing plain gut.
16. Apply ointment to eye and wound.

Postoperative Procedure

1. Apply antibiotic ointment to eye and wound twice per day for 2 days.
2. Use ice pack to decrease swelling.
3. Elevate head of bed 30 degrees to decrease swelling.

Complications

1. Ptosis
2. Exposure of weight
3. Infection
4. Allergy to gold implant
5. Weight migration

50

Ectropion Repair

■ Introduction

Involutional ectropion results, in general, from aging changes of the lid and, in particular, from generalized laxity and descent of the eyelid structures and midface. Seventh nerve palsy will manifest a similar but more pronounced appearance. Numerous procedures and variations have been designed to correct ectropion. The specific operation undertaken depends on the anatomic etiology of a particular case and the personal preference of the surgeon.

Following are some of the commonly used procedures for correcting routine cases of involutional, cicatricial, and paralytic ectropion.

Indications

Repair of Punctal Ectropion

This technique may be used alone or in combination with another ectropion procedure to reposition a punctum that is everted from the globe secondary to medial ectropion.

Full-Thickness Eyelid Shortening by Wedge Resection

Horizontal lid shortening (described in Chapter 46, "Repair of Full Thickness Lid Margin Lacerations and Defects") is easy to carry out and is occasionally useful for central lower lid ectropion. It may be combined with a blepharoplasty-type skin excision in cases where, in addition to horizontal lid laxity, excess skin is present (see Chapter 52).

Full-Thickness Eyelid Shortening by Lateral Tarsal Strip

The lateral tarsal strip technique is indicated for generalized ectropion and horizontal lid laxity, lateral ectropion, and ectropion with lateral canthal tendon laxity. It may be used in

cases of seventh nerve palsy—although the long-term result varies from patient to patient.

Treatments of Cicatricial Ectropion

Patients with ectropion and vertical deficiency of skin may benefit from full-thickness eyelid shortening with midface elevation with or full-thickness eyelid shortening with skin graft skin. These patients may have a general history of actinic damage and skin cancer. Some patients have a specific history of removal of lower eyelid or cheek skin cancers, prior lower eyelid transcutaneous blepharoplasty, or facial trauma. In most cases, examination shows smooth, relatively unwrinkled skin. Pull the ectropic lateral eyelid up to a normal position at the lateral canthal angle. If there is significant pull at the angle of the mouth or below, there may be descent of the midfacial structures or deficiency of skin. Cicatricial ectropion is worse in upgaze, as the skin cannot allow superior movement of the eyelids.

Midface Elevation with Tarsal Strip to Treat Involutional and Cicatricial Ectropion

Select patients with ectropion may benefit from elevations of the midfacial structures together with full-thickness eyelid tightening.

Skin Graft with Tarsal Strip to Treat Cicatricial Ectropion

Patients with ectropion and vertical deficiency of skin may benefit from full-thickness eyelid shortening with skin graft skin. This treatment is usually curative, but the mismatch of skin between the donor and recipient beds may be objectionable to some patients.

For all procedures, discontinue aspirin and nonsteroidal anti-inflammatory agents for 10 days before surgery. Discontinue warfarin 2–3 days preoperatively, if medically possible.

Query patient on bleeding tendencies. A useful screening question is asking if the patient had unusual bleeding after dental extraction. Obtain hematological evaluation if bleeding tendency is suspected.

■ Repair of Punctal Ectropion

Indications

See Introduction section at the beginning of this chapter.

1. Treatment of epiphora secondary to everted inferior punctum.
2. May be combined with other ectropion procedures in cases with prominent punctal eversion.

Preoperative Procedure

See Chapter 3.

1. Document medical indications for surgery.
2. For oculoplastic procedures, discontinue aspirin and nonsteroidal anti-inflammatory agents for 10 days before surgery. Discontinue warfarin 2–3 days preoperatively, if medically possible.

Instrumentation

- Lacrimal probe
- Scleral shield
- Toothed forceps
- Chalazion clamp
- Needle holder
- Sutures (7–0 Vicryl)
- Scalpel (e.g., # 15 Bard-Parker blade)
- Scissors (e.g., Westcott).

Operative Procedure

1. Apply topical anesthetic.
2. Subconjunctival infiltration in the medial lower eyelid beneath the canaliculus:
   a. 50:50 mixture of lidocaine 2% plus 1:100,000 epinephrine and 0.75% bupivacaine.
3. Prep and drape in the usual sterile manner.
4. Place scleral shield.
5. Place "0" lacrimal probe in inferior canaliculus to identify canaliculus during procedure.
6. Evert lid with chalazion clamp or forceps. (Plate of chalazion clamp may facilitate initial incisions.)

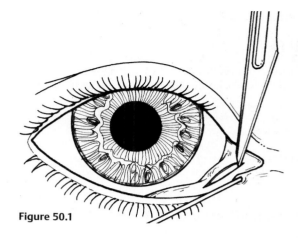

Figure 50.1

7. Excise a horizontal ellipse of tissue including conjunctiva and a portion of the underlying lid retractor complex using scalpel or scissors (**Fig. 50.1**).
   a. Center excision below punctum.
   b. Apex of superior incision should be 2 mm below inferior canaliculus.
   c. Excision should be ~5 mm long and 3 mm wide.
8. Remove lacrimal probe.

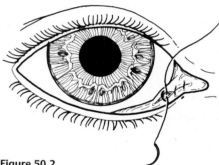

Figure 50.2

9. Close defect with interrupted 7–0 Vicryl sutures (**Fig. 50.2**).
   a. Pass suture deep enough to imbricate the edges of the tarsus and lower lid retractors.
   b. Bury knots in wound.
10. Remove scleral shield.
11. Apply antibiotic ointment.
12. Apply chilled compress.

Postoperative Procedure

1. Apply ice packs to decrease swelling.
2. Elevate head of bed 30 degrees to decrease swelling.
3. Apply topical antibiotic ointment twice daily for 3 days or until patient has no conjunctival discomfort or irritation.

Complications

■ Overcorrection
■ Undercorrection

■ Ectropion Repair: Lateral Tarsal Strip

Indications

See Introduction section at the beginning of this chapter.

■ Generalized ectropion with horizontal lid laxity.
■ Lateral ectropion.
■ Ectropion secondary to seventh nerve palsy.

Preoperative Procedure

See Chapter 3.
  Document medical indications for surgery.

Instrumentation

■ Scleral shield
■ Needle holder
■ Sutures (5–0 Dexon on half-circle (SS-2) needle, 6–0 Vicryl, 6–0 Prolene)
■ Scissors (e.g., Stevens)
■ Toothed forceps
■ Blaire retractor or double skin hook
■ Cautery
■ Scalpel with #15 Bard-Parker blade.

Operative Procedure

1. Apply topical anesthetic
2. Subcutaneous and subconjunctival infiltration with a 50:50 mixture of lidocaine 2% plus 1:100,000 epinephrine and 0.75% bupivacaine.
3. Prep and drape in the usual sterile manner.
4. Keep both eyes exposed for comparison during procedure.
5. Place scleral shield.

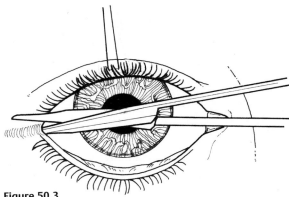

Figure 50.3

6. Perform lateral canthotomy, horizontally dividing the lateral canthal tendon with scissors (**Fig. 50.3**).

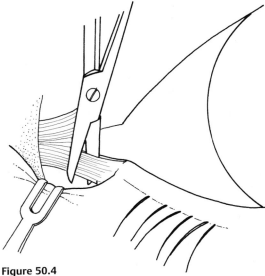

Figure 50.4

7. Divide the inferior limb of lateral canthal tendon (**Fig. 50.4**).
   a. Aim inferotemporally.
   b. Pull laterally on lower lid with forceps and completely release fibers of inferior limb of the canthal tendon with scissors.
   c. When inferior limb of tendon is cut, the lower lid should become markedly loose.
8. Bluntly spread and dissect a preperiosteal pocket just inside the orbital rim, exposing the periosteum (**Fig. 50.5**).
   a. Pocket will determine position of new canthal angle.
   b. Aim to match opposite eye or, if bilateral, to make lateral canthal angle 2 mm higher than medial canthal angle.

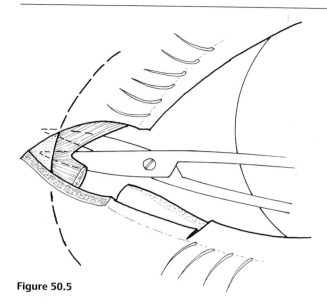

Figure 50.5

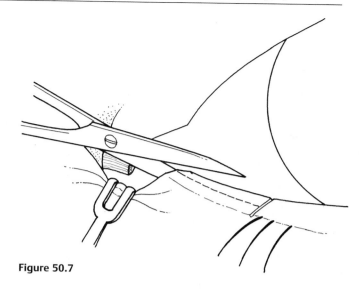

Figure 50.7

9. Pull lower lid temporally into the lateral preperiosteal pocket.
   a. Mark the point at which the lid meets the lateral periosteum. width of necessary lid.
   b. This is the approximate length of the tarsal tongue to be subsequently prepared.

11. Form a flap of skin and orbicularis by incising skin horizontally at gray line with scissors (**Fig. 50.7**).

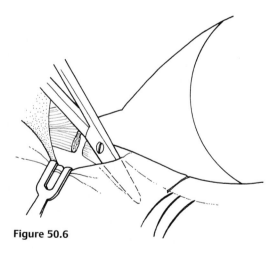

Figure 50.6

10. Bluntly separate skin and orbicularis from tarsus with scissors (**Fig. 50.6**).

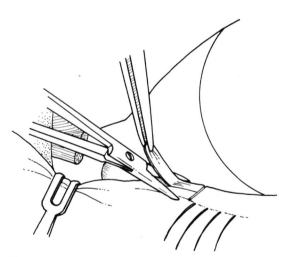

Figure 50.8

12. Shave lid margin over the developing tarsal tongue with scissors (**Fig. 50.8**).
13. Scrape conjunctiva from posterior surface of tarsus with a scalpel.

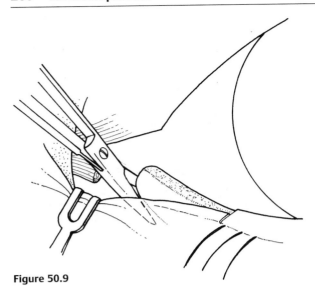

Figure 50.9

14. Finish forming tarsal strip by incising horizontally just below tarsus for length of the strip (**Fig. 50.9**).

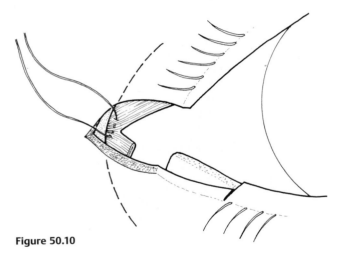

Figure 50.10

15. Place double-armed sutures of 5–0 Dexon through periosteum of orbital rim (**Fig. 50.10**).
    a. Use a cotton-tipped swab or have the assistant use a double skin hook or rake to retract the tissues medially away from the periosteum.
    b. It is helpful to engage the periosteum with the needle and then pull it anteriorly (toward the skin) rather than attempting to rotate the needle through the tissues.

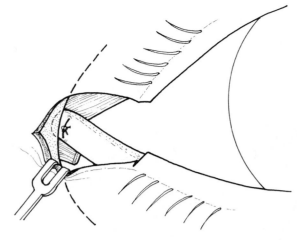

Figure 50.11

16. Bring double-armed sutures through the tarsal strip and tie in slip knot. Check tension of the eyelid. Tighten or loosen knot as needed before final throws are placed. May fashion additional length of tarsal strip as needed. Tie knot securely (**Fig. 50.11**).

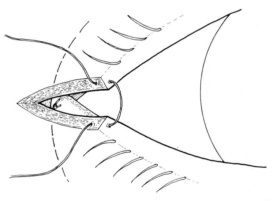

Figure 50.12

17. Reform lateral canthal angle with horizontal mattress suture of 6–0 Prolene between upper eyelid and lower eyelid (**Fig. 50.12**).
18. Advance lateral skin and muscle superotemporally.
19. Excise lateral dog ear.
20. Suture muscle layer with 6–0 Vicryl with attention to bury the knot through the tarsal strip.
21. Sutures the skin with 6–0 Prolene or 6–0 fast-absorbing plain gut.
22. Remove scleral shield.
23. Apply antibiotic ointment to suture line.
24. Cover wound with chilled eye pad.

■ Midface Lift

Indications

See Introduction section at the beginning of this chapter.

■ Cicatricial ectropion (especially following previous cosmetic lower blepharoplasty when trying to avoid skin graft)
■ Facial nerve palsy
■ Cosmetic elevation of midface and cheek fat pads.

Preoperative Procedure

See Chapter 3.

1. Document medical indications for surgery.
2. For oculoplastic procedures, discontinue aspirin and nonsteroidal anti-inflammatory agents for 10 days before surgery. Discontinue warfarin 2–3 days preoperatively, if medically possible.
3. Query patient about bleeding tendencies. A useful screening question is asking if the patient had unusual bleeding after dental extraction. Obtain hematological evaluation if bleeding tendency is suspected.

Instrumentation

■ Scleral shield
■ Needle holder
■ Sutures (4–0 pds)
■ Jaeger lid plate
■ Scissors (e.g., Stevens)
■ Freer periosteal elevator
■ Electrocautery with needle tip (e.g., straight Colorado needle)
■ Senne retractor
■ Scalpel (#15 Bard-Parker blade)
■ Headlight

Operative Procedure

1. Apply topical anesthetic.
2. Infiltrate with a 50:50 mixture of lidocaine 2% plus 1:100,000 epinephrine and 0.75% bupivacaine. Inject subcutaneously and subconjunctivally at lateral canthus, into lower fornix, along infraorbital foramen and deeply across entire cheek.
3. Prep and drape in the usual sterile manner. Keep both eyes exposed for comparison during procedure.

4. Place scleral shield.
5. Perform lateral canthotomy, horizontally dividing the lateral canthal tendon with scissors (**Fig. 50.3**).
6. Divide the inferior limb of lateral canthal tendon (**Fig. 50.4**).
   a. Aim ~45 degrees inferiorly from canthotomy.
   b. Pull laterally on lower lid with rake retractor or forceps and directly palpate fibers of inferior limb with scissors before cutting.
   c. Incise tendon with scissors.
   d. When inferior limb of tendon is cut, the lower lid should become much more lax.

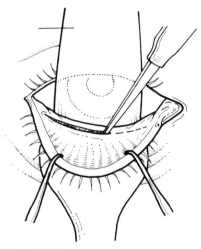

Figure 50.13

7. Evert eyelid with use of two double hooks held by assistant at inferior tarsal border (**Fig. 50.13**).
8. Incise across the conjunctival and lower eyelid retractors, 2 mm below lower tarsal border using cutting cautery (**Fig. 50.13**).
9. Place traction suture through the lower eyelid retractors, and use Stevens scissors to dissect just anterior to the orbital septum, to the level of the orbital rim.
10. Continue the suborbicularis plane of dissection past the orbital rim for 4–5 mm.
11. Use cutting cautery or #15 Bard-Parker blade to incise down to the bone of the orbital rim, leaving a cuff of 3–4 mm of intact tissue inferior to the arcus marginalis.

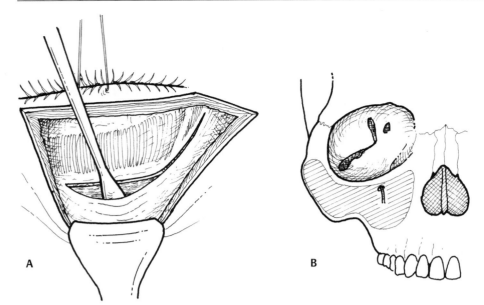

Figure 50.14

12. Perform subperiosteal dissection across the malar eminence using freer periosteal elevator (**Fig. 50.14A**). Dissect lateral to the infraorbital nerve (avoid compromise of this nerve) (**Fig. 50.14B**).

Note: To achieve greater elevation, dissection medial to the infraorbital nerve may be indicated.

13. Use cautery or a #15 Bard-Parker blade to incise the periosteum at medial, inferior, and lateral aspects of dissection to allow cheek to ride upward.
    a. Use a retractor or your finger to widely release and stretch the cheek tissues.
14. Suspend the periosteum of the cheek to the cuff of remaining tissue at the orbital rim and to the lateral orbital periosteum using three sutures of 4–0 pds (**Fig. 50.15**).
15. Complete lateral tarsal strip repair (see Ectropion Repair: Lateral Tarsal Strip section in this chapter, p. 258).

16. Apply antibiotic ointment to suture line.
17. Cover eye with chilled eye pad.

Postoperative Procedure

1. Apply chilled compresses for 24 hours.
2. Elevate bed to 30 degrees to decrease swelling.
3. Apply eye ointment to wounds for 5 days.
4. Expect weeks to months of cheek swelling.

Complications

1. Numbness across cheek and upper gums (V 2 injury)
2. Facial nerve weakness (VII injury)
3. Prolonged swelling
4. Pucker of skin at site of cheek fixation sutures

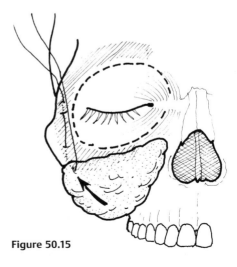
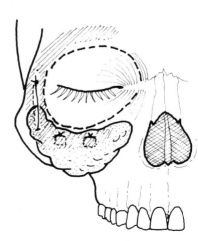

Figure 50.15

■ Skin Graft

Indications

See Introduction section at the beginning of this chapter.

■ Cicatricial ectropion due to skin loss (e.g., trauma, skin cancer).
■ Cicatricial ectropion due to skin shrinkage (e.g., actinic damage, cicatrizing skin disease).

Preoperative Procedure

See Chapter 3.

1. Document medical indications for surgery.
2. For oculoplastic procedures, discontinue aspirin and nonsteroidal anti-inflammatory agents for 10 days before surgery. Discontinue warfarin 2–3 days preoperatively, if medically possible.
3. Query patient about bleeding tendencies. A useful screening question is asking if the patient had unusual bleeding after dental extraction. Obtain hematological evaluation if bleeding tendency is suspected.

Instrumentation

■ Scleral shield
■ Needle holder
■ Sutures (6–0 fast absorbing gut, 6–0 silk)
■ Scissors (e.g., Stevens)
■ Toothed forceps
■ Blaire retractor or double skin hook
■ Cautery
■ Scalpel (e.g., #15 Bard-Parker blade)

Operative Procedure

1. Apply topical anesthetic.
2. Infiltration with a 50:50 mixture of lidocaine 2% plus 1:100,000 epinephrine and 0.75% bupivacaine.
   a. Inject subcutaneously and subconjunctivally at lateral canthus, lower eyelid and potential graft sites (e.g., behind ear, eyelid, supraclavicular).
3. Prep and drape; include all potential donor sites.
4. Keep both eyes exposed for comparison during procedure.
5. Place scleral shield.
6. Place 6–0 silk traction suture across eyelid margin centrally just posterior to the lash line. Clamp to forehead drape.

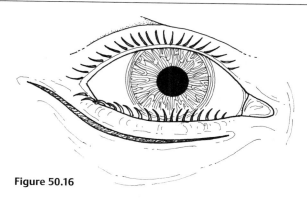

Figure 50.16

7. Make subciliary incision across eyelid and into lateral canthal area (**Fig. 50.16**).

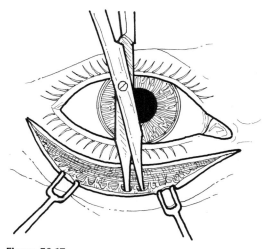

Figure 50.17

8. Dissect skin only flap to level of orbital rim inferiorly (**Fig. 50.17**).
9. *Optional (but usually required):* Perform full-thickness shortening by:
   a. Excising and repairing a pentagon of lower eyelid, at the junction of the middle third and lateral third of the eyelid (see Chapter 46, "Repair of Full-Thickness Lid Margin Lacerations and Defects"). Or,
   b. Performing lateral tarsal strip (see Chapter 50, "Ectropion Repair: Lateral Tarsal Strip").
10. Place lower eyelid in normal anatomic position. Measure horizontal and vertical dimensions of defect.
11. Graft should be 25% longer vertically than measured.
12. Harvest graft from appropriate site (e.g., upper eyelid, retroauricular, supraclavicular).
    a. Eyelid skin is the best match. The technique is similar to upper eyelid blepharoplasty (see Chapter 52, "Blepharoplasty").
13. Do not open orbital septum (reduces chances of bleeding). Orbicularis muscle may be either left in donor site or removed with donor skin.

14. If entire width of upper eyelid is not needed, leave medial upper eyelid undisturbed (less chance of problems with closure).
15. Remove subcutaneous elements (including orbicularis muscle) from posterior aspect of skin graft.

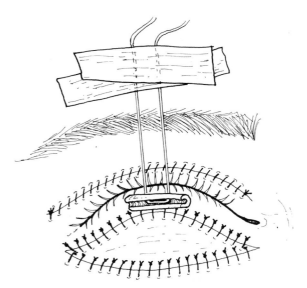

Figure 50.18

16. Sew into position with 6–0 fast-absorbing cat gut or silk with running and interrupted sutures (**Fig. 50.18**).
17. Tape eyelid marginal suture to forehead (keeps skin graft on stretch (**Fig. 50.18**).
18. Dress with ophthalmic ointment, Telfa dressing, and pressure patch.

Postoperative Procedure

1. Apply ice packs to decrease swelling.
2. Elevate head of bed to 30 degrees to decrease swelling.
3. Remove patch in 2–3 days.
4. Remove sutures in 7 days.

Complications

1. Undercorrection
2. Failure of graft
3. Mismatch between graft and recipient tissues
4. Hematoma
5. Infection

51

Entropion Repair

■ Introduction

Involutional entropion results from aging changes in the lid. Such changes include: (1) horizontal lid laxity, (2) lower lid retractor disinsertion and laxity, and (3) overriding of the pretarsal by preseptal orbicularis. Numerous procedures and variations have been designed to correct entropion by ameliorating one or more of these pathological conditions. The specific operation undertaken will depend upon the individual case and the personal preference of the surgeon.

The less commonly encountered entropion due to cicatricial conjunctival disease (e.g., cicatricial ocular pemphigoid) will require a lid splitting procedure or mucous membrane graft.

Note: These chapters will deal only with the surgical correction of involutional entropion. The management of cicatricial entropion will not be discussed.

The following describes the most commonly used procedures for the correction of routine cases of involutional entropion.

Indications

Entropion sutures prevent overriding of the orbicularis while reinforcing the lower lid retractors. This technique is useful in cases where permanent repair may not be necessary (e.g., spastic entropion) or where a simple procedure is desired (e.g., debilitated patients). Entropion sutures may also be used as an adjunct to other lid procedures.

Horizontal Lid Splitting and Lid Shortening

Combined horizontal lid splitting and lid shortening is useful for entropion with horizontal lid laxity. This technique tightens the lid while reinforcing the lower lid retractors and preventing orbicularis override.

Reinsertion of Lower Eyelid Retractors (with full-thickness horizontal tightening)

Most involutional entropion results from horizontal eyelid laxity and generalized laxity or dehiscence of the lower eyelid retractors from the normal tarsal attachments. Tightening of the lower eyelid retractors may be accompanied by horizontal shortening of the eyelid by tarsal strip procedure or by wedge resection.

■ Entropion Sutures

Indications

See Introduction in this chapter.

- Temporary correction of mild or intermittent ectropion (e.g., spastic ectropion)
- Correction of ectropion in debilitated patients who are unable to undergo a more complex and time-consuming procedure
- May be used as an adjunct to other entropion procedures.

Preoperative Procedure

See Chapter 3.

1. Discontinue aspirin and nonsteroidal anti-inflammatory agents for 10 days before surgery. Discontinue warfarin 2–3 days preoperatively, if medically possible.
2. Query patient about bleeding tendencies. A useful screening question is asking if the patient had unusual bleeding after dental extraction. Obtain hematological evaluation if bleeding tendency is suspected.

Instrumentation

- Suture (double-armed 4–0 chromic gut with long needles)
- Needle holder
- Toothed forceps

Operative Procedure

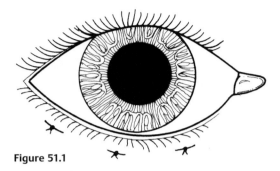

Figure 51.1

1. Locate suture placement (**Fig. 51.1**):
   a. Place medialmost mattress suture at junction of medial third and lateral two thirds of lower lid (avoid eversion of punctum).
   b. Proceed laterally, separating each mattress suture by ~5 mm, for a total of three sutures.
   c. The lateralmost suture should end ~5 mm from the lateral canthus.

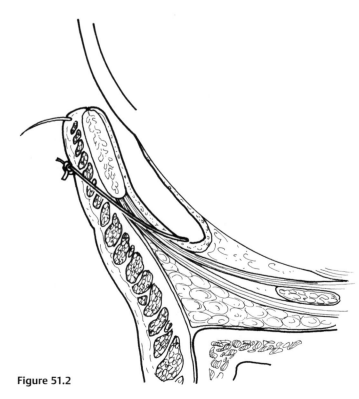

Figure 51.2

2. Technique of suture placement (**Fig. 51.2**):
   a. Grasp lid with forceps and pass each end of double-armed 4–0 chromic gut suture
      i. through conjunctiva deep in inferior fornix
      ii. upward toward inferior edge of tarsus, imbricating lower lid retractors and passing just below inferior edge of tarsus, and
      iii. out through skin ~2 mm below lash line (pull skin inferiorly when passing needle through it).
   b. Separate the two arms of the suture by 3 mm.
   c. Titrate tightness of suture to provide for slight over-correction (slight ectropion).
3. Mechanism of suture action.
   a. Formation of adherence of pretarsal orbicularis to lower eyelid retractors preventing the preseptal muscle from overriding the pretarsal orbicularis.
   b. Tightening of lower lid retractors and transfer of their pull to the anterosuperior tarsus, causing tarsal eversion.
4. Apply antibiotic ointment into lower conjunctival fornix and onto external sutures .

Postoperative Procedure

1. Apply ice packs to decrease swelling.
2. Keep head of bed elevated 30 degrees to decrease swelling.
3. Apply antibiotic ointment twice daily to suture line.
4. Remove sutures in 2 to 3 weeks.

Complications

1. Undercorrection
2. Loss of correction with time

Note: Entropion sutures may be repeated as necessary.

■ Horizontal Lid Splitting/Lid Shortening

Indications

See Introduction section at the beginning of this chapter.

1. Entropion with horizontal lid laxity.
2. Horizontal lid splitting and reinsertion of the lower lid retractors, without lid shortening, may be performed in cases of entropion without horizontal lid laxity.

Preoperative Procedure

See Chapter 3.

1. For oculoplastic procedures, discontinue aspirin and nonsteroidal anti-inflammatory agents for 10 days before surgery. Discontinue warfarin 2–3 days preoperatively, if medically possible.

2. Query patient about bleeding tendencies. A useful screening question is asking if the patient had unusual bleeding after dental extraction. Obtain hematological evaluation if bleeding tendency is suspected.

Instrumentation

- Scleral shield
- Needle holder
- Sutures (4–0 silk, 6–0 Vicryl, 6–0 silk, double-armed 4–0 chromic gut or 5–0 silk)
- Toothed forceps
- Tissue scissors (e.g., Westcott, Stevens)
- Scalpel with #15 Bard-Parker blade

Operative Procedure

1. Apply topical anesthetic.
2. Inject local infiltrative anesthetic solution.
   a. Subcutaneous infiltration with a 50:50 mixture of lidocaine 2% plus 1:100,000 epinephrine and 0.75% bupivacaine.
   b. Inject subcutaneously and subconjunctivally at lateral canthus.
3. Prep and drape. Keep both eyes exposed for comparison during procedure.
4. Place scleral shield.
5. Place 4–0 silk upper lid suture for lid retraction during procedure.
   a. Position ~2–3 mm above lid margin
   b. Place suture through skin and partial-thickness tarsus.
6. Perform a full-thickness vertical incision through the lid centrally with scissors, extending incision just below tarsal plate.

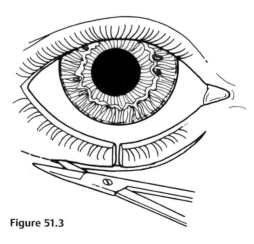

Figure 51.3

7. Perform a full-thickness horizontal incision just below the tarsus (**Fig. 51.3**).

   a. Extend medially from the previously performed vertical incision to a point ~3 mm lateral to the lower punctum.
   b. Extend laterally from the vertical incision to the level of the lateral canthus, keeping incision horizontal (do not follow upward arc of lid contour).
8. Secure hemostasis with cautery.
9. Overlap the lateral and medial lid flaps to estimate the required amount of lid shortening.
   a. Mark the section of lid to be resected on the lateral flap.
   b. May incise lid margin with a scalpel or crush lid margin with forceps to mark distance.

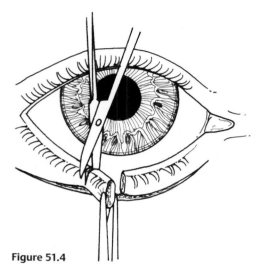

Figure 51.4

10. Resect the measured portion of lid flap with scissors (**Fig. 51.4**).
11. Close the two lid flaps (see Chapter 46, "Repair of Full-Thickness Lid Margin Lacerations and Defects").
    a. Approximate tarsus with two or three interrupted, partial-thickness, absorbable sutures (e.g., 6–0 Vicryl).
    b. Approximate lid margin with interrupted sutures (e.g., 6–0 silk) through (1) gray line, (2) lash line, and (3) posterior lid margin.
12. Excise any excess skin and orbicularis below horizontal incision.

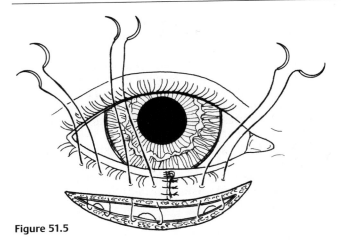

Figure 51.5

13. Close horizontal incision and reinsert lower lid retractors with double-armed 4–0 chromic gut or 5–0 silk lid eversion sutures (**Fig. 51.5**).
    a. Identify retractors by observing their movement as patient looks downward.
    b. Pass each end of suture (1) through conjunctiva ~2 mm below lower margin of incision, (2) through lower lid retractors, (3) through superior margin of incision just anterior to tarsus, and (4) out through skin ~2 mm below lash line.
    c. Place three such sutures through the incision laterally, centrally, and medially (avoid eversion of punctum).
    d. Titrate tightness of sutures to slightly evert lid.

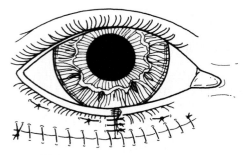

Figure 51.6

14. Close skin with running or interrupted 6–0 or 7–0 nylon sutures (**Fig. 51.6**).
15. Remove scleral shield.
16. Apply antibiotic ointment to suture line.
17. Apply dressing.

Postoperative Procedure

1. Apply ice packs to decrease swelling.
2. Elevate head of bed to 30 degrees to decrease swelling.
3. Apply antibiotic ointment twice daily to suture line.
4. Remove skin sutures in 5 to 7 days.
5. Remove lid eversion sutures in 2 weeks.

Complications

1. Undercorrection and overcorrection
2. Hematoma
3. Infection
4. Lid notching

■ Entropion Repair with Insertion of Lower Eyelid Retractors

Indications

See Introduction section earlier in this chapter.

- ■ Involutional or "spastic" entropion with horizontal lid laxity
- ■ Absence of cicatricial conjunctival component

Preoperative Procedure

See Chapter 3.

1. For oculoplastic procedures, discontinue aspirin and nonsteroidal anti-inflammatory agents for 10 days before surgery. Discontinue warfarin 2–3 days preoperatively, if medically possible.
2. Query patient about bleeding tendencies. A useful screening question is asking if the patient had unusual bleeding after dental extraction. Obtain hematological evaluation if bleeding tendency is suspected.

Instrumentation

- ▩ Scleral shield
- ▩ Needle holder
- ▩ Sutures (6–0 Prolene, 6–0 fast-absorbing cat gut)
- ▩ Scissors (e.g., Westcott, Stevens)
- ▩ Toothed forceps
- ▩ Blaire retractor or double skin hook
- ▩ Desmarres retractor
- ▩ Scalpel (e.g, #15 Bard-Parker blade)

Operative Procedure

1. Apply topical anesthetic.
2. Inject local infiltrative anesthetic solution.
   a. Subcutaneous infiltration with a 50:50 mixture of lidocaine 2% plus 1:100,000 epinephrine and 0.75% bupivacaine.
   b. Inject subcutaneously and subconjunctivally at lateral canthus.
3. Prep and drape.
4. Keep both eyes exposed for comparison during procedure.
5. Place scleral shield.

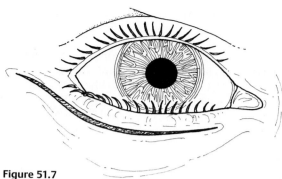

Figure 51.7

6. Incise skin with scalpel across lower eyelid from punctum to beyond the lateral canthus (**Fig. 51.7**).

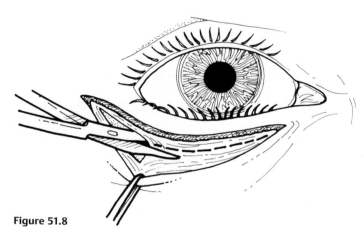

Figure 51.8

7. Open orbicularis muscle horizontally (**Fig. 51.8**).

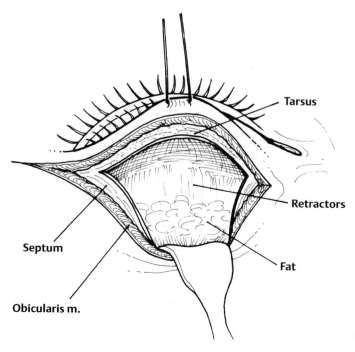

Figure 51.9

8. Button hole and then open orbital septum horizontally, and retract orbital fat inferiorly with Desmarres retractor to expose white lower eyelid retractors (**Fig. 51.9**).

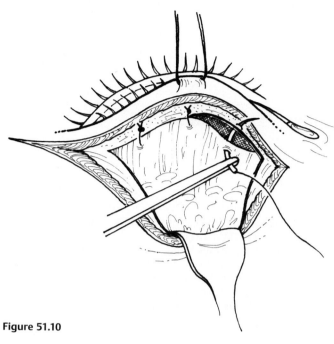

Figure 51.10

9. Inspect the lower eyelid retractors.
   a. If disinserted, reattach the free edge to the tarsal plate with three interrupted sutures of 6–0 Prolene (**Fig. 51.10**).
   b. If not disinserted, advance the retractors to the tarsal plate superiorly 4–6 mm.
10. If the lower eyelid is horizontally lax (as is usually the case):
   a. Excise and repair a pentagon of lower eyelid, at the junction of the middle third and lateral third of the eyelid (see Chapter 46, "Repair of Full-Thickness Lid Margin Lacerations and Defects"); or
   b. Perform lateral tarsal strip (see Chapter 50, "Ectropion Repair: Lateral Tarsal Strip").

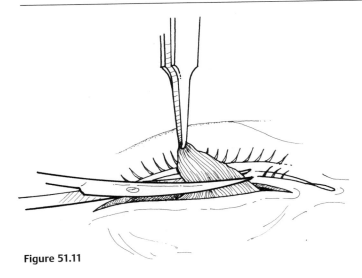

Figure 51.11

11. Excise a strip of orbicularis from the inferior aspect of the incision (**Fig. 51.11**).
    a. This weakens overriding orbicularis and helps create adherence to keep entropion from recurring.
12. May resect skin from inferior aspect of wound.
    a. Drape lower eyelid skin over wound.
    b. Have the patient open the mouth and look up.
    c. Conservatively trim excess skin.

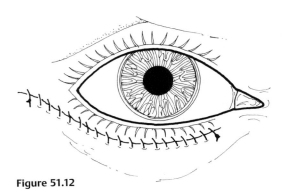

Figure 51.12

13. Suture skin with 6–0 fast absorbing plain gut or Prolene (**Fig. 51.12**).
14. Apply antibiotic ointment to suture line.

Operative Procedure: Transconjunctival Entropion Repair

1. Make an incision with scissors or cutting cautery inferior to the tarsal plate across the entire lower eyelid.
2. Grasp the lower eyelid retractors and conjunctiva as a unit and gently tease them from the orbicularis muscle.
3. Dissect the lower eyelid retractors from the conjunctiva for several millimeters.
4. Excise a strip of pretarsal orbicularis across the lower eyelid using scissors or cutting cautery.
5. Sew the lower eyelid retractors to the inferior aspect of the tarsal plate using buried 6–0 Vicryl sutures.
6. Perform tarsal strip procedure if indicated (see Chapter 50, "Ectropion Repair: Lateral Tarsal Strip").

Postoperative Procedure

1. Apply ice packs to decrease swelling.
2. Keep head of bed elevated 30 degrees to decrease swelling.
4. Apply antibiotic ointment twice daily to suture line.
5. Remove skin sutures in 5 to 7 days.

Complications

1. Undercorrection and overcorrection
2. Hematoma
3. Infection
4. Lid notching

52

Blepharoplasty

■ Upper Eyelid

Indications

- Removal of redundant skin that is obstructing visual field or causing symptoms of heaviness and fatigue
- Cosmetic improvement
- Upper blepharoplasty may be used as an adjunct to ptosis surgery in patients with lid droop and excess upper lid skin.
- Upper blepharoplasty may be used to harvest skin for reconstructive skin graft.

Preoperative Procedure

See Chapter 3.

1. Complete lid and eye examination to determine detailed operative plan.
2. Measure position of lid crease. (If lid crease is indistinct or malpositioned, placement of supratarsal fixation sutures may be indicated.)
3. Evaluate presence and location of herniated orbital fat. (Cosmetically unacceptable fat prolapse is often located medially.)
4. Evaluate brow position. (A brow lift may be required if brow droop is present.)
5. Evaluate lid position. (A ptosis procedure may be indicated in combination with the blepharoplasty.)
6. Check corneal sensation, corneal staining, Bell phenomenon, and Schirmer test to evaluate potential impact of any postoperative lagophthalmos.
7. Perform a visual field examination to document any field cut (usually superior) secondary to dermatochalasis if required by insurance.
8. Obtain photographs in frontal and side view to document preoperative appearance.

9. Discontinue aspirin and nonsteroidal anti-inflammatory agents for 10 days before surgery. Discontinue warfarin 2–3 days preoperatively, if medically possible.
10. Query patient about bleeding tendencies. A useful screening question is asking if the patient had unusual bleeding after dental extraction. Obtain hematological evaluation if bleeding tendency is suspected.

Instrumentation

- Scleral shield
- Marking pen
- Toothed forceps
- Scalpel (e.g., #15 Bard-Parker blade)
- Stevens scissors
- Westcott scissors
- Cautery
- Needle holder
- Hemostat
- Sutures 6–0 Prolene or 6–0 fast absorbing plain gut

Operative Procedure

1. Mark location of desired lid crease with tissue marking pen usually at the upper border of the tarsal plate.
   a. In general, use the existing lid crease because it is easier to make symmetric marks.

Note: Creases are lower in men than in women, and lower in most Asian individuals than in Caucasians.

   b. The eyelid crease is ~6 mm above lashes at the lateral canthus, 7–9 mm centrally, and 5 mm nasally.

2. Ascertain upper border of planned skin resection, noting the preoperative appearance of eyelids and size of desired eyelid fold. Use one of the following methods:

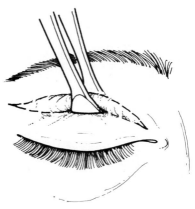

Figure 52.1

a. Place lower tooth of forceps on the premarked lid crease line, pinch excess skin just enough to evert lid margin slightly. Repeat this maneuver over the full extent of the upper lid, marking upper border of skin to be resected with marking pen. (This maneuver suggests the most skin that can be removed without developing lagophthalmos) (**Fig. 52.1**).

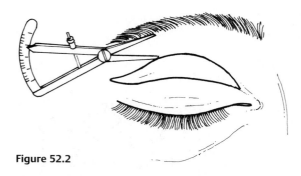

Figure 52.2

b. Measure from inferior aspect of eyebrow to upper aspect of planned excision on each side. In functional blepharoplasty, it is rare to leave less than 8–10 mm from inferior brow to upper aspect of the incision. In cosmetic blepharoplasty, leaving 12–17 mm of skin is typical. Note, by inspection and palpation, the junction of thin eyelid skin and thicker skin below eyebrow; do not extend excision into the thicker skin (**Fig. 52.2**).

3. Extend marks medially to level of superior punctum and temporally beyond lateral canthus.

a. Lateral extent of blepharoplasty is determined by redundancy of skin beyond canthus. If skin is to be excised laterally, gently slope excision superiorly from the canthus following the normal skin crease pattern.

b. Angle upward if extending medial past punctum to avoid webbing.

4. Apply topical anesthetic.

5. Subcutaneous infiltration with a 50:50 mixture of lidocaine 2% plus 1:100,000 epinephrine and 0.75% bupivacaine.

6. Prep and drape (keep full face exposed for comparison during procedure).

7. Place scleral shield.

8. Incise skin along marks with scalpel.

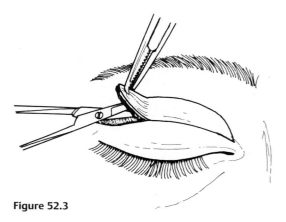

Figure 52.3

9. Use Westcott scissors, Stevens scissors, cutting cautery, or CO_2 laser to remove a skin muscle flap along the marked lines, exposing the orbital septum (**Fig. 52.3**). (CO_2 laser requires metal eye shields for patients, protective lenses for all operating room personnel, avoidance of supplemental oxygen.)

10. If desired, the skin and muscle may be removed as separate layers.

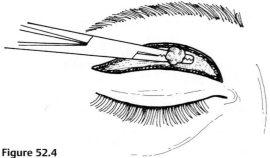

Figure 52.4

11. Remove prolapsed orbital fat (**Fig. 52.4**).

Note: Not all patients have prolapsing orbital fat. Overzealous removal of fat tends to make the lids look overly surgical and can make the patient look aged.

a. Open the orbital septum horizontally to expose prolapsing orbital fat. Keep the incision relatively high in the preseptal area to avoid violating the levator aponeurosis.

b. Apply gentle pressure over the lower lid to prolapse fat from the wound. To prevent hemorrhage, avoid direct traction on orbital fat.

c. Clamp fat at its base with hemostat.

d. Excise fat over hemostat (scalpel or Westcott scissors).

e. Cauterize stump.

f. Before unclamping the hemostat, grasp the fat under the clamp with toothed forceps.

g. Release the hemostat and, securing the fat with forceps, inspect for any bleeding and cauterize as necessary.

h. Release the fat, allowing it to retract back into the orbit.

12. Secure hemostasis with cautery.

13. Close wound in single layer.

a. Do not suture the septum back together.

b. *Optional:* Reform or enhance eyelid crease with interrupted sutures.

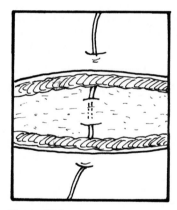

Figure 52.5

i. Place ~4 supratarsal fixation sutures to enhance lid crease (**Fig. 52.5**).

ii. Use 6–0 Prolene or Vicryl.

iii. Technique.

   1. Enter skin near cut edge.

   2. Pass suture through the levator aponeurosis in the location of the desired lid crease (near lower border of wound).

   3. Exit through the apposing cut edge of the skin.

iv. Check contour of lid crease and lid margin, replacing sutures as necessary.

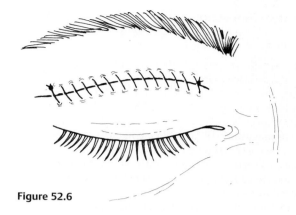

Figure 52.6

  v. Close skin with running 6–0 sutures (**Fig. 52.6**).

c. *Optional:* Reform or enhance eyelid crease with running skin closure.

   i. Run skin suture across eyelid.

   ii. Pick up wisps of levator aponeurosis or tarsus with every other running bite.

14. Remove scleral shield.

15. Apply topical antibiotic ointment to suture line.

Postoperative Procedure

1. Apply ice packs to decrease swelling.
2. Keep head of bed elevated 30 degrees to decrease swelling.
3. Apply antibiotic ointment to suture line twice daily.
4. Remove skin sutures in 4 to 6 days.

Complications

1. Orbital hemorrhage with possibility of consequent blindness
2. Exposure keratopathy secondary to lagophthalmos
3. Malpositioned or indistinct lid crease
4. Ptosis secondary to levator damage

■ Lower Eyelid

Indications

■ Cosmetically objectionable prolapse of lower eyelid fat.

■ Lower transconjunctival blepharoplasty has minimal risk of postoperative lower eyelid retraction compared with external (transcutaneous) lower blepharoplasty.

■ Lower blepharoplasty may be combined with ectropion or entropion repairs by lateral tarsal strip or eyelid wedge resection.

■ Lower blepharoplasty may be combined with laser resurfacing procedures (see Chapter 53) or pinch removal of lower lid skin (described later).

Preoperative Procedure

See Chapter 3.

1. A complete lid and eye examination will determine the detailed operative plan.
2. Evaluate lower eyelid position (a tarsal strip or other canthal procedure may be indicated for ectropion or horizontal laxity).
3. Evaluate magnitude of fat prolapse in each of three fat-containing compartments.
4. Evaluate skin excess (patients with redundant skin or lines may be candidates for skin pinch or laser resurfacing procedure).
5. Evaluate midfacial and cheek anatomy (may be candidate for midfacelift).
6. If possible, discontinue aspirin and nonsteroidal anti-inflammatory agents for 10 days before surgery. Discontinue warfarin preoperatively, if medically possible.
7. Query patient about bleeding tendencies. A useful screening question is asking if the patient had unusual bleeding after dental extraction. Obtain hematological evaluation if bleeding tendency is suspected.
8. Obtain preoperative photographs.

Instrumentation

- Jaeger lid plate
- Cutting cautery with needle tip or CO_2 laser
- Toothed forceps
- Needle driver
- Desmarres retractors
- Fine double skin hooks
- Westcott scissors
- Hemostat
- 4–0 silk traction suture.

Operative Procedure

1. Use local anesthetic or local anesthetic with intravenous sedation.
   a. Apply topical anesthetic to the operative eyes.
   b. Inject local infiltrative anesthetic solution transconjunctivally.
   c. Subconjunctival infiltration with a 50:50 mixture of lidocaine 2% plus 1:100,000 epinephrine and 0.75% bupivacaine.
2. Prep and drape in the usual sterile manner. Keep both eyes exposed for comparison during procedure.
3. Place double skin hooks medially and laterally to retract lower eyelid.

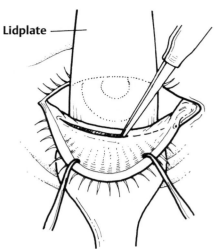

Figure 52.7

4. Using lid plate to retract and protect eye, use cutting cautery to incise 4–5 mm below lower tarsal border from lateral commissure to level of punctum (**Fig. 52.7**).
5. Use lid plate to apply pressure to globe until knuckle of fat prolapses.
6. Remove skin hooks and place Desmarres retractor. Place 4–0 silk traction suture through lower lid retractors and clamp to drape over forehead (brings lower lid fat into view).

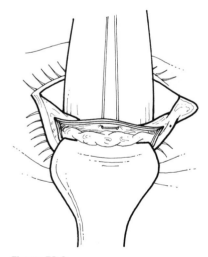

Figure 52.8

7. Incise eyelid tissues along level of incision (through conjunctiva and lower eyelid retractors) until medial, central, and lateral fat pads are fully exposed (**Fig. 52.8**).
   a. *Optional:* Note inferior oblique muscle between medial and central fat pads. Do not violate
   b. May cut arcuate expansion between central and lateral fat pads to aid in exposure.

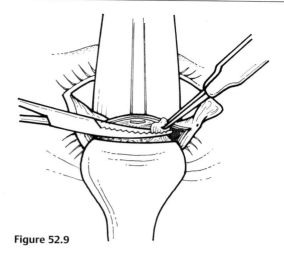

Figure 52.9

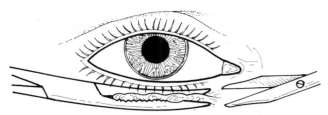

Figure 52.11

8. Excise lower eyelid fat with cautery or with clamp, cut, cauterized technique (see Upper Eyelid section earlier in this chapter) (**Fig. 52.9**).
9. Judge amount of fat to remove from each compartment of each eye.
   a. Remove fat until flush with the orbital rim with gentle pressure to globe.
      1. May have patient sit upright to judge contour of eyelid.
   b. Measure quality of excised fat.
      1. Use marking pen to place five vertical lines on gauze pad to represent six fat pads (medial, central, and lateral fat pads of left and right lower eyelids).

11. *Optional:* May crush 1–3 mm lower lid skin just below ciliary margin with hemostat and excise with Westcott forceps to improve excess skin. Close skin with 6–0 fast-absorbing plain gut or 6–0 Prolene (**Fig. 52.11**).

Postoperative Procedure

1. Apply ice packs to decrease swelling.
2. Keep head of bed elevated 30 degrees to decrease swelling.
4. Apply antibiotic ointment to external suture line (if present) twice daily.
5. Remove skin sutures in 4–6 days.

Complications

1. Lower lid retraction
2. Asymmetry
3. Diplopia
4. Orbital hemorrhage and possibility of subsequent blindness

Lateral Central   Medial

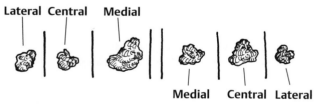

Medial   Central Lateral

Figure 52.10

   2. Place excised fat on marked gauze pad oriented as to which pad was excised (**Fig. 52.10**).
   3. Allows assessment of magnitude of fat removal and symmetry.
   4. Usually equal amounts of fat are removed from similar compartments on each side (e.g., equal amount of fat removed from medial compartments of left and right lower eyelids).
10. Remove traction sutures. Pull up on lower lid retractors (no suture needed). Apply Steri-Strips horizontally across lower eyelid.

53

Laser Skin Resurfacing

Laser resurfacing procedures with CO_2 or erbium laser technology use the ability of these lasers to cause tissue ablation with minimal thermal damage. Superficial skin is ablated and new collagen formation is stimulated. CO_2 technology uses either a pulsed beam or a rapid scanner to deliver fluence greater than 5 J/cm^2 with a tissue-dwelling time well under 1 millisecond. Erbium:YAG lasers rely on a pulsed technology and, because of erbium's greater absorption by water. Erbium:YAG lasers cause minimal thermal damage to underlying tissues.

Although these technologies require similar preoperative, intraoperative, and postoperative skills, the treatment parameters may vary. Safe resurfacing requires consideration of patient skin type, type of laser and settings, and intraoperative observations that require hands-on training and experience.

CO_2 and erbium may be combined with transconjunctival blepharoplasty but not external blepharoplasty because of risk to the skin flap.

The principles described here may be applied to newer techniques of fractional CO_2 resurfacing.

Indications

- Facial rhytidosis
- Periocular hyperpigmentation/actinic changes

Preoperative Procedure

See Chapter 3.

1. Prescribe Retin-A, 0.05% cream to be applied nightly.
2. Prescribe pigment cream (hydroquinone 4% or kojic acid) to select patients nightly for 1 month before treatment.
3. Start antiviral agents to suppress herpetic infection and reactivation. Begin the day before surgery and until epithelialization is complete.
4. Prescribe oral antibiotics from the day before surgery and continue until epithelialization is complete.

Instrumentation

- CO_2 or erbium laser
- Metal eye shields

Operative Procedure

1. Local or general anesthesia.
2. Inject local infiltrative anesthesia (e.g., lidocaine 2% with or without epinephrine) in areas to be treated.
3. Implement laser safety procedures:
   a. Place metal shields beneath eyelids.
   b. Operating room personnel need to wear laser-specific goggles.
   c. Turn off oxygen.
   d. Moist towels around surgical field.
4. Test laser on tongue blade off of surgical field.

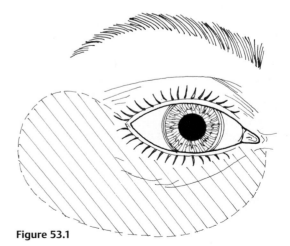

Figure 53.1

5. Mark boundaries for proposed treatment (**Fig. 53.1**).

6. Treat skin with laser at laser-specific parameters (e.g., fluence and number of passes).
7. Laser specifics:
   a. For CO_2 laser:
      i. Wipe accumulated skin products from tissue.
      ii. Perform second pass as clinically indicated.
      iii. Wipe tissues with gauze.
      iv. End point as clinically indicated.
   b. For erbium laser:
      i. Do not remove tissue between passes.
      ii. End point as clinically indicated.
8. Considerations for end point:
   a. Fluence and number of laser passes.
   b. Appearance of skin (e.g., contraction, appearance of "chamois" color).
   c. Patient skin type.
9. Remove scleral shields.
10. Cover treated tissues with Aquaphor ointment.

   Alternatively, Vigilon or other semiocclusive dressing applied.

Postoperative Care

1. Instruct patient to apply cold compresses to treated area with chilled water or saline. When skin is not soaked, apply Aquaphor ointment. Soak and remove crusts at least four times a day. If crusting is persistent, use a solution of 1 tablespoon white vinegar in one quart water solution to soak skin.
2. Continue antibiotics until skin has epithelialized.
3. When skin is epithelialized, begin sun screens and moisturizers.

Complications

1. Ectropion and eyelid retraction
2. Hypopigmentation
3. Hyperpigmentation
4. Scarring
5. Persistent erythema
6. Failure to achieve desired effect
7. Mismatch between treated skin and untreated skin

54

Ptosis Repair

■ Introduction

Numerous approaches to ptosis surgery have been described. The optimal procedure is determined by the etiology, severity, and characteristics of the ptotic eyelids and the personal preference of the surgeon.

Ptosis may be broadly classified:

- Neurogenic (e.g., third nerve palsy, Horner syndrome)
- Myogenic (e.g., most congenital ptosis, chronic progressive ophthalmoplegia)
- Aponeurotic (involutional due to levator aponeurotic thinning, stretching, dehiscence, and disinsertion)
- Mechanical (e.g., eyelid masses)
- "Pseudo"-ptosis (e.g., enophthalmos, phthisis bulbi, contralateral eyelid retraction).

Treatment based on the specific etiology will give the best results.

Obtain a complete history to appropriately classify ptosis. The type and severity of ptosis will dictate the appropriate surgical management. Perform a complete lid and eye examination to determine a detailed operative plan. Evaluation of levator function and magnitude of ptosis are the most important determinants of the type of surgery to be performed.

Preoperative Procedure

1. Evaluate lid position and levator function.
   a. Measure palpebral fissure width.
   b. Ascertain amount of ptosis by measuring the margin to pupillary reflex distance (MRD) (the distance from the upper eyelid margin to the pupillary light reflex).
      i. Mild ptosis: 1–2 mm of lid droop (MRD = 2–3 mm)
      ii. Moderate ptosis: 3 mm of lid droop (MRD = 1 mm)
      iii. Severe ptosis: 4 mm or more (lid margin at or below visual axis)
   c. Measure levator function.
      i. Good: More than 8 mm.
      ii. Fair: 5–7 mm.
      iii. Poor: 4 mm or less.
   d. Note lid position on downgaze.
      i. Congenital ptosis is associated with lid lag.
      ii. In acquired ptosis, lid remains ptotic on downgaze.
   e. Compare lid symmetry.
2. Measure position of lid crease.
   a. A high lid crease suggests disinsertion or dehiscence of the levator aponeurosis.
3. Check corneal sensation, Bell phenomenon, and Schirmer test to evaluate potential impact of any postoperative lagophthalmos.
4. Perform an external examination with eversion of the upper eyelids to look for eyelid or orbital masses.
   a. Pseudoptosis is a consideration (from enophthalmos of involved eye, or proptosis of contralateral eye.
5. Perform neuromuscular examination.
   a. Examine pupils to rule out Horner syndrome or third nerve palsy.
   b. Check extraocular muscle function to rule out third nerve palsy or lack of Bell phenomenon.
   c. Rule out hypotropia as cause of pseudoptosis.
   d. Rule out myasthenia gravis.
6. Perform a visual field examination to document any field cut secondary to ptosis.
7. Take straight-on photographs to document presurgical presence of ptosis.

■ Müller Muscle–Conjunctival Resection

The posterior Müller muscle–conjunctival resection procedure is useful for mild ptosis (less than 3.0 mm lid droop) with good levator function (8 mm or more). It gives excellent symmetry and contour when performed bilaterally.

Indications

- Mild ptosis (less than 3.0 mm lid droopy) with good levator function (10 mm or greater).
- Significant reversal of ptosis with administration of 2.5% phenylephrine hydrochloride in superior conjunctival fornix.

Preoperative Procedure

See Chapter 3.

1. Discontinue aspirin and nonsteroidal anti-inflammatory agents for 10 days before surgery. Discontinue warfarin 2–3 days preoperatively, if medically possible.
2. Query patient about bleeding tendencies. A useful screening question is asking if the patient had unusual bleeding after dental extraction. Obtain hematological evaluation if bleeding tendency is suspected.

Instrumentation

- Scalpel (e.g., #15 Bard-Parker blade)
- Putterman ptosis clamp (Karl-Ilg)
- Sutures (6-0 plain gut)
- Needle holder
- Toothed forceps
- Locking toothed forceps

Operative Procedure

1. Apply topical anesthetic.
2. Anesthesia: Local infiltrative anesthetic or general anesthetic in children and uncooperative patient.
   a. Inject 2.5 ml of 2% lidocaine without epinephrine in the frontal nerve distribution and pretarsal area
   b. Avoid epinephrine since it stimulates the Müller muscle and may influence results of surgery.
3. Prep and drape in the usual sterile manner.
   a. Keep both eyes exposed for comparison of two eyes during procedure.

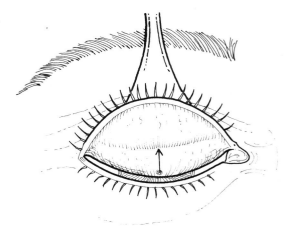

Figure 54.1

4. Evert eyelid over Desmarres retractor and mark conjunctiva with gentle cautery (monopolar or bipolar) 8.0 mm (for 2 mm of lift) above upper tarsal border centrally above the pupil (**Fig. 54.1**).

   See step 5 for table of magnitude of resection.

5. Mark 4 mm above the tarsal border in the medial and lateral eyelid, approximately 15 mm apart centered on the pupil (**Table 54.1**).

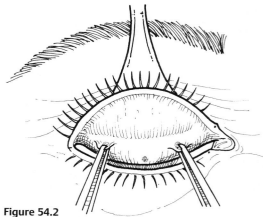

Figure 54.2

6. Apply locking Castroviejo forceps (6-0 mm long silk traction sutures may be substituted) to medial and lateral marks (**Fig. 54.2**).

Table 54.1 Müller Muscle–Conjunctival Resection

Desired lift of lid	Placement of central mark above upper tarsal border	Placement of medial and lateral forceps	Total advancement of conjunctiva and Müller muscle
1 mm	4 mm	2	4
1.5	6	3	6
2	8	4	8
2.5	10	5	10

7. Remove Desmarres retractor.

A

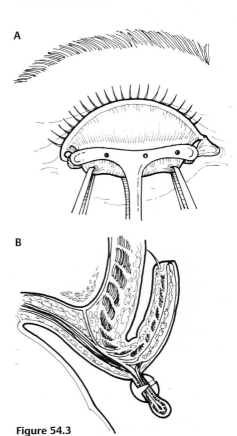

Figure 54.3

A

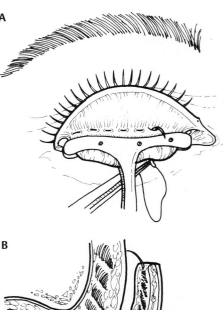

B

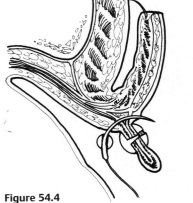

Figure 54.4

8. With the assistant tenting up tissues within the locking Castroviejo forceps, apply the ptosis clamp with the top of the clamp to the previously placed mark 8 mm above tarsal border (**Fig. 54.3**).
    a. Clamp includes 8 mm of conjunctiva and adherent Müller muscle.
    b. Clamp advances the levator aponeurosis internally.
9. Sew 6-0 plain suture lateral to medial across eyelid in horizontal fashion approximately 1 mm below clamp (**Fig. 54.4**).

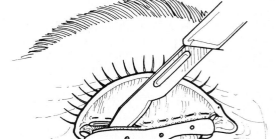

Figure 54.5

10. Use scalpel (e.g. #15 Bard-Parker blade) to excise tissue within clamp (**Fig. 54.5**).
    a. Angle scalpel toward metal clamp to prevent cutting of suture.

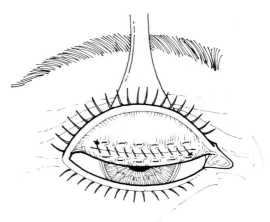

Figure 54.6

11. Sew medial to lateral in simple running fashion (**Fig. 54.6**).
    a. Expect fine oozing from tissues (absence of epinephrine). Have assistant wipe ahead of surgeon with cotton applicators.
12. Tie two ends of suture together.
13. Apply antibiotic ointment to eye.
14. Apply iced compresses.

Postoperative Procedure

1. Apply ice packs to decrease swelling.
2. Apply antibiotic ointment 4 times daily to eye for lubrication.

Complications

1. Lid swelling and ecchymosis
2. Corneal abrasion secondary to suture irritation
3. Lid hemorrhage
4. Over- and undercorrections
5. Lid asymmetry
6. Poor lid contour
7. Malpositioned or indistinct lid crease
8. Exposure keratopathy secondary to lagophthalmos

■ Fasanella-Servat Procedure

Like the posterior Müller muscle–conjunctival resection procedure, the Fasanella-Servat procedure is useful for mild cases of ptosis (2 mm or less) with good levator function (8 mm or more). It is the most technically straightforward of the ptosis procedures performed. Because the tarsal plate is vertically shortened, there is increased risk of central "peaking" of the eyelid compared to the Müller muscle–conjunctival resection procedure. Additionally, the vertical shortening of the tarsal plate that results from this procedure may make additional ptosis surgeries more difficult.

Indications

■ Mild congenital ptosis (less than 2 mm lid droop), with good levator function (8 mm or more)
■ Select cases of mild acquired involutional ptosis
■ Mild ptosis associated with Horner syndrome

Preoperative Procedure

See Chapter 3.

1. If possible, discontinue aspirin and nonsteroidal anti-inflammatory agents for 10 days before surgery. Discontinue warfarin 2–3 days preoperatively, if medically possible.
2. Query patient about bleeding tendencies. A useful screening question is asking if the patient had unusual bleeding after dental extraction. Obtain hematological evaluation if bleeding tendency is suspected.

Instrumentation

■ Tissue marking pen
■ Scleral shell
■ Scalpel
■ Small curved hemostats
■ Sutures (double-armed 6-0 plain gut)
■ Needle holder
■ Stevens scissors
■ Toothed forceps

Operative Procedure

1. Apply topical anesthetic.
2. Anesthesia: Local infiltrative anesthetic or general anesthetic in children and uncooperative patient.
3. Prep and drape.
   a. Keep both eyes exposed for comparison of two eyes during procedure.
4. Place scleral shell to protect globe (not shown in illustrations).

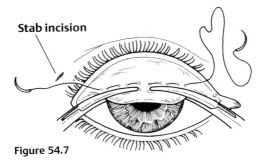

Figure 54.7

5. Use scalpel (e.g., #11 Bard-Parker blade) to make small stab incision through skin at lateral border of lid crease (**Fig. 54.7**).

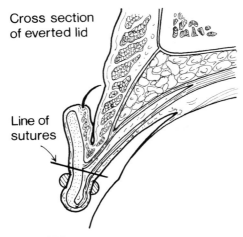

Figure 54.8

6. Evert upper lid (**Figs. 54.7 and 54.8**).
7. Clamp two small curved hemostats across upper tarsal border encompassing superior tarsus, the inferior edge of the Müller muscle, and overlying conjunctiva.
   a. Place 2–3 mm from superior edge of tarsus.
   b. Ensure that the clamps are positioned so the width of engaged tarsus is constant along the entire length of the clamps. This avoids resecting too much tarsus centrally.
   c. Ensure that neither skin nor levator aponeurosis has been imbricated by the clamp.
8. Run one end of a double-armed 6-0 plain gut suture in mattress fashion, approximately 1 mm above the hemostats.
   a. Place full thickness through all tissues (inferior conjunctiva-tarsus Müller muscle–superior conjunctiva).
   b. Start medially and take approximately 4–6 bites, proceeding laterally.
9. Remove hemostats (**Fig. 54.9**).

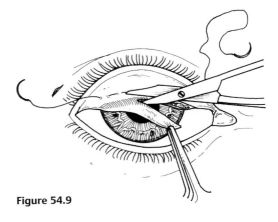

Figure 54.9

10. Cut through crush marks with Stevens scissors.
    a. Only upper tarsus, inferior portion of the Müller muscle, and conjunctiva should be removed. No more than one half of tarsus should be resected.
    b. Do not cut through levator aponeurosis and skin.

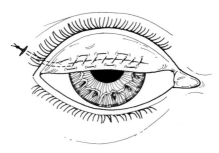

Figure 54.10

11. Using the medial free arm of the suture placed in step 8 as a running suture, rejoin superior tarsal edge and inferior border of the Müller muscle while approximating the cut conjunctival edges (**Fig. 54.10**).
12. Carry both arms of the suture through the preplaced skin stab incision, tie the ends, and bury the knot beneath skin.
13. The skin incision usually does not need suturing.
14. Remove scleral shell.
15. Apply antibiotic ointment to eye.
16. Apply chilled compress.

Postoperative Procedure

1. Apply ice packs to decrease swelling.
2. Apply antibiotic ointment 4 times daily for corneal lubrication.

Complications

1. Lid swelling and ecchymosis
2. Corneal abrasion secondary to suture irritation
3. Asymmetry of lids
4. Poor lid contour

■ Ptosis Repair by External Levator Aponeurosis Advancement

Levator aponeurotic advancement or repair is useful in cases of uncomplicated congenital or acquired ptosis of any magnitude with 5 or more mm of levator function. With poorer levator function, a levator resection or frontalis suspension should be considered.

Indications

■ Acquired (involutional, traumatic) ptosis secondary to thinning, stretching, dehiscence, or disinsertion of the levator aponeurosis
■ Select cases of congenital ptosis with good levator function
■ Select cases of neurogenic ptosis with good levator function

Preoperative Procedure

See Chapter 3.

1. If possible, discontinue aspirin and nonsteroidal anti-inflammatory agents for 10 days before surgery. Discontinue warfarin 2–3 days preoperatively, if medically possible.
2. Query patient about bleeding tendencies. A useful screening question is asking if the patient had unusual bleeding after dental extraction. Obtain hematological evaluation if bleeding tendency is suspected.

Instrumentation

■ Tissue marking pen
■ Scleral shield
■ Sutures (6-0 Prolene, 6-0 fast-absorbing catgut, 5-0 silk)
■ Needle holder
■ Scalpel (e.g., #15 Bard-Parker blade)
■ Toothed forceps
■ Stevens scissors
■ Westcott scissors
■ Rake retractors (e.g. Blaire)
■ Desmarres retractor

Operative Procedure

1. Mark the location of desired lid crease with tissue marking pen (usually 8–10 mm above lash line and symmetric with contralateral lid.)
   a. If the lid crease is indistinct or malpositioned, placement of supratarsal fixation sutures may be indicated (see step 21).
   b. In unilateral repairs, attempt to match lid crease of unoperated eye.
2. Apply topical anesthetic.
3. Anesthesia: Local infiltrative anesthesia with no or light sedation.
   a. Local anesthesia is preferred to allow for voluntary levator movements by the patient when identifying aponeurosis and positioning the eyelid.
   b. Subcutaneous infiltration into pretarsal eyelid with a 50:50 mixture of lidocaine 2% plus 1:100,000 epinephrine and 0.75% bupivacaine
4. Prep and drape in the usual sterile manner.
   a. Keep both eyes exposed for comparison of two eyes during procedure.
   b. Place scleral shield to protect globe.

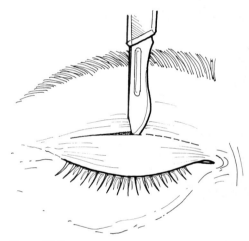

Figure 54.11

5. Incise skin along lid crease mark with scalpel (e.g., #15 Bard-Parker blade) (**Fig. 54.11**).
6. *Optional:* Place 5-0 silk traction suture through inferior margin of upper lid and secure to drape inferiorly with hemostat.
7. Grasp upper and lower edges of wound opposite each other centrally, and buttonhole muscle horizontally with tissue scissors (Stevens or Westcott).
8. Using sharp dissection, cut orbicularis horizontally parallel with skin incision to reveal orbital septum.
9. Secure hemostasis with cautery.

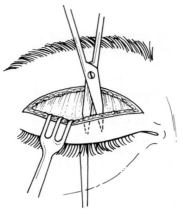

Figure 54.12

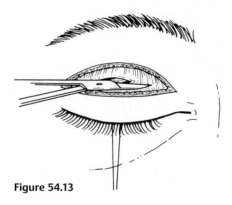

Figure 54.13

10. At inferior aspect of incision, sharply dissect down to tarsus with scissors. May retract skin inferiorly with retractor (**Fig. 54.12**).
11. Clean residual tissue from anterior surface of tarsus with sharp dissection:
    a. Dissect to expose superior 3 mm of tarsus.
    b. Always stop dissection if lash roots visualized.
12. While tenting superior skin and orbicularis with forceps, use sharp and blunt dissection to buttonhole orbital septum.

13. Incise orbital septum horizontally (toothed forceps, Stevens or Westcott scissors) (**Fig. 54.13**). Stay superior so as to encounter orbital fat and not cut into levator aponeurosis.

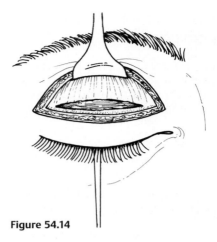

Figure 54.14

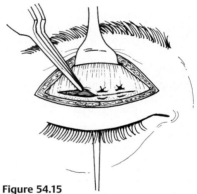

Figure 54.15

14. Retract preaponeurotic fat with Desmarres retractor. (**Fig. 54.14**).
15. Identify aponeurosis defect or edge of disinserted aponeurosis. Aponeurosis will move as patient looks up, facilitating its identification.

16. Suture disinserted aponeur\osis to tarsal plate with 6-0 horizontal mattress suture of Prolene (**Fig. 54.15**).
    a. Place first suture centrally just above pupil to establish eyelid height.
    b. Begin superiorly at cut edge of levator
    c. Place sutures horizontally through partial thickness tarsus, approximately 1–2 mm from its superior edge.
    d. Evert tarsal plate and replace suture if it has violated the conjunctiva and gone full thickness. Then come back superiorly into levator.
17. Tie suture in slip knot fashion.
18. Inspect lid height while patient looks straight, up, and down, and reposition sutures as necessary. The final intraoperative eyelid height should be 1–1.5 mm higher than desired postoperative elevation.
19. Repair aponeurosis medially and laterally with additional interrupted or mattress sutures to shape contour of eyelid.

20. In some cases it may be desirable to have the patient sit upright to check eyelid position.
21. *Optional:* Remove excess skin from lid (see Chapter 52).
   a. Mark upper lid skin to be removed with marking pen.
   b. Remove crescent of skin and orbicularis with sharp scissors.
   c. If desired, clamp prolapsed aponeurotic fat, cut on clamp, and cauterize stump before removing clamp.

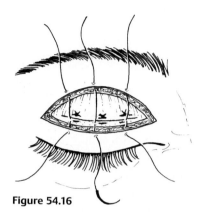

Figure 54.16

22. Place approximately three supratarsal fixation sutures to enhance lid crease (**Fig. 54.16**).
   a. Use 6-0 Prolene or fast-absorbing plain gut interrupted sutures.
   b. Place one suture near the lateral canthal border of the incision, and the others centrally and medially.
   c. Technique:
      i. Enter skin near cut edge; include cut edge of orbicularis muscle. Pass suture through the levator aponeurosis in the location of the desired lid crease near lower border of wound.
      ii. Exit through the apposing cut edge of the skin.
      iii. Close skin with interrupted or running 6-0 Prolene or fast-absorbing plain sutures.
23. Apply antibiotic ointment to suture line.
24. Apply ice compresses.

Postoperative Procedure

1. Apply ice packs to decrease swelling.
2. Keep head of bed elevated 30 degrees to decrease swelling.
3. Apply antibiotic ointment to wound twice daily.
4. Use aggressive ocular lubrication to eye because of expected postoperative lagophthalmos.
5. Remove skin sutures in 4–6 days.

6. If eyelid is too high or too low in the first 3–10 days postoperatively, you may return patient to treatment room. Wound may be teased open with no to minimal anesthetic infiltration and steps 15–24 repeated.

Complications

1. Orbital hemorrhage with possibility of consequent blindness
2. Lid hemorrhage
3. Over- and undercorrections
4. Lid asymmetry
5. Poor lid contour
6. Malpositioned or indistinct lid crease.
7. Exposure keratopathy secondary to lagophthalmos

■ Levator Resection

Levator resection is useful in cases of moderate to severe ptosis with 4–8 mm of levator function. This procedure is similar to aponeurotic advancement or repair, but useful in cases of more severe ptosis (by magnitude of ptosis or deficiency of levator function). The levator muscle is resected. With even poorer levator function, a frontalis suspension should be considered.

Preoperative Procedure

See Chapter 3.

1. Complete history to appropriately classify ptosis. The type and severity of ptosis will dictate the appropriate surgical management.
2. Complete lid and eye examination to determine detailed operative plan.
3. Evaluate lid position and levator function. Plan necessary amount of resection.

The length of levator to be resected may vary between approximately 10 and 26 mm. The specific amount depends on two criteria: (1) the severity of ptosis and (2) the levator function. For instance, a moderate ptosis with fair levator function may respond to 18–22 mm of resection, but only a 14–17 mm resection may be necessary in the presence of good levator function. A number of published guidelines are available relating to the suggested amount of resection to the degree of ptosis and levator function.

   a. One method for determining resection is based on intraoperative appearance (after Berke).
      i. For fair levator function, set the intraoperative lid level at the desired postoperative position.
      ii. For good levator function, undercorrect by 1–2 mm.
      iii. For poor levator function, overcorrect by 1–2 mm.

b. Another method for determining resection is based on magnitude of levator resection (after Beard).
   i. In patients with 1–2 mm of ptosis, resect 10–13 mm of levator if function is 8 mm or better.
   ii. In patients with 3 mm of ptosis, resect 14–17 mm if levator function is 8 mm or more; resect 18–22 mm if levator function is 5–7 mm.
   iii. In patients with 4 mm or ptosis or more, resect 14–17 mm if levator function is 8 mm or more; resect 18 mm or more if levator function is less than 7 mm.

Instrumentation

- Tissue marking pen
- Scleral shell
- Hemostat
- Sutures (5-0 silk, 6-0 plain gut, 5-0 double-armed Dexon, 6-0 silk, 4-0 silk, 6-0 fast-absorbing cat gut)
- Scalpel (e.g., 15 Bard-Parker blade)
- Toothed forceps
- Stevens scissors
- Westcott scissors
- Blaire retractors
- Desmarres retractor
- Ptosis clamp (e.g., Berke)
- Needle holder
- Castroviejo calipers
- Silicone bolster (e.g., silicone retinal buckling band)

Operative Procedure

1. Apply topical anesthetic.
2. Mark location of desired lid crease with tissue marking pen (usually 7–10 mm above lash line and symmetric with contralateral lid).
3. Anesthesia: General or local infiltrative anesthesia.
   a. Local anesthesia is preferred to allow for voluntary levator movements by the patient when identifying aponeurosis and positioning lid.
   b. Subcutaneous infiltration with a 50:50 mixture of lidocaine 2% plus 1:100,000 epinephrine and 0.75% bupivacaine
4. Prep and drape. Keep both eyes exposed for comparison of two eyes during procedure.
5. Place scleral shell to protect globe.
6. Place 5-0 silk traction suture through inferior margin of upper lid and secure to drape inferiorly with hemostat.

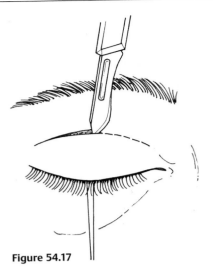

Figure 54.17

7. Incise skin along lid crease mark with scalpel (e.g., #15 Bard-Parker blade) (**Fig. 54.17**).
8. Tent orbicularis with toothed forceps holding inferior and superior aspects of wound and buttonhole muscle horizontally with sharp scissors (Stevens or Westcott).
9. Using blunt dissection, undermine orbicularis and incise it horizontally along skin incision.
10. Secure hemostasis with cautery.

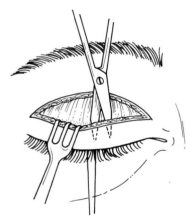

Figure 54.18

11. Perform sharp and blunt dissection down to tarsus with scissors. May retract skin with rake retractor (**Fig. 54.18**).
12. Clean residual tissue from anterior-superior tarsus with sharp and blunt dissection.

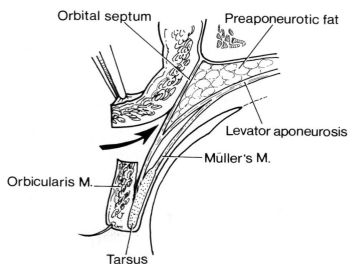

Figure 54.19

13. While tenting superior skin and orbicularis with forceps, expose anterior surface of orbital septum using sharp and blunt dissection (**Fig. 54.19**).

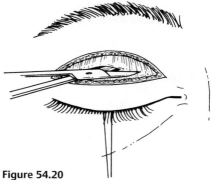

Figure 54.20

14. Buttonhole orbital septum and incise horizontally with toothed forceps, Stevens or Westcott scissors (**Fig. 54.20**).
15. Identify levator aponeurosis.
    a. Retract preaponeurotic fat with Desmarres retractor.
    b. Have patient look superiorly while observing for movement of aponeurosis.

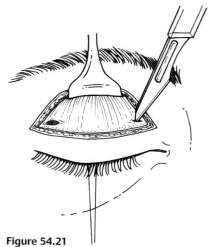

Figure 54.21

16. Buttonhole full-thickness lid at nasal and temporal borders of lid crease with scalpel or scissors (**Fig. 54.21**).

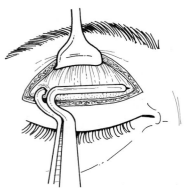

Figure 54.22

17. Insert ptosis clamp (**Fig. 54.22**).
18. Close ptosis clamp just above superior border of tarsus.
19. Incise full-thickness lid below clamp with scissors or scalpel. Clamp contains conjunctiva, Müller muscle, levator aponeurosis, and sometimes orbital septum.

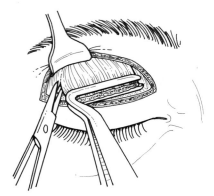

Figure 54.23

20. If necessary, cut horns of levator posteriorly to release levator for resection (**Fig. 54.23**).

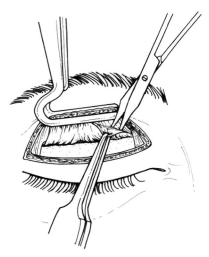

Figure 54.24

21. Dissect conjunctiva free from Müller muscle and ptosis clamp (**Fig. 54.24**).
    a. Inject lidocaine plus epinephrine subconjunctivally for hemostasis.
    b. Start dissection approximately 5 mm from the clamp for greater ease.
    c. Use scissors to perform sharp and blunt dissection.
    d. The two corners of the cut conjunctiva may be marked with 6-0 silk sutures to be used for retraction during dissection.
    e. Dissection of conjunctiva from Müller muscle must be continued posteriorly enough to allow for levator resection without conjunctival damage.
22. For large levator resection, resect approximately 5 mm of conjunctiva to avoid redundancy upon its reattachment to tarsus.

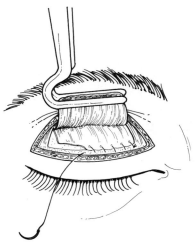

Figure 54.25

23. Reattach free end of conjunctiva to tarsus with interrupted or running 6-0 plain gut suture (**Fig. 54.25**).
24. Lyse any remaining adhesions of orbital septum to levator and clean anterior resect of levator, freeing enough for desired resection.
25. Measure length of desired resection with calipers.

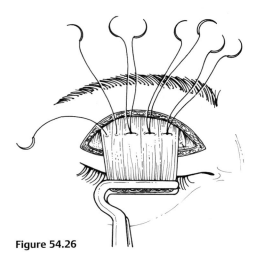

Figure 54.26

26. At a distance of approximately 2 mm proximal to desired level of resection, place four double-armed 5-0 Dexon mattress sutures through full-thickness muscle (**Fig. 54.26**).
    a. Space sutures equally.
    b. Place through backside of muscle and tie anteriorly.
    c. Leave both ends long with needles attached.
27. Resect muscle just distal to the sutures.
28. Remove scleral shell.

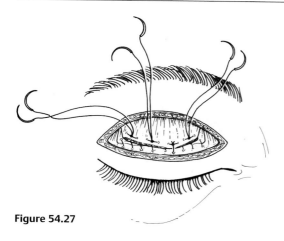

Figure 54.27

29. Use preplaced sutures to secure levator to tarsal plate approximately 1 mm below superior tarsal border (**Fig. 54.27**).
    a. Place sutures through partial thickness tarsus approximately 1–2 mm from its superior border.
    b. First tie only one loop and check lid contour. May have patient look up and down to better evaluate positioning.
    c. Reposition tarsal bites as needed to restore desired lid contour.
30. If necessary, remove excess skin from lid (see Chapter 52).
    a. Mark upper lid skin to be removed with marking pen.
    b. Remove crescent of skin and orbicularis with sharp scissors.

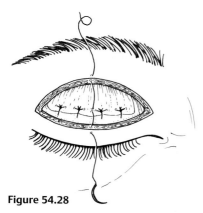

Figure 54.28

31. Place three or more supratarsal fixation sutures to form lid crease (**Fig. 54.28**).
    a. Use 6-0 silk interrupted sutures.
    b. Place one suture near the lateral canthal border of the incision, and the others centrally and medially.
    c. Technique I:
        i. Enter skin near cut edge.
        ii. Pass suture through levator in the location of the desired lid crease near lower border of wound.

iii. Exit through the apposing cut edge of the skin.
    d. Technique II:
    If dissolving sutures use 6-0 Vicryl or other absorbable suture.
        i. Place suture subcuticularly through one border of the wound.
        ii. Place subcuticularly through apposing border.
        iii. Pass suture through levator in the location of the desired lid crease.
        iv. Tie and bury knot under orbicularis.
32. Close skin with interrupted or running 6-0 silk sutures or 6-0 fast-absorbing cat gut.
33. Remove traction suture.

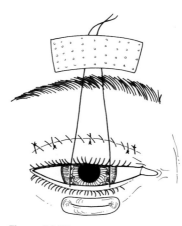

Figure 54.29

34. *Optional:* Place 4-0 silk Frost suture to protect cornea from exposure (**Fig. 54.29**).
    a. Place in mattress fashion through gray line of lower lid and out through a bolster (e.g., silicone retinal buckling band).
    b. Tape suture ends to brow to close eye without placing tension on upper lid postoperatively.
35. Apply antibiotic ointment to suture line.

Postoperative Procedure

1. Apply ice packs to decrease swelling.
2. Keep head of bed elevated 30 degrees to decrease swelling.
3. Remove Frost suture in 1 or 2 days.
4. Apply antibiotic ointment twice daily wound.
5. Use aggressive ocular lubrication to eye because of expected postoperative lagophthalmos.
6. Remove skin sutures in 4–6 days (unless dissolvable sutures used).

Complications

1. Orbital hemorrhage with possibility of consequent blindness
2. Lid hemorrhage
3. Under- and overcorrection
4. Asymmetry of lids
5. Poor lid contour
6. Malpositioned or indistinct lid crease
7. Conjunctival prolapse
8. Entropion and ectropion
9. Exposure keratopathy secondary to lagophthalmos

■ Frontalis Suspension

In cases with little or no levator function (4 mm or less), a frontalis suspension using autogenous fascia lata, silicone rods, or other synthetic materials is the procedure of choice.

Indications

■ Select cases of congenital ptosis with poor levator function.
■ Select cases of neurogenic or myopathic ptosis with poor levator function.

Preoperative Procedure

See Introduction section at the beginning of this chapter.
  See Chapter 3.

Instrumentation

■ Scleral shield
■ Sutures 6-0 Vicryl, 6-0 fast-absorbing catgut
■ Needle holder
■ Scalpel (e.g., #15 Bard-Parker blade)
■ Toothed forceps
■ Stevens scissors
■ Westcott scissors
■ Cautery
■ Rake retractors (e.g., Blaire)
■ Desmarres retractor
■ Jaeger lid plate
■ Watzke sleeve spreader
■ 1mm silicone rod
■ Watzke silicone sleeve

Operative Procedure

1. Anesthesia: General anesthesia for children. General anesthesia or local anesthesia for cooperative adults.
2. Apply topical anesthetic.
3. Prep and drape. Keep both eyes exposed for comparison of two eyes during procedure.
4. Soak 1 mm silicone rod and Watzke sleeve in antibiotic solution.
5. Place scleral shield beneath lids to protect globe.

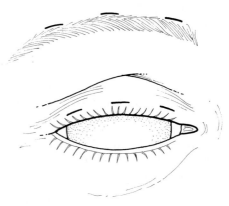

Figure 54.30

6. Mark incision sites for eyelid (**Fig. 54.30**):
   a. One 6 mm medial to lateral canthus, 1–2 mm above lashes.
   b. One above pupil, 1–2 mm above lashes.
   c. One 6 mm lateral to medial canthus, 1–2 mm above lashes.
7. Mark incision sites at upper aspect of eyebrow (**Fig. 54.30**).
   a. One above lateral canthus 3 mm in length.
   b. One above pupil 3 mm in length.
   c. One above medial canthus 3 mm in length.

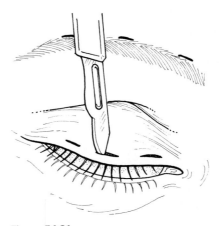

Figure 54.31

8. Make incisions in eyelid with scalpel through skin and orbicularis onto tarsal plate (**Fig. 54.31**).

9. Make incisions in eyebrow down to periosteum.
10. Through the medial and lateral brow stab incisions, spread to create a large pocket beneath the frontalis muscle superiorly using Stevens scissors to allow for easy placement of Watzke sleeve and silicone at end of operation.
11. Remove scleral shield and place Jaeger lid plate under eyelid to protect globe. Press superiorly against orbital rim to protect orbital and ocular contents.
12. Advance Wright fascia needle from lateral eyelid incision to central eyelid incision.

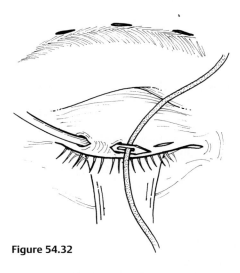

Figure 54.32

13. Thread silicone rod through eye of Wright fascia needle (**Fig. 54.32**).
14. Withdraw threaded Wright fascia needle passing silicone rod beneath skin and muscle.

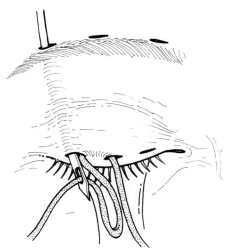

Figure 54.33

15. Insert Wright fascia needle through lateral brow stab incision and advance it through the lateral eyelid incision (**Fig. 54.33**).

16. Thread silicone through eye of Wright fascia needle.
17. Withdraw fascia needle advancing the silicone out the lateral brow incision.

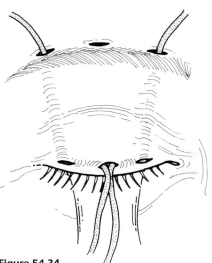

Figure 54.34

18. Similarly, use the Wright fascia needle to thread a separate piece of silicone from central eyelid incision to the medial eyelid incision and then up through the medial eyebrow (**Fig. 54.34**).
19. Insert unloaded Wright fascia needle from central brow incision to the central eyelid incision.

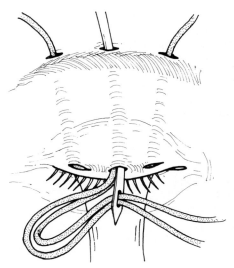

Figure 54.35

20. Thread both silicone rods into the eye of the Wright fascia needle (**Fig. 54.35**) and withdraw needle back through the brow incision (**Fig. 54.36**).

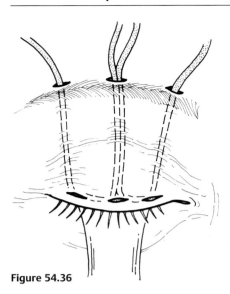

Figure 54.36

21. Advance empty Wright fascia needle from lateral brow incision to central brow incision.

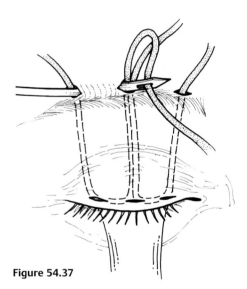

Figure 54.37

22. Thread the silicone rod that was placed through the lateral rhomboid (**Fig. 54.37**).
23. Withdraw Wright fascia needle and recover silicone in lateral brow incision.
24. Do identical maneuver for medial rod, recovering the ends of the silicone rod through the medial brow incision.

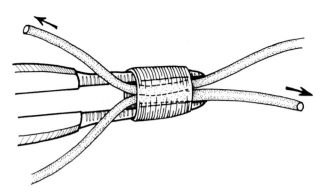

Figure 54.38

25. Load Watzke sleeve on to sleeve spreader (**Fig. 54.38**).
26. Thread two ends of silicone rod through Watzke sleeve. The ends of the silicone enter the sleeve in opposing directions.
27. Close eyelid incisions with 6-0 fast-absorbing catgut before tightening the silicone rods.
    a. When silicone rods are tightened, the eyelid is brought upward and the eyelid incisions are difficult to close.

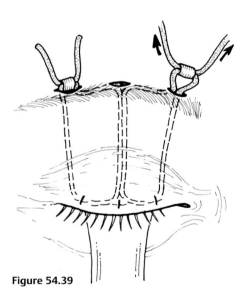

Figure 54.39

28. Pull up and tighten silicone rods until height and position of eyelid are optimal (**Fig. 54.39**).
29. Trim silicone rod leaving 10–20 mm excess (allow for adjusting position post operatively).
30. Position the Watzke sleeves within wound.
    a. Confirm height and contour of eyelids.
    b. Place the free ends of the sleeves in the deep pockets made superior to the brow incisions.

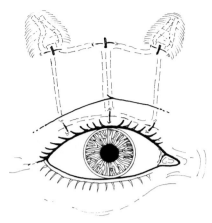

Figure 54.40

31. Close brow incisions with buried 6-0 Vicryl and reabsorbable 6-0 fast-absorbing catgut (**Fig. 54.40**).

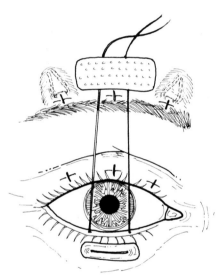

Figure 54.41

32. Optional:

Place 4-0 silk Frost suture to protect cornea from exposure (**Fig. 54.41**).

a. Place in mattress fashion through gray line of lower lid and out through a bolster (e.g., silicone retinal buckling band).

b. Tape suture ends to brow to close eye without placing tension on upper lid postoperatively.

33. Options and variations to Frontalis suspension:

a. May be combined with blepharoplasty with epitarsal fixation to form eyelid crease and remove bulky eyelid tissues.

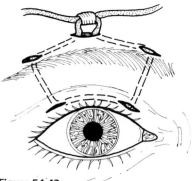

Figure 54.42

b. May be performed a simple pentagon in small children using a single piece of silicone (**Fig. 54.42**).

Postoperative Procedure

1. Use ice packs to decrease swelling.
2. Keep head of bed elevated 30 degrees to decrease swelling.
3. Apply antibiotic ointment to cornea every 2 hours until certain that cornea can tolerate exposure. Antibiotic to incision sites 2 times a day.

Complications

1. Orbital hemorrhage with possibility of consequent blindness
2. Lid hemorrhage
3. Over- and undercorrections
4. Lid asymmetry
5. Poor lid contour
6. Malpositioned or indistinct lid crease
7. Exposure keratopathy secondary to lagophthalmos
8. Exposure of implant material
9. Breakage of sling
10. Loss of results with time due to cheese wiring of sling material
11. Cellulitis

55

Endoscopic Forehead/Brow Lift

Indications

- Eyebrow ptosis that is interfering with vision
- Eyebrow ptosis or laxity of forehead and temporal tissues that is cosmetically undesirable

Preoperative Procedure

See Chapter 3.

1. Assess the eyebrow position from functional and cosmetic standpoint:
   a. Many patients mask eyebrow ptosis with volitional efforts. Ask the patient to close the eyes and massage the eyebrows to a resting position. Are the brows low?
   b. Look at old photographs. Often brow ptosis has been present since a patient's teens or early twenties. Old photographs may reveal the patient's baseline eyebrow position.
   c. Analyze the current and desired height and contour of the eyebrow.

   Note: Lateral eyebrow ptosis is most commonly associated with visual and aesthetic problems. Lateral eyebrow ptosis increases with age.

   d. Determine the action of the corregator and procerus muscles. Decide whether to and how much to weaken these at surgery.
   e. Analyze and document preexisting asymmetries and differences in frontalis function.
   f. For significant asymmetries, be sure to ask about and examine for dysfunction of the seventh cranial nerve.
2. Discuss alternative methods of brow elevation (direct, mid-forehead, pretrichial, coronal lifts). Discuss alternative methods of making the eyes appear more open (blepharoplasty).

3. Make a full assessment of upper eyelid and tear function, including the presence or absence of true eyelid ptosis and the presence and magnitude of redundant eyelid skin.
4. Consider administering Botox into the corregator and procerus muscles 2 weeks preoperatively to reduce their downward pull on the eyebrow during the postoperative period

Instrumentation

- Thirty degree endoscope
- Endoscopic browlift sheath specific for each manufacturer of endoscopes
- Video endoscopy setup including: xenon light source, high-resolution video monitor, and endoscopic camera
- Scalpel (e.g., #15 bard parker blade)
- Endobrow dissectors and elevators
- Endobrow scissors
- Endobrow grasping forceps
- Endotine forehead fixation device, drill bits and insertion tool (Coapt Systems, Inc., Palo Alto, CA). Other systems may also be used by surgeon preference.
- Surgical stapler
- Suture: 4–0 Vicryl
- Self-retaining toothed retractor
- Needle holder
- Adson forceps

Operative Procedure

Endoscopic brow/forehead lift may be combined with upper blepharoplasty.

Underlying premise: Complete undermining of the forehead and fixation of the tissues in a more superior anatomic position will lead eyebrow elevation without lengthy incisions.

1. Review relevant anatomy of the temporal and glabellar areas.

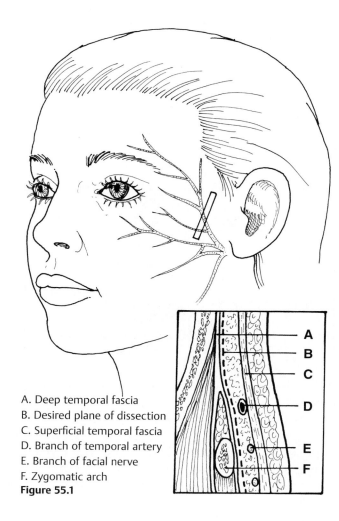

A. Deep temporal fascia
B. Desired plane of dissection
C. Superficial temporal fascia
D. Branch of temporal artery
E. Branch of facial nerve
F. Zygomatic arch
Figure 55.1

a. The safe dissection plan is along the deep temporal fascia. In this surgical plane the facial nerve is anterior to the plane of dissection (**Fig. 55.1**).

b. The supraorbital nerve emerges from a notch or foramen. The corrugator muscle traverses superotemporally from its bony origin (**Fig. 55.2**).

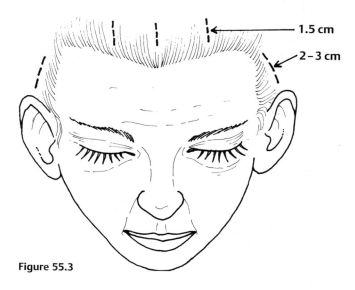

Figure 55.3

2. Mark the patient preoperatively (**Fig. 55.3**).
   a. Mark sagittal central and paracentral incisions 1.5 cm in length behind the hairline.
   b. Mark 2–3 cm temporal incisions curvilinear and placed 2–5 cm behind he hairline.
   c. Conservatively shave the scalp where scalpel will be cutting. Tie back hair with rubber bands to prevent hair migrating into surgical space.
3. Test instrumentation before initiating anesthesia.
4. Monitored or general anesthesia. The patient requires more sedation than with standard eyelid procedures, and communication with the anesthesia staff is particularly important.
5. Inject Xylocaine 0.5% with 1:200,000 epinephrine into the planned sites of incision, across the forehead, and temporal to the orbital rims.
6. Prep with Betadine solution.

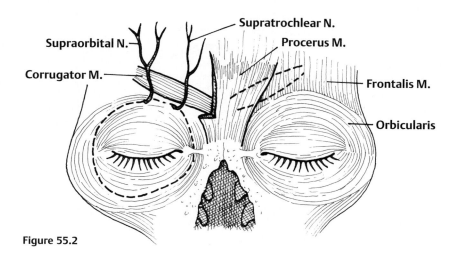

Supratrochlear N.
Supraorbital N.
Procerus M.
Corrugator M.
Frontalis M.
Orbicularis

Figure 55.2

7. Incise along central and lateral marks down to periosteum.
8. Incise temporal incision down to glistening deep temporal fascia.
9. Subperiosteal dissection:
   a. Place retractor to open the incisions.
   b. With or without endoscopic visualization, introduce the periosteal elevators through the central and paracentral incisions.

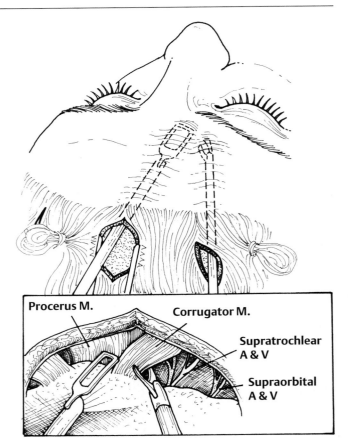

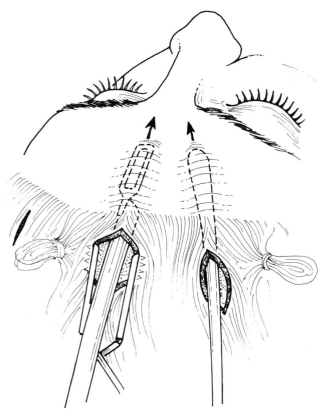

Figure 55.5

Figure 55.4

c. With a scraping motion, free the periosteum from the bony skull and dissect toward the orbital rims (**Fig. 55.4**).
10. Under endoscopic visualization, complete the dissection to the orbital rims.
   a. Lift the endoscope away from the skull to create an optic cavity that allows for visualization of the surgical area.
   b. Use endoscopic scissors or endoscopic dissector to release the periosteum fully at the orbital rims moving lateral to medial.
   c. During the medial dissection, preserve the supraorbital and supratrochlear nerves.
11. Under endoscopic visualization, use endoscopic forceps to avulse the corregator and procerus muscles as needed (**Fig. 55.5**).

12. Through the temporal incision, use the dissector to break through the temporal crest and join up with the subperiosteal dissection created earlier (**Fig. 55.6**).

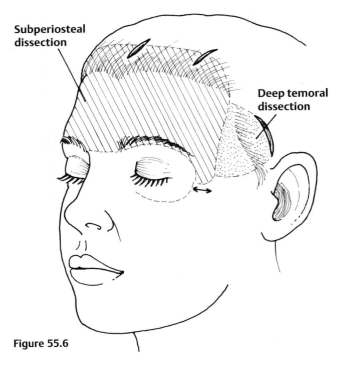

Figure 55.6

a. Then dissect along the deep layer of the temporal fascia.
b. Release the conjoint tendon, which limits mobilization of the brow.
c. Free along orbital rim to level of the lateral canthal tendon.
d. Near the frontozygomatic suture, a branch of the zygomaticotemporal vein (the sentinel vein) is seen. It may be retracted or cauterized.

13. Drill holes into cranial bone at the paracentral incisions for placement of endotine fixation devise.

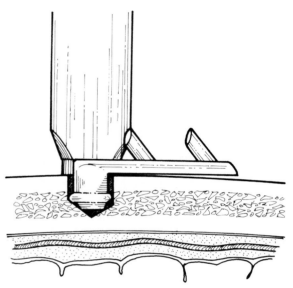

Figure 55.7

14. Insert endotine fixation devise into holes in bone (**Fig. 55.7**).

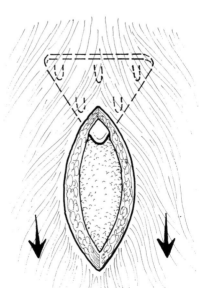

Figure 55.8

15. Pull back scalp over the fixation devise (**Fig. 55.8**).

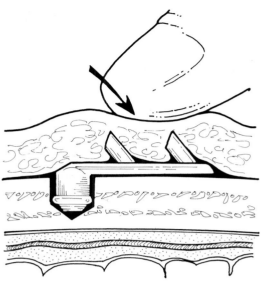

Figure 55.9

16. Press down onto scalp to engage endotine devise (**Fig. 55.9**). Adjust the tension based on the amount of elevation desired.
17. Resect redundant temporal scalp.
18. Place Vicryl sutures from anterior temporal scalp into the deep temporal fascia to reinforce temporal lift.
19. Close incisions with staples.
20. No drain is necessary unless unusual bleeding is encountered.
21. Wrap with occlusive dressing.

Postoperative Care

1. Change dressing on postoperative day 1.
2. Apply antibiotic ointment to incisions.
3. May use systemic antibiotics.
4. Use iced compresses for 24–48 hours postoperatively.

Complications

1. Facial nerve paralysis (usually temporary and reflects traction on the nerve during surgery)
2. Paresthesias and sensory disturbance from disruption and manipulation of sensory nerves
3. Asymmetry
4. Hematoma (may require evacuation, or, rarely, direct cauterization)
5. Infection

56

Dacryocystorhinostomy

Indications

- Chronic epiphora secondary to acquired stenosis of the nasolacrimal duct.
- Select cases of recurrent or chronic dacryocystitis.
- Select cases of congenital dacryostenosis that are unresponsive to more conservative medical and surgical interventions.
- In cases of nasolacrimal duct obstruction without canalicular abnormality, the dacryocystorhinostomy (DCR) may be performed intranasally under endoscopic or direct visualization (this procedure is not discussed).
- Note: the location of obstruction to tear drainage will dictate particular variations in the procedure to be performed. For example, cases with obstruction of the canaliculi will require a procedure to bypass the entire lacrimal drainage system. An in-depth discussion of each variation lies beyond the scope of this book. Instead, this chapter will describe a basic DCR with silicone intubation of the lacrimal system.

Preoperative Procedure

See Chapter 3.
  Rule out other causes of epiphora.

1. Ocular irritation secondary to blepharitis.
2. Reflex tearing in response to dry eye.
    a. Perform Schirmer test.
    b. Measure tear break-up time.
3. Eyelid malposition or dysfunction.
    a. Lid laxity.
    b. Ectropion.
    c. Punctal ectropion.
4. Punctal stenosis.
5. Canaliculitis.

6. Perform medical evaluation of lacrimal system anatomy to locate the site of obstruction to tear drainage.
    a. Jones primary and secondary dye tests.
    b. Probing and irrigation.
    c. Dacryocystography if indicated.
    d. Evaluation of nasal anatomy.
    e. Orbital imaging if mass lesion is suspected.
7. Control any active infection with appropriate antibiotic therapy before proceeding with surgery.
8. If possible, discontinue aspirin and nonsteroidal anti-inflammatory agents for 10 days before surgery. Discontinue warfarin preoperatively, if medically possible.

Instrumentation

- Fiber optic headlight
- Cocaine 4% solution
- Nasal speculum
- Tissue marking pen
- Calipers
- Rake retractors
- Lacrimal speculum or Alm self-retaining retractor
- Scleral shield
- Scalpel (e.g., # 15 and #11 or #12 Bard-Parker blade)
- Suction
- Cautery
- Periosteal elevator (e.g., Freer)
- Hemostat
- Bone rongeurs (e.g., 2 mm and 3 mm 90 degree Kerrison punch), and small-tipped, direct-acting rongeurs (e.g., Belz Lacrimal Sac rongeur)
- Punctum dilator
- Lacrimal probes
- Steven tenotomy scissors
- Westcott scissors
- Double skin hook
- Lacrimal irrigating cannula
- Bayonette forceps

- Silastic lacrimal tubing on Quickert-Dryden, Jackson, Crawford, or similar lacrimal probes
- Grooved director
- Sutures (4–0 chromic gut on half-circle cutting needle, 6–0 Vicryl, 4–0 Mersilene on half circle needle, 6–0 Prolene or fast absorbing plain gut)

Operative Procedure

1. Anesthesia: General or local anesthetic with sedation. Reduce blood pressure to lowest tolerated level.
2. *Optional:* Administer intraoperative prophylactic antibiotic.
3. Pack middle and inferior meatuses of nose 1 × 3 inch neurologic cottonoids in 4% cocaine.

Note: A fiber optic headlight will facilitate visualization during the procedure.

   a. Use nasal speculum for visualization.
   b. Use bayonet forceps to facilitate packing. Grab the distal end of the neurologic cottonoid and advance into nose.
   c. The cocaine causes anesthesia and vasoconstriction of nasal mucosa, resulting in shrinkage and decreased bleeding.

4. Apply topical anesthetic to eye.
5. Inject 50:50 mixture of lidocaine 2% plus 1:100,000 epinephrine and 0.75% bupivacaine into site of planned skin incision, adjacent soft tissues, and anterior medial wall of orbit to decrease operative bleeding and for analgesia.
6. Prep and drape in the usual sterile manner.
7. Insert scleral shield to protect globe.
8. Mark incision with tissue marking pen.
   a. Place 10 mm medial to the medial canthus to avoid angular vessels and postoperative web formation.
   b. Begin just below the medial canthal tendon and extend inferiorly 15 mm.
   c. Incision should be straight, proceeding inferiorly toward the nasal alar fold.
   d. Distances may be measured with calipers.

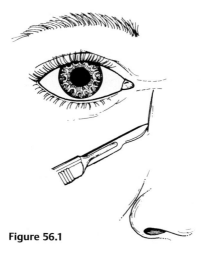

Figure 56.1

9. Incise skin with scalpel (**Fig. 56.1**).
10. Use sharp and blunt dissection through muscle layer to reach periosteum immediately below incision site, anterior to the anterior lacrimal crest.
   a. May retract skin with rake retractors, lacrimal speculum, or 4–0 silk skin traction sutures.
   b. Avoid angular vessels if visualized. However, if the angular vessels are violated secure hemostasis with suction, cautery, and ligation as necessary.
11. When the periosteum is adequately exposed, incise it parallel with the incision with a scalpel or periosteal elevator.
12. Reflect the periosteum posteriorly over the anterior lacrimal crest with a periosteal elevator to expose the lacrimal fossa.

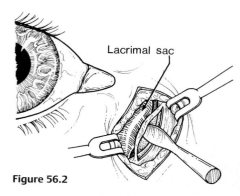

Figure 56.2

13. Use periosteal elevator to mobilize the lacrimal sac, exposing the posterior lacrimal crest posteriorly, the medial canthal tendon superiorly, and the nasolacrimal duct inferiorly (**Fig. 56.2**).

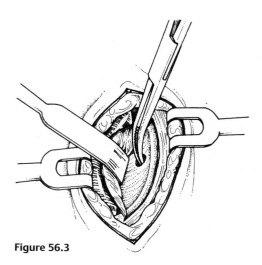

Figure 56.3

14. Retract the lacrimal sac and use tip of hemostat to carefully break through bone just posterior to anterior lacrimal crest (**Fig. 56.3**).

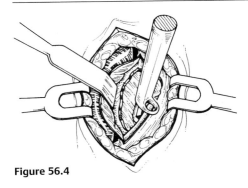

Figure 56.4

15. Use rongeurs to enlarge the osteotomy (**Fig. 56.4**).
    a. Final size of osteotomy should be ~10 mm × 15 mm extending anterior to the anterior lacrimal crest.
    b. Take precautions not to damage the underlying nasal mucosa.
16. Dilate puncta with punctum dilator.
17. Pass a lacrimal probe through the upper and lower canaliculi, respectively, to ensure patency from the puncta to the medial wall of the lacrimal sac.

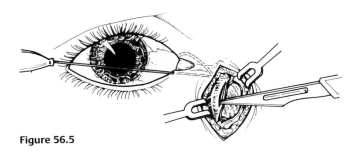

Figure 56.5

18. Incise the posteromedial wall of the lacrimal sac longitudinally with a scalpel (e.g., #11 or 12 Bard-Parker blade) (**Fig. 56.5**).
    a. May cut over lacrimal probes placed through canaliculi to ensure correct anatomical location.
    b. Initial scalpel incision may be enlarged with scissors and "H"-shaped anterior and flaps created.
    c. If done properly, the lacrimal probe should be visible through the incision.
19. Remove nasal packing.
20. Place cotton tip soaked with cocaine or lidocaine with epinephrine passed up through nose to palpate and identify nasal mucosa through previously fashioned osteotomy.

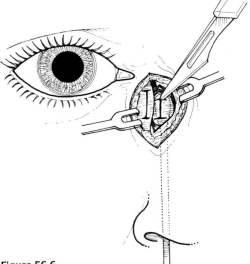

Figure 56.6

21. Use scalpel or scissors to fashion anterior and posterior nasal mucosal flaps (**Fig. 56.6**).
22. Suture the posterior lacrimal sac flap to the posterior nasal mucosal flap using one or two interrupted 4–0 chromic gut sutures (acutely curved needles will facilitate suture placement).

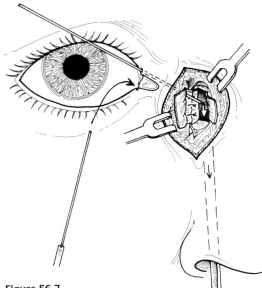

Figure 56.7

23. Intubate the lacrimal system with silicone tubing (**Fig. 56.7**).
    a. Use Quickert-Dryden, Jackson, Crawford, or similar lacrimal probes.
    b. Through upper and lower canalicular system, respectively, thread the tubing through the lacrimal sac, through the opening in the nasal mucosa, and

out through the nose (may use a grooved director to facilitate passage of the tubing).

  c. Remove wire probes from the end of the Silastic tubing and tie a knot in the tubing ~5–10 mm up in the nostril.

Assistant may hold a muscle hook beneath tubing in medial canthus to prevent excessive tension and later tearing of punctum and canaliculus. Use many throws for security.

  d. Secure the tubing to the nasal mucosa.
    i. Use 4–0 Mersilene on a half-circle needle or other permanent, interrupted suture.
    ii. Suture to lateral alar mucosa to prevent the tubing from slipping superiorly out of reach.

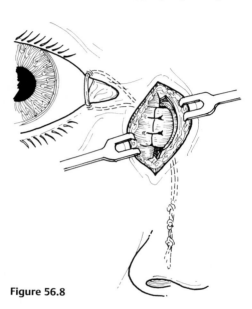

Figure 56.8

24. Suture the anterior lacrimal sac flap to the anterior nasal mucosa flap using one or two interrupted 4–0 chromic gut sutures (**Fig. 56.8**).

25. Close muscle layer with 6–0 Vicryl interrupted sutures.
26. Close skin with interrupted sutures of 6–0 Prolene, or fast-absorbing plain gut.
27. Apply ointment to wound and small dressing over incision site. Use cut eye pad or other gauze to place moustache dressing to capture any bleeding from the nose.

Postoperative Procedure

1. Apply ice packs to reduce swelling.
2. Keep head of bed at 30 degrees to reduce swelling.
3. Change dressing daily or as needed (may remove when patient stable).
4. Apply antibiotic ointment to incision site and conjunctival fornix twice daily for 1 week.
5. Continue systemic antibiotics if indicated.
6. Patient should not blow nose for a few days postoperatively to avoid lid emphysema.
7. Remove skin sutures in 5–7 days.
8. Keep Silastic tubing in place ~3–6 months if tolerated.
9. *Optional:* Irrigate lacrimal system to ensure patency of the surgical anastomosis.

Complications

1. Hemorrhage
2. Infection
3. Closure of ostomy
4. Scarring of incision site
5. Tube erosion of punctum and canaliculus

57

Punctoplasty

Indications

Punctal stenosis with tearing

Preoperative Procedure

1. Evaluate the tearing patient for etiology of condition.
2. Use the dye disappearance test.
3. Do corneal and conjunctival staining.
4. Perform Schirmer testing.
5. Make evaluation for punctal stenosis and position.
6. Lacrimal irrigation.

Instrumentation

- Punctum dilator
- Toothed forceps
- Westcott scissors with sharp tips

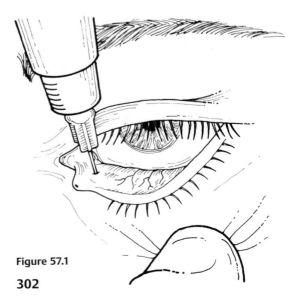

Figure 57.1

302

Operative Procedure

1. Instill topical anesthetic drop into corneal fornix.
2. Inject 2% lidocaine with 1:100,000 epinephrine entering conjunctiva 4 mm inferior to punctum (**Fig. 57.1**).

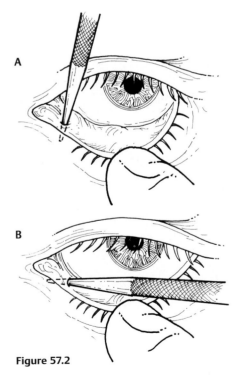

Figure 57.2

3. Dilate punctum widely with punctum dilator (**Fig. 57.2A and 57.2B**).

a. First direct the dilator inferiorly to get into canaliculus.
b. Then direct punctal dilator medially along the normal course of the canaliculus.

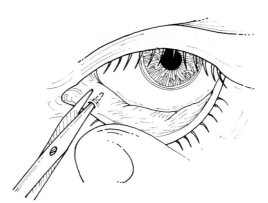

Figure 57.3

4. With the eyelid slightly everted, place one blade of scissors inside of punctum at its most medial aspect and vertically snip punctum (**Fig. 57.3**).

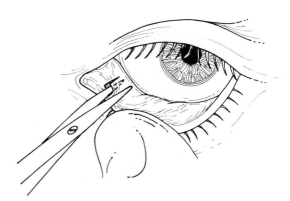

Figure 57.4

5. Place one blade of scissors inside of punctum at its most lateral aspect and vertically snip punctum (**Fig. 57.4**).

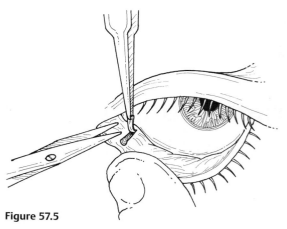

Figure 57.5

6. Grasp incised tissue with the forceps and cut horizontally across its base to complete the punctoplasty (**Fig. 57.5**).

Postoperative Procedure

1. No medications needed.
2. Have patient return in 2 weeks for dilation of punctum (**Figs. 57.2A and 57.2B**) to prevent adhesions and repeat stenosis.

58

Introduction to Evisceration, Enucleation, and Exenteration

The loss of the eye is sometimes inevitable despite the best medical care.

Evisceration is the removal of the contents of the eye, including the retina, uveal tissue, and lens. The cornea is generally removed to minimize the potential for postoperative irritation to the socket. The remaining scleral pocket is filled with an implant and covered with the Tenon capsule and conjunctiva. Evisceration has significant reconstructive advantages over enucleation and exenteration. The procedure is technically straightforward. Because the socket is not disrupted, the implant is stable and resists migration. The movement is excellent. Evisceration carries a minimal risk of sympathetic ophthalmia to the unoperated eye, which has previously limited the appeal of evisceration as a surgical procedure.

Enucleation is removal of the entire eye, including sclera. The empty socket is filled with an ocular implant, which is covered meticulously with Tenon layer and conjunctiva. Various techniques help resist implant migration with time and to optimize movement of the ocular prosthesis. Implant migration and relatively poor motility are problems with enucleation as opposed to evisceration.

Traditional implants for evisceration and enucleation are nonporous spheres composed of methylmethacrylate or silicone. These produce a viable solution for many patients. Newer, more costly implants of hydroxyapatite and porous polyethylene (Medpor) are porous and allow for vascular ingrowth. Advantages of these porous implants are resistance to infection and migration. They also have the potential for improved motility by allowing late (after 6 months) placement of a peg, which can be coupled to the patient's prosthesis.

Exenteration is removal of the entire eye and its soft tissues, including conjunctiva, eyelids, and extraocular muscles. This deforming procedure is reserved for patients with life-threatening neoplasia or infection, chronic otherwise unremitting pain, or significant deformity. After an exenteration, the patient has a large soft tissue defect that may be masked by a patch or eyelid containing oculofacial prosthesis. Remember, however, that the prosthesis made for a patient after exenteration does not blink, and the skin does not match the adjacent skin.

59

Enucleation

Indications

See Chapter 58.

- Intraocular tumors
- Blind eyes following severe penetrating injuries
- Blind eyes with recalcitrant infections
- Blind, painful eyes unresponsive to medical treatment

Preoperative Procedures

See Chapter 3.

1. Treat any infectious processes as necessary.
2. If possible, discontinue aspirin and nonsteroidal anti-inflammatory agents for 10 days prior to surgery. Discontinue warfarin 2–3 days preoperatively, if medically possible.
3. Query patient about bleeding tendencies. A useful screening question is asking if the patient had unusual bleeding after dental extraction. Obtain hematological evaluation if bleeding tendency is suspected.

Instrumentation

- Lid speculum
- Toothed forceps
- Sutures (6–0 Vicryl, 6–0 plain, 5–0 Vicryl)
- Needle holder
- Cautery
- Scissors (Westcott, Stevens)
- Muscle hooks
- Spherical implant (silicone or methylmethacrylate for Technique One and Medpor SST implant for Technique II; see below)
- Sizer set of spheres
- Methylmethacrylate conformer

Operative Procedures

1. Determine method to be used for enucleation:
   a. Technique I: Silicone or methylmethacrylate sphere
   b. Technique II: Medpor sphere

Note: Text will indicate where techniques vary.

2. General anesthesia in most cases.
3. Verify eye to be enucleated.
4. Prep and drape in sterile manner.
5. Place lid speculum.
6. Perform 360 degree limbal peritomy taking care to preserve all conjunctiva (Westcott scissors).

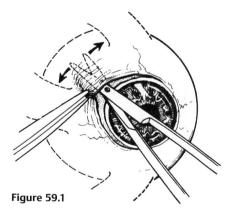

Figure 59.1

7. Bluntly spread between rectus muscles in all quadrants (**Fig. 59.1**).
   a. Use Westcott or Stevens scissors to bluntly buttonhole through the Tenon capsule down to bare sclera.
   b. Aim scissors 45 degrees between rectus muscles.
   c. Spread scissors.

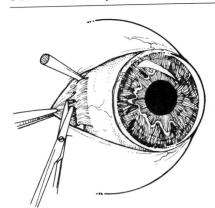

Figure 59.2

8. Isolate medial and lateral rectus muscle with muscle hooks (**Fig. 59.2**).
9. Use Q-tip or scissors to conservatively strip the Tenon capsule.

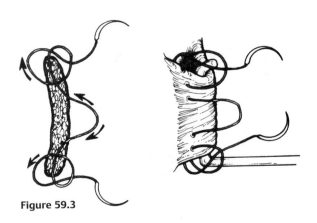

Figure 59.3

10. Whiplock medial and lateral rectus muscles at the insertion with double-armed 6–0 Vicryl sutures with S-14 needles (**Fig. 59.3**).
11. Sever medial and lateral rectus muscles at their insertions (Westcott scissors).
    a. Pull up on muscle hook and sutures to prevent cutting sutures.
    b. Leave ~5 mm stump at medial rectus insertion to enable surgeon to hold and rotate globe.

Technique I: Silicone or Methylmethacrylate Sphere

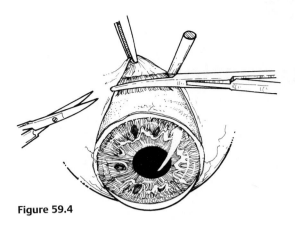

Figure 59.4

1. Hook inferior and superior rectus muscles (**Fig. 59.4**).
2. Strip muscles from the Tenon capsule modestly.
3. Cut muscles flush with globe and allow to retract.

Technique II: Medpor Sphere

1. Whiplock superior and inferior rectus muscles at the insertion with double-armed 6–0 Vicryl sutures.
2. Sever superior and inferior rectus muscles at their insertions (Westcott scissors).

Both Techniques

1. Optional: Isolate and sever superior and inferior oblique muscles.
    a. Superior oblique:
        i. Retract conjunctiva and Tenon capsule posteriorly.
        ii. Grasp superior rectus stump and pull eye inferotemporally.
        iii. Under direct visualization, isolate the superior oblique tendon posterior to the superior rectus stump with muscle hook.
        iv. Clamp tendon with hemostat.
        v. Sever tendon with scissors.
    b. Inferior oblique.
        i. Direct eye superonasally.
        ii. Retract conjunctiva and Tenon capsule posteriorly.
        iii. Isolate oblique muscle between the inferior and lateral recti with muscle hooks.
        iv. Clamp muscle near globe with two hemostats.
        v. Sever muscle between hemostats with scissors.
        vi. Cauterize muscle stumps before removing clamps.

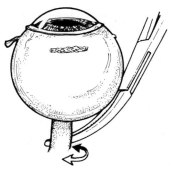

Figure 59.5

2. Strum the optic nerve with side-swiping movement (**Fig. 59.5**) using hemostat.
3. Grasp medial rectus stump with hemostat or forceps.
   a. Use cotton swap to clear residual adhesions to globe.
   b. Palpate the optic nerve with a hemostat.
4. Stabilize the globe and rotate it laterally using an instrument on the medial rectus stump.
5. Clamp optic nerve ~1 minute.
   a. If the nerve is fully clamped, movement of the clamp should be transmitted to orbit.
   b. Do not clamp optic nerve if intraocular tumor is suspected, as clamping of optic nerve increases intraocular pressure and may seed tumor into circulation.
   c. Do not clamp optic nerve if the globe is ruptured since increased intraocular pressure caused by clamping nerve might lead to extrusion of intraocular contents.
6. Remove the clamp.

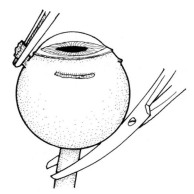

Figure 59.6

7. Cut the optic nerve with enucleation scissors (**Fig. 59.6**).
   a. Apply upward traction on the globe with hemostat or forceps on the medial rectus muscle stump.
   b. Before cutting, press the enucleation scissors posteriorly into the orbit to avoid cutting the nerve too close to the globe.
8. Pull on medial rectus clamp to remove globe.
9. Sever oblique muscles if not previously done in step 1.
10. Lyse any residual adhesions to the globe.

11. Secure hemostasis.
    a. Pack socket with gauze or neurologic 1 cm × 3 cm cottonoids soaked in lidocaine with 1:100,000 epinephrine.
    b. Apply firm pressure for 5 minutes. Use finger or plunger from a syringe.
    c. If bleeding continues, use orbital retractors to cauterize bleeders, usually the artery within the optic nerve stump.
12. Inspect globe to ensure that it has not been transected and that it is completely removed.
13. Use Stevens scissors to open posterior Tenon's layer.

Technique I: Silicone or Methylmethacrylate Sphere

1. Place silicone or methylmethacrylate sphere posterior to posterior Tenon's capsule in the muscle cone.
2. Choose implant size so the Tenon can be closed over it without tension; 18–20 mm is most common.

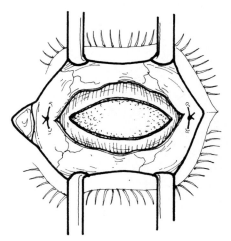

Figure 59.7

3. Sew the previously placed sutures in the medial rectus muscle through the Tenon capsule and conjunctiva, 5–10 mm from the medial commissure and tie. Similarly advance and tie lateral rectus muscle (**Fig. 59.7**).

Technique II: Medpor

1. Determine correct size implant with sizer set.
2. Insert implant into orbit with eight holes in implant facing anteriorly to allow for suturing of muscles to implant.

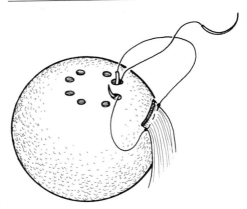

Figure 59.8

3. The Medpor SST implant has connecting channels for passing sutures. Pass suture with S-14 needle attached through tunnel in implant and recover the needle. Beginning at the hole from which the first suture was recovered, pass the other end of this double-armed suture through the implant (**Fig. 59.8**).

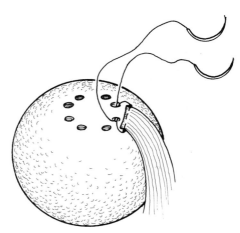

Figure 59.9

4. Pull up on sutures to advance the rectus muscle to the anterior surface of the implant (**Fig. 59.9**).
5. Tie double-armed suture.

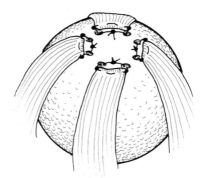

Figure 59.10

6. Suture the other three rectus muscles to the implant in similar fashion (**Fig. 59.10**).

Both Techniques

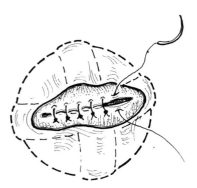

Figure 59.11

1. Close the Tenon capsule meticulously in deep and superficial layers with interrupted 5–0 Vicryl sutures (**Fig. 59.11**).
2. Inspect for any remaining gaps in the Tenon capsule using Q-tip or tip of muscle hook as a probe. Close with additional interrupted sutures. A complete and secure Tenon closure is essential.
3. Run conjunctiva with 6–0 plain gut.
4. Place conformer.
5. Apply antibiotic ointment.
6. Apply firm dressing.

Postoperative Procedure

1. Use oral antibiotics for 5 days.
2. Remove pressure dressing after 24–48 hours.
3. Discharge patient when able to tolerate oral pain meds, generally day after surgery.
4. Apply antibiotic ointment 3 times per day for 3 weeks.
5. Fit for custom prosthesis in 8 weeks.
6. For Medpor, a peg may be placed into the implant to improve motility once implant is vascularized (select cases).

Complications

1. Sectioning of the posterior globe rather than optic nerve, leaving ocular structures in the orbit. In such cases residual tissues should be identified and removed.
2. Hemorrhage
3. Infection
4. Implant extrusion, migration, and exposure
5. Ptosis

60

Evisceration

Indications

See Chapter 58.

- Select cases of intraocular infection in blind eyes.
- Debilitated patients for whom a short procedure or local anesthetic is preferred.
- Patients for whom cosmetic outcome is of particular importance and can accept risk of sympathetic ophthalmic.

Contraindications

- Intraocular tumor
- Ocular condition for which histopathologic examination is necessary
- Severely traumatized eye

Preoperative Procedure

See Chapter 3.

1. Treat any infectious processes as necessary.
2. Make certain eye is not harboring malignancy.
   a. Perform ultrasound examination or magnetic resonance imaging scan if entire fundus cannot be visualized.
3. Select type of implant to be used. Silicone and methylmethacrylate are low cost and relatively inert. Hydroxyapatite and porous polyethylene (Medpor) allow for vascularization and later pegged prosthesis if better prosthetic movement is desired.

Instrumentation

- Lid speculum
- Toothed forceps
- Sutures (6–0 Vicryl, 6–0 plain)
- Needle holder
- Corneoscleral and Westcott scissors
- Cautery
- Microsurgical knife
- Evisceration spoon
- Spherical implant (e.g., silicone, methylmethacrylate, hydroxyapatite, porous polyethylene (Medpor)
- Set of spheres (sizing)
- Methylmethacrylate conformer
- Cyclodialysis spatula
- Absolute alcohol

Operative Procedure

1. Anesthesia: General or retrobulbar (see Chapter 4).
2. Verify eye to be eviscerated.
3. Prep and drape in the usual sterile manner.
4. Place lid speculum.
5. Perform 360 degree conjunctival peritomy at the limbus (Westcott scissors).
6. Enter anterior chamber at the limbus (microsurgical knife).

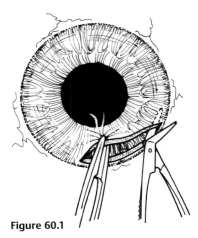

Figure 60.1

7. Remove cornea at the limbus (Westcott or corneoscleral scissors) (**Fig. 60.1**).

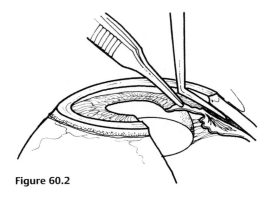

Figure 60.2

8. Disinsert uvea from scleral spur using a cyclodialysis spatula (**Fig. 60.2**).

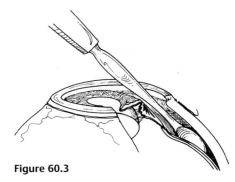

Figure 60.3

9. Carefully shell out intraocular contents with evisceration spoon, attempting to deliver the contents in toto from scleral shell (**Fig. 60.3**).
10. Secure hemostasis.
   a. Directly cauterize bleeding vessels most commonly at optic nerve head.

11. Remove any residual uveal tissue in the scleral cavity with evisceration spoon and moistened cotton-tipped applicators.
12. Scrub scleral cavity with cotton-tipped applicators soaked in absolute alcohol (remove residual uveal cells and denature residual proteins).
13. Irrigate scleral shell with normal saline to remove any residual alcohol.
14. Carefully inspect scleral shell for any remaining tissue.
15. Irrigate scleral shell with antibiotic solution if evisceration is performed for intraocular infection.

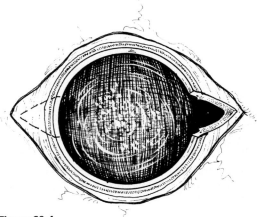

Figure 60.4

16. Excise small triangles of sclera at 3 and 9 o'clock to allow placement of implant and to avoid dog ears when sclera is closed (**Fig. 60.4**).
17. Determine size of implant to be inserted (14, 16, or 18 mm are most common) using sizer set.

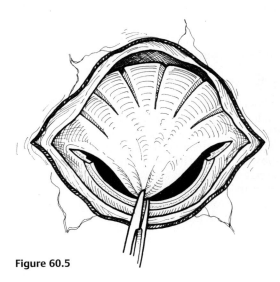

Figure 60.5

18. Ensure that sclera closes over the implant without tension. If not, make vertical or horizontal sclerotomies posterior to equator of globe to allow larger implant and to avoid postoperative enophthalmos (**Fig. 60.5**).

19. Insert chosen implant material.

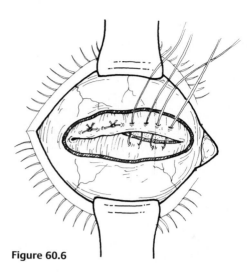

Figure 60.6

20. Close sclera with 4–5 imbricated horizontal mattress sutures of 5–0 Vicryl (barrier to extrusion) (**Fig. 60.6**).
21. Reinforce sclera with additional simple interrupted Vicryl sutures. Close the Tenon capsule with interrupted or running 6–0 Vicryl sutures.

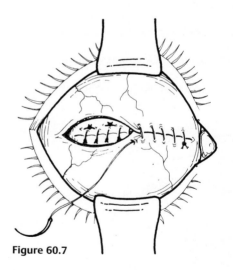

Figure 60.7

22. Close conjunctiva with running 6–0 plain gut (**Fig. 60.7**).

23. Inject subconjunctival antibiotic if there has been a previous infection.
24. Place conformer sized to fill the upper and lower fornices, but allow gentle closure of eyelids.
25. Apply antibiotic ointment.
26. Apply a firm pressure patch.

Postoperative Procedure

1. Continue intravenous or oral antibiotics for several days postoperatively in infected cases to prevent orbital spread. Use oral antibiotics for 5 days for patients without preoperative infection.
2. Remove dressing after 24–48 hours.
3. Discharge patient when pain can be managed with oral medications.
4. Apply antibiotic ointment 3 times per day for 3 weeks.
5. Custom prosthesis is fit in 8–10 weeks.

Complications

1. Risk of sympathetic ophthalmia
2. Intraoperative discovery of unsuspected intraocular tumor
3. Orbital infection
4. Loss of tissue for pathologic examination
5. Exposure or extrusion of implant

61

Orbital Exenteration

Indications

See Chapter 58.

Preoperative Procedure

1. Complete the relevant systemic and regional evaluation. Is disease confined to the orbit? Is there evidence of spread to regional lymph nodes, the continuous paranasal sinuses, brain, or other distant sites?
2. Review the indications for this highly disfiguring procedure with the patient. If the goal of surgery is to "cure" the patient of malignancy, discuss how likely recurrent disease might be. If the surgery is palliative or for control of local disease (as is often the case when disease has shown regional or distant spread), explain the benefits of the procedure over alternatives such as radiation or doing no surgery.
3. Decide if and how the patient thinks he might like to cover the surgical defect. A patient who will have an oculofacial prosthesis will benefit from the deeper socket obtained with complete exenteration. A patient with a superficial orbital process, such as conjunctival malignancy, and who does not want to wear a prosthesis or patch, might benefit from keeping the orbital defect shallow—as is possible with a more limited anterior exenteration.

Instrumentation

- Toothed forceps
- Sutures (4–0 silk traction)
- (5–0 or 6–0 chromic suture)
- Needle holder
- Freer periosteal elevator
- Cautery: monopolar and bipolar
- Malleable retractors
- Scissors (Stevens, Enucleation)

Operative Procedure

1. General anesthesia is preferred. Supplement with a 50:50 mixture of lidocaine 2% plus 1:100,000 epinephrine and 0.75% bupivacaine injected along orbital rim and in retrobulbar or peribulbar fashion.
   a. Conscious sedation may be used in patients at increased anesthetic risk.
   b. Epinephrine decreases soft tissue bleeding.
   c. Local anesthetic helps with post-operative analgesia.
2. Sew eyelids closed.
   a. Sutures are left long to allow mobilization of the specimen.
3. Mark the bony orbital margin with surgical pen.

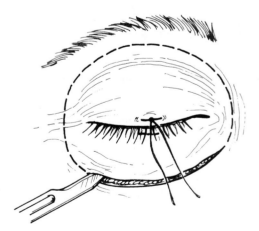

Figure 61.1

4. Incise the periorbital skin with a scalpel (**Fig. 61.1**).

   Optional: Eyelid skin and orbicularis muscle can be preserved by incising skin just above (for upper eyelid) or below (for lower eyelid) lashes. In this variant, eyelid skin and orbicularis muscle are undermined to the level of the orbital rim creating myocutaneous flaps that are draped into the empty orbit at the end of the procedure.

5. If the periocular skin and muscle are involved with tumor, obtain disease-free margins using frozen section or Mohs techniques.

6. Use the scalpel or cutting cautery to incise orbital tissues and periosteum down to the bony orbital rim.

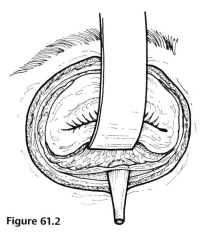

Figure 61.2

7. Separate the periorbita from the bony orbit along the entire circumference of the cavity with a periosteal elevator and retractors (**Fig. 61.2**).

   a. The periorbita is closely fixed to bone at the inferior and superior orbital fissures, trochlea, lateral orbital tubercle, and at the origin of the inferior oblique muscle. Free periorbita with careful dissection.

   b. Special care is taken in the superior orbit, as violation of the superior bony orbit may predispose to cerebrospinal fluid leak, and at the thin lamina papyracea of the medial orbit, since penetration may result in a fistulous tract with the ethmoid sinus.

   c. Avoid monopolar cautery to roof of orbit since it has been associated with cerebrospinal fluid leak.

8. Cut the nasolacrimal duct as it enters the bony nasolacrimal canal. The canal can be followed surgically into the nose, if tumor has involved the lacrimal drainage system.

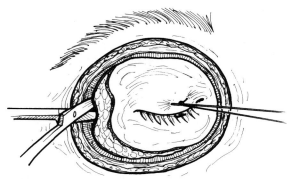

Figure 61.3

9. Divide the specimen from the orbital apex with an enucleation scissors (**Fig. 61.3**). If the disease process does not extend deeply into the orbit, the specimen can be cut just behind the globe—leaving a shower orbital cavity.

10. Remove the specimen and pack the orbital cavity with gauze to achieve hemostasis.

    a. Remove the packing after 5 minutes and cauterize any bleeding vessels.

    b. Excise the most apical tissue, which is difficult to remove, with the scalpel or scissors. Cautery is only conservatively used, as it will prevent histopathologic examination of apical.

11. Harvest a split-thickness skin graft from the anterior thigh using a dermatome set to a 0.015 inch thickness. Cover the donor site with topical ointment or an occlusive membranous dressing.

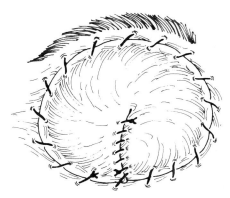

Figure 61.4

12. Sew the graft to the patient's remaining periocular skin at the orbital margin with 5–0 or 6–0 chromic sutures. Drape the graft into the depths of the orbit. Trim overlapping tissue and sew graft together with chromic sutures (**Fig. 61.4**).

    a. Pack the socket with lubricated gauze.

    b. *Optional:* Do not obtain skin graft, but just pack the socket with lubricated gauze. Healing will occur by secondary intention. This will take longer to heal than if a skin graft is used.

Postoperative Procedure

1. Systemic antibiotics are initiated.

2. One to 2 weeks later, the packing is removed and the socket has largely epithelialized. Split-thickness grafts provide for speedier healing than does healing by granulation.

3. The cavity may be covered by a patch or prosthesis and recurrent disease may be detected by inspection.

4. *Optional:* If the socket is allowed to granulate rather than being grafted, daily wet to dry dressing will be needed until epithelization is complete in 4–7 weeks.

    a. Healing by granulation will result in a shallower socket than healing with split-thickness skin grafting.

b. Healing by granulation may result in retraction on surround tissues including the eyebrow.

5. *Optional:* Select patients may benefit from regional transfers, such as transposition of the temporalis muscle into the orbit, or freeze flaps, such as a latisimus dorsi free flap to eradicate the orbital cavity.

Complications

1. Bleeding from the ophthalmic artery and its branches
2. Fistulae between the sinuses and orbit causing chronic hygiene problems, malodorous discharge, difficulty in blowing the nose, or change in voice
3. Cerebrospinal fluid leaks

62

Botox (Botulinum Toxin, Type A) Chemodenervation

Botox comes as a sterile, vacuum-dried form of purified botulinum toxin, type A, produced from a culture of *Clostridium botulinum*. Botox causes a temporary localized muscle paralysis by chemical denervation.

Indications

- Benign essential blepharospasm (FDA approved)
- Hemifacial spasm (FDA approved)
- Cosmetically objectionable glabellar lines in patients younger than 65 years (FDA approved)
- Cosmetically objectionable forehead wrinkles or laugh lines (also called crow's feet) (not FDA approved)
- Many other functional and cosmetic applications are in clinical use, though not FDA approved

Contraindications

Allergy to human albumen; pregnancy; preexisting neuromuscular disease, current use of aminoglycosides

Preoperative Procedure

1. Discuss with patient the indications and use of Botox. A patient's response to specific doses is highly variable. Several treatments may be required before determining optimum dosing and toxin placement.
2. Botox is not currently FDA approved for cosmetic purposes, except for treatment of glabellar lines.

Instrumentation

- Botox (botulinum toxin, type A) purified neurotoxin complex.

- Unpreserved 0.9% sodium chloride injection (preserved saline is commonly used because it stings less when injected, although this practice is not recommended by the manufacturer).
- A 3 mm syringe with 18–22 gauge needle; 0.5–1 ml insulin or TB syringe with 27, 29, or 30 gauge needle (e.g., B-D ultra-fine U-100 insulin syringe pre-wedged onto 0.5 ml with 29 gauge needle).

Operative Procedure

1. *Optional:* Topical anesthetic cream may be applied to skin 15 minutes before injection.
2. Reconstitute vacuum-dried Botox.
   a. Withdraw 1 ml of 0.9% sodium chloride injection without preservative in 1 or 3 ml syringe.
   b. Carefully inject saline solution into vacuum-dried Botox bottle.
   c. Avoid bubbles or turbulence.

Note: This makes a concentration of 10 units per 0.1 ml.

Note: Another popular dilutions is 5 units per 0.1 ml (mixed with 2 ml normal saline into the vial).

   d. The toxin, once mixed, should be used within 4 hours according to the manufacturer. (In clinical practice, the drug continues to be effective when stored in the refrigerator for several days after reconstitution.)
3. Wipe involved facial areas with alcohol and allow to dry, as alcohol may inactivate Botox.
4. Proceed with injections:
   a. Injections are subcutaneous to avoid diffusion past the orbital septum into the orbit, where ptosis or diplopia may occur.

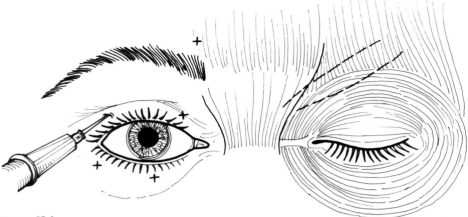

Figure 62.1

b. In the glabellar area, injections are deeper—onto the surface of the glabellar musculature—because the skin is thicker than in the eyelids.
5. For hemifacial spasm, inject 1.25–2.5 units per site on the involved side as depicted (**Fig. 62.1**).
6. For essential blepharospasm, inject 2.5–5.0 units per site as depicted (**Fig. 62.2**).
7. For cosmetic indications:
   a. Reduction of cosmetically objectionable glabellar lines (**Fig. 62.2**).
      i. Inject 5 units at head of eyebrow 1 cm above the orbital rim, then angle the needle superiorly for 7 mm and inject an additional 5 units. This weakens the corrugators (vertical lines). Repeat on the opposite side.
      ii. Inject 5 units in midline to weaken for procerus (horizontal glabellar lines).
   b. For smile lines, inject 2–4 units in 3 sites in the lateral laugh line (crow's feet) area.
   c. For horizontal brow furrows inject 2 units in 4 places across brow.

Postoperative Instructions

1. Botox may take 2–10 days for maximum effect.
2. Most patients with blepharospasm or hemifacial spasm have symptoms of ocular dryness and benefit from artificial tears.

Complications

1. Double vision
2. Ptosis
3. Dry eye
4. Tearing
5. Brow ptosis
6. Brow asymmetry
7. Localized bruising

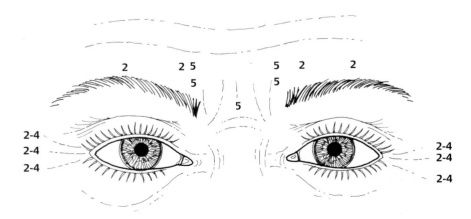

Figure 62.2

IX

Vitreoretinal

63

Posterior Segment Vitrectomy

Indications

The goals of posterior vitrectomy are varied. Most important among these are:

- Removal of media opacities.
- Management of tractional or traction-rhegmatogenous retinal detachment (e.g., detachments associated with proliferative vitreoretinopathy [PVR] or proliferative diabetic retinopathy [PDR]).
- Repair of rhegmatogenous retinal detachment.
- Alleviation of tangential traction on the retina (e.g., epiretinal membrane [ERM]).
- Repair of macular hole.
- Submacular surgery to remove subfoveal blood (e.g., with retinal arterial macroaneurysm-induced hemorrhage) or subfoveal choroidal neovascularization (e.g., associated with the presumed ocular histoplasmosis syndrome) in carefully selected patients.
- Removal of intraocular foreign bodies (IOFB).
- Biopsy of the vitreous to identify infectious organisms in cases of endophthalmitis or cancer cells in cases of intraocular large cell lymphoma.
- Biopsy of the retina and/or choroid in cases of ocular inflammatory disease of uncertain origin (e.g., nocardia endophthalmitis).
- Removal of cataractous lens with zonular dehiscence using pars plana approach.
- Repositioning of subluxed intraocular lens (IOL) implant.
- As an adjunct to drainage of hemorrhagic or serous choroidal detachment.

Specialized techniques include segmentation and/or excision of vitreoretinal membranes, internal drainage of subretinal fluid, application of endolaser photocoagulation or endocryotherapy, use of heavier-than-water perfluorocarbon liquids, use of illuminated intraocular instruments (e.g., forceps, scissors), gas-fluid exchange to name a few. An in-depth treatment of these techniques is beyond the scope of this book. Rather, this chapter will describe the essential features of the posterior vitrectomy procedure.

Preoperative Procedure

See Chapter 3.
1. Complete retinal evaluation with ultrasound examination if necessary.
2. Dilate pupil (e.g., cyclopentylate 1% plus phenylephrine 2.5% every 15 minutes × 3 starting 1 hour before surgery).

Instrumentation

- Lid speculum
- Fine-toothed tissue forceps (e.g., 0.12 mm straight Castroviejo and/or Colibri)
- Westcott and Stevens scissors
- Muscle hooks
- Cautery with attachments both for external and intraocular use
- Castroviejo calipers
- Marking pen (optional)
- 20-gauge microvitreoretinal (MVR) blade
- Fine-tipped needle holder (preferably locking)
- Infusion cannula, 2.5, 4, or 6 mm depending on: (1) size of eye (e.g., 2.5 mm for pediatric cases) and (2) the visibility of the cannula tip after insertion into the vitreous cavity and/or the presence of choroidal detachment (e.g., 6 mm cannula for cases with choroidal detachment)
- Sutures (4–0 white silk or 6–0 Vicryl, 7–0 Vicryl, and 8–0 Vicryl or 6–0 plain gut)
- Vitrectomy suction/cutting instrumentation

Note: In this chapter, the Alcon Accurus vitrectomy machine and settings are used for illustrative purposes. The authors recognize that other excellent machines are available. The authors have no financial interest in the Accurus system.

- Fiber optic endoilluminator (some surgeons use chandelier illumination, which is inserted through a sclerotomy and sutured in position rather than held in the nondominant hand)
- Corneal ring and high refractive index contact lenses (20 degree and 30 degree prism), wide field (48 degree), macula (34 degree), and biconcave (90D) lenses; or, the wide-angle viewing lens system (wide-angle system lenses: macula, 66D lens; equator, 91D lens; wide field, 155D lens)
- Scleral plugs
- Cotton-tipped applicators
- Indirect ophthalmoscope
- 20 D and/or 28 D lenses
- Intraocular forceps (e.g., Tano asymmetric forceps, De Juan forceps), scissors (e.g., Sutherland vertical and horizontal, 25 gauge), pick (e.g., serrated tip, fine tip), diamond-dusted flexible tip cannula (Tano). Some instruments (e.g., scissors, forceps) accommodate fiber optic light and are illuminated.
- Fluted needle with or without (Charles) silicone tip
- Laser (endo- and/or indirect)
- Cryo unit (transscleral cryotherapy) plus appropriate probes
- Gas pump (provided as part of the Alcon Accurus vitrectomy machine)
- Silicone oil infusion syringe (provided as part of the Alcon Accurus vitrectomy machine pack)
- Flexible iris retractors and 15 degree blade (for patients with small pupils)
- Perfluorocarbon liquid and/or silicone oil (depending on the case)
- Gas: SF_6, C_3F_8
- Inverting system for the wide-angle vitrectomy lenses (e.g., ROLS by Volk)
- Several companies manufacture such inverting systems, including Volk, Ocular, and Avi. Any of these inverting systems can be used with the wide-angle contact lenses manufactured by any of these companies (e.g., use Volk lenses with Avi inverter).
- BD Visitec 20 gauge × 1 inch cannula with 30 gauge × 3/16 inch tip extension for viscodissection (optional)
- Instruments for subretinal surgery: subretinal forceps, pick, and 33 gauge infusion cannula (optional)

Operative Procedure

1. Anesthesia: General, or retrobulbar + sedation + anesthesia monitoring ± lid block.
2. Prep and drape eye. Adhesive-backed plastic is preferred to keep eyelashes out of the surgical field. If there is a concern about patient head movement under local anesthesia, consider taping the patient's head to the stretcher.
3. Place lid speculum.
4. Perform conjunctival peritomy (Westcott scissors, tissue forceps).
   a. Perform fornix-based localized conjunctival peritomy over the planned entry sites (**Fig. 63.1A**).
   b. Alternatively, perform small focal peritomies over the planned sclerotomy sites (**Fig. 63.1B**).

Note: If a scleral buckle is to be placed, perform a 360 degree limbal peritomy.

5. *Optional:* Cauterize bleeding vessels and planned sclerotomy sites.
6. Isolate and sling rectus muscles with 2–0 black silk suture if a scleral buckle is to be placed (**Figs. 63.2 and 63.3**).
   a. Buttonhole Tenon capsule and intermuscular septum between muscles with Stevens scissors (may use cotton-tipped applicator to bluntly dissect between and expose muscles).
   b. Isolate muscle with muscle hook (see Chapter 37).
   c. Sling each rectus muscle with a 2–0 silk suture threaded through a fenestrated muscle hook.
      i. Suture is placed through fenestrated muscle hook, which is then passed under muscle. Suture is then pulled from the hook with forceps, slinging the muscle.
      ii. Sling superior rectus muscle last, using the other traction sutures to achieve adequate exposure. Muscle hook should be passed in a temporal to nasal direction to avoid slinging the superior oblique tendon.
7. Plan location of entry sites.
   a. Place sclerotomies 3 mm posterior to limbus in aphakic/pseudophakic eyes and 4 mm posterior to limbus in phakic eyes (measure with calipers).

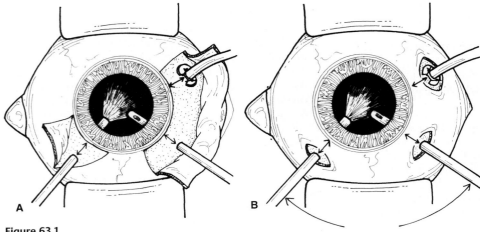

Figure 63.1

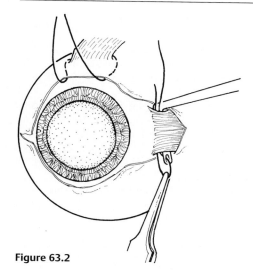

Figure 63.2

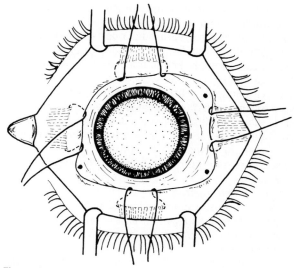

Figure 63.3

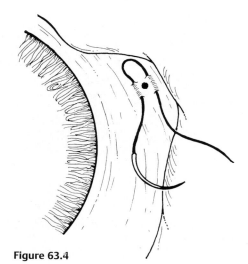

Figure 63.4

b. Place infusion cannula inferotemporally (unless there is a contraindication) and place sites for bimanual manipulation superotemporally and superonasally.

c. Sclerotomy sites should be parallel to the limbus.

d. *Optional:* Mark sites with marking pen or cautery.

8. First prepare infusion site.

a. Place inferotemporally in most cases.

b. Pre-place 4–0 white silk or 6–0 or 7-0 Vicryl mattress suture through partial thickness sclera spanning the sclerotomy site (**Fig. 63.4**).

c. Enter eye with MVR blade (**Fig. 63.5A**).

   i. Hold blade perpendicular to scleral surface, aiming toward anatomical center of globe.

   ii. Place blade tip on scleral surface, enter eye with controlled firm pressure, and penetrate pars plana completely.

   iii. Visualize knife tip through pupil to verify penetration, if media are clear.

   iv. Directing probe into the anterior vitreous can result in lens damage (**Fig. 63.5B**).

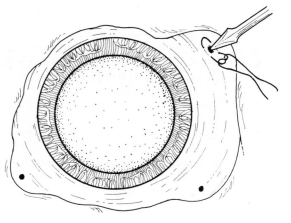

A

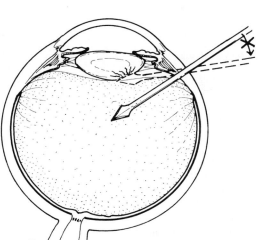

B

Figure 63.5

d. Place infusion cannula through sclerotomy. (A twisting motion facilitates entry of cannula.)
e. View cannula directly through pupil externally.
   i. Can direct the fiber optic endoilluminator light beam through the pupil toward the infusion cannula to improve view, or
   ii. Use indirect ophthalmoscope to verify proper cannula position and penetration through pars plana. If infusion cannula does not completely penetrate the pars plana, infusion fluid may detach the retina and/or choroid.
f. Secure infusion cannula to sclera with the preplaced suture.
9. Prepare the two superior entry sites.
   a. Place incisions in superotemporal and superonasal quadrants near superior borders of rectus muscles for comfortable bimanual manipulation (e.g., at 10 and 2 o'clock).
   b. Use MVR blade in similar fashion to Step 8c: Final instrument positioning according to type of peritomy.
   c. Close sclerotomies with silver scleral plugs. Gold-colored plugs have a larger diameter than silver plugs.
10. 23 gauge and 25 gauge: Transconjunctival entrance is performed for sclerotomy; conjunctival peritomy is not needed.
   a. Use a caliper to mark the site of sclerotomy. The sclerotomy for the infusion line usually is made in the inferotemporal quadrant.
   b. Slightly displace the conjunctiva over the marked site using a forceps or a cotton tip applicator.
   c. Take the sharp inserter-cannula system (a pre-loaded sharp trocar or a stiletto blade with a cannula; manufacturers include Alcon, Bausch & Lomb, or DORC) to make a beveled incision for the sclerotomy.

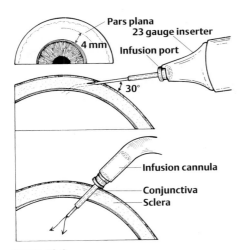

Figure 63.6

d. Insert the pre-loaded trocar at a 30 degree angle through the conjunctiva and the sclera for approximately 1 mm and then angle directly toward the optic nerve. (For the 25 gauge vitrectomy, some surgeons prefer to make a nonbeveled transconjunctival, incision perpendicular to the sclera.) (**Fig. 63.6**)

e. Stabilize the cannula with a forceps and remove the trocar.
f. Connect the infusion line to the cannula. Confirm the location of the cannula tip in the vitreous cavity.
g. Perform superior sclerotomies at 2 and 10 o'clock positions similarly.
11. If pupil is inadequately dilated, place flexible iris retractors.
   a. Incise limbus at 2, 4, 8, and 10 o'clock with 15 degree blade.
   b. Use 0.12, 0.3, or 0.5 mm toothed forceps or McPherson tying forceps to guide flexible iris retractors through the limbal incisions and capture the pupillary margin.

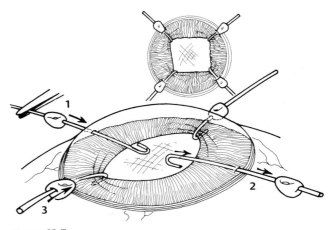

Figure 63.7

c. Advance the sleeve around the flexible iris retractors, thus opening the pupil (**Fig. 63.7**).
12. Suture corneal ring in position and place contact lens on cornea.
   a. Secure ring with superficial suture bites ~2–3 mm posterior to the limbus at 6 and 12 o'clock, or 3 and 9 o'clock meridians.
   b. Place viscous coupling medium on cornea (e.g., Healon or Goniosol).
13. Place contact lens on cornea.
   a. For those using the traditional Machemer lens system:
      i. Usually begin with the wide field (48 degree) lens.
      ii. For dissection over the macula (e.g., internal limiting membrane [ILM] stripping, membrane dissection), use macula lens.
      iii. For peripheral vitreous dissection, use prism (20 degree, 30 degree) lens.
   b. For those using the contact wide-angle lens system (Volk, Oculus, or Avi):
      i. The inverter should be connected in the microscope.
      ii. Usually begin with the wide-angle lens (Ocular 155D, or Volk's Mini Quad/Quad XL).
      iii. For macular dissection, use the macula lens (~66D).
      iv. For equatorial dissection, use the equator lens (~91D).

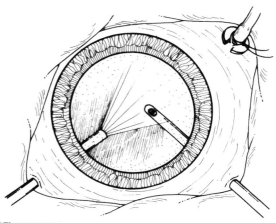

Figure 63.8

14. Insert fiber optic endoilluminator and vitrectomy instrument after removing scleral plugs (**Fig. 63.8**).
15. Turn off room and microscope lights.
16. Set vitrectomy instrument parameters: Alcon provides different vitrectomy probes that have different cutting rates and different mechanisms of action. For example, the Accurus 800 and 2500 probes have guillotine action, and the InnoVit probe has rotary action. This machine features a dual mode foot pedal. At initiation of foot pedal depression, the machine activates to a high preset cutting rate (e.g., InnoVit 1800 cpm) and 0 mm Hg vacuum. As foot pedal depression proceeds further, the cutting rate gradually decreases and the vacuum increases to preset levels (e.g., InnoVit 1200 cpm, 200 mm Hg). The settings outlined below are just suggestions. Different surgeons prefer different settings.
   a. Accurus 800 probe:
      i. Core vitrectomy: cutting rate 800 cpm, vacuum 150 mm Hg, infusion pressure 25–35 mm Hg.
      ii. Vitreous base: cutting rate 800 cpm, vacuum 50 mm Hg, infusion pressure 25 mm Hg.
      iii. Extraction of dense membranes or induction of posterior vitreous detachment (PVD): low cutting rate of 200–400 cpm (0 cpm for PVD induction), vacuum 100–250 mm Hg, infusion pressure 35 mm Hg. With high vacuum, may need to increase infusion pressure to prevent globe collapse.
      iv. If close to detached retina: high cutting rate 800 cpm, vacuum 50 mm Hg, infusion pressure 25 mm Hg.
   b. InnoVit probe:
      i. Core vitrectomy: cutting rate 1000 cpm, vacuum 150–200 mm Hg, infusion pressure 35 mm Hg.
      ii. Vitreous base: cutting rate 1800 cpm, vacuum 50–75 mm Hg, infusion pressure 25–35 mm Hg.
      iii. Extraction of dense membranes or PVD induction: low cutting rate of 400–600 cpm (0 cpm for PVD induction), vacuum 100–250 mm Hg, infusion pressure 35 mm Hg. With high vacuum, may need to increase infusion pressure to prevent globe collapse.

      iv. If close to detached retina: cutting rate 1800 cpm, vacuum 30 mm Hg, infusion pressure 25–50 mm Hg.
   c. Accurus 2500 probe:
      i. Core vitrectomy: cutting rate 1500 cpm, vacuum 75–150 mm Hg, infusion pressure 35 mm Hg.
      ii. Vitreous base: cutting rate 2500 cpm, vacuum 50 mm Hg, infusion pressure 30 mm Hg.
      iii. Extraction of dense membranes or PVD induction: low cutting rate of 400–600 cpm (0 cpm for PVD induction), vacuum 100–250 mm Hg, infusion pressure 35 mm Hg. With high vacuum, may need to increase infusion pressure to prevent globe collapse.
      iv. If close to detached retina: cutting rate 2500 cpm, vacuum 50 mm Hg, infusion pressure 30 mm Hg.
   d. Accurus 23 gauge 2500 cpm probe:
      i. Core vitrectomy: 1500 cpm, vacuum 400 mm Hg, infusion pressure 35 mm Hg.
      ii. Vitreous base: cutting rate 2500 cpm, vacuum 150 mm Hg, infusion pressure 25 mm Hg.
      iii. Induction of posterior vitreous detachment: increase suction to 500 mm Hg.
   e. Accurus 25 gauge 1500 cpm probe:
      i. Core vitrectomy: 1100 cpm, vacuum 600 mm Hg, infusion pressure 40 mm Hg.
      ii. Vitreous base: 1500 cpm. vacuum 250 mm Hg, infusion pressure 25 mm Hg.
      iii. Induction of posterior vitreous detachment: increase suction to 600 mm Hg.
17. Perform vitrectomy.
   a. Remove lens if opacity precludes adequate visualization for procedure (see Chapter 66).

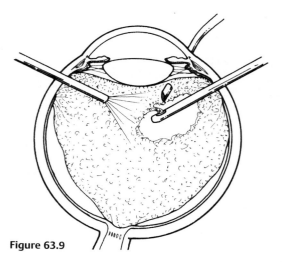

Figure 63.9

   b. Remove central vitreous (**Fig. 63.9**).

Do not touch posterior surface of crystalline lens with intraocular instruments.

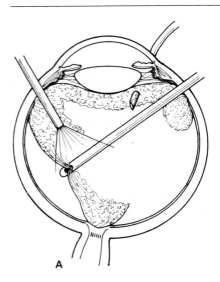 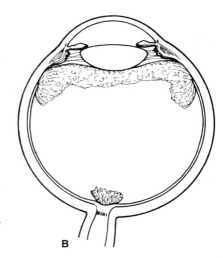

A   B

Figure 63.10

c. "Backlighting" rather than direct illumination with fiber optic probe facilitates visualization of the vitreous.

d. Identify posterior hyaloid face (PHF) and proceed with posterior vitrectomy, removing posterior cortical vitreous (**Figs. 63.10A and 63.10B**).

e. If posterior hyaloid is attached to the optic nerve and posterior pole retina, lift the PHF using vitrector in the aspiration mode with high vacuum 200–250 mm Hg over the edge of the optic disc. If unsuccessful, incise and elevate PHF with the tip of a bent MVR blade: (1) use active suction over the edge of the optic disc; (2) with the vitreous engaged in the cutting port, elevate the hyaloid by slightly withdrawing the vitrector away from the retina surface and insinuate the tip of the MVR blade into the junction of the retina and PHF at the edge of the optic disc; (3) elevate the MVR blade to peel the PHF away from the retina.

   i. Once edge of a Weiss ring (white glial ring at the edge of the optic disc) is visible, use active suction with the vitrector or use a pick to peel the PHF off the posterior and peripheral retina out to the equator.

   ii. Must be alert for creation of retinal breaks during this maneuver.

   iii. If retina is detached and PHF is attached to retinal surface, one can infuse perfluorocarbon liquid into the eye, provided that there are no posterior retinal breaks, to maintain posterior retinal attachment during the PHF dissection.

f. Perform a 360 degree peripheral vitrectomy. Remove the vitreous base as completely as possible without touching the posterior surface of the crystalline lens.

   i. Can use prism lenses to visualize peripheral vitreous in phakic eyes. If wide-angle viewing system is not available, the far peripheral vitreous can be visualized using scleral indentation and the coaxial illumination of the operating microscope. Alternatively, in selected case, one can combine use of the prism lens and scleral

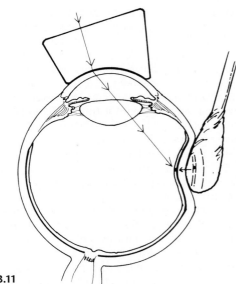

Figure 63.11

indentation to visualize the peripheral vitreous (**Fig. 63.11**).

   ii. If using wide-angle viewing system, use the Ocular 155D, or Volk's Mini Quad/Quad XL lens for peripheral vitrectomy.

g. Relieve vitreomacular traction.

   i. Use pick or bent MVR blade to identify/develop cleavage plane between retina and ERMs and cut tissue with intraocular scissors and/or peel tissue with intraocular forceps (**Fig. 63.12**).

   ii. If retina is detached and/or quite atrophic, Healon® can be infused (using a BD Visitec 20 gauge × 1 inch cannula with 30 gauge × 3/16-inch tip extension) into the potential space between epiretinal tissue and retina to develop a cleavage plane atraumatically (viscodissection).

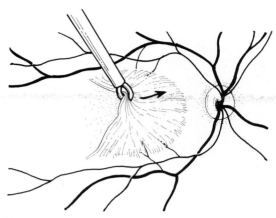

Figure 63.12

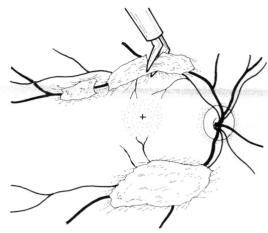

Figure 63.14

iii. Depending on tightness of adhesion, the free edge of epiretinal tissue can be grasped with intraocular forceps and stripped from retinal surface (e.g., ERM peeling) (ERM stripping with forceps, **Fig. 63.12**), or

19. Remove instruments from eye.

Some surgeons stop infusion before instrument removal to prevent vitreous incarceration in sclerotomies.

a. Any vitreous that prolapses through sclerotomy sites should be cut flush with sclera using Westcott scissors.

b. Usually one uses the vitrectomy probe just inside the vitreous cavity at a high cutting rate (e.g., Accurus 800: 800 cpm; InnoVit: 1800 cpm; Accurus 2500: 2500 cpm), low vacuum (e.g., 50 mm Hg), and low infusion pressure (e.g., 25 mm Hg) to excise vitreous that is incarcerated in the sclerotomy site.

Note: The latter maneuver can be dangerous if the retina is detached (inadvertent cutting of detached peripheral retina); generally the maneuver is executed once the retina is attached fully.

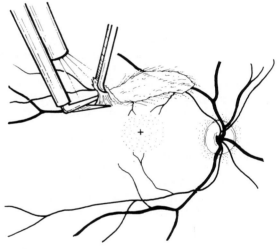

Figure 63.13

iv. Intraocular scissors can be introduced between the retina and epiretinal tissue, and the connecting tissue can be severed in an en bloc fashion (delamination) (**Fig. 63.13**), or

v. With segmentation, islands of tightly adherent epiretinal tissue are left in place with all surrounding vitreous adhesions severed (segmentation) (**Fig. 63.14**).

18. Perform specialized manipulations as indicated for particular vitreoretinal pathology (e.g., retinal reattachment with expression of subretinal fluid through peripheral retinal breaks using perfluorocarbon liquid, air–fluid exchange, segmentation of intraocular membranes, endophotocoagulation, intraocular foreign body removal, etc.).

20. Place scleral plugs in open sclerotomy sites to prevent globe decompression.

21. Examine peripheral retina for retinal breaks and treat them if present.

a. Examine the fundus with indirect ophthalmoscope using a 20 D or a 28 D lens after the instruments are removed from the eye.

b. For wide-angle viewing system users, one can examine the peripheral retina under the microscope just before all the instruments are removed from the eye. Use light pipe through one of the sclerotomy ports and place scleral plug in the other remaining superior port. Scleral depress with the other hand and look for any peripheral tears under the microscope.

c. When inspecting for retinal breaks or detachment, search carefully behind sclerotomy of the surgeon's dominant hand (site of most frequent passage of instruments into and out of eye).

d. Treat retinal breaks with laser photocoagulation (including indirect laser ophthalmoscope and/or endolaser) if retina has been reattached or with transscleral cryoretinopexy, especially if media opacity or blood precludes laser uptake or if retina is detached at the time of treatment.

e. To flatten the peripheral retina (once all membrane dissection is complete and, in selected cases, after the scleral buckle has been placed) prior to laser photocoagulation, perform fluid–air exchange.
  i. Turn on air infusion (25–35 mm Hg) while draining subretinal fluid using the Charles fluted needle or using active suction (e.g., silicone-tipped cannula attached to vitrectomy machine to achieve maximum vacuum of 100–150 mm Hg) over the retinal tear.
    I. Operating microscope-guided technique.
      A. Place biconcave lens (90 D) or, if using wide-angle system, Ocular 155 D, or Volk's Mini Quad/Quad XL lens on cornea.
      B. Focus retina at maximum magnification.
      C. Select drainage retinotomy (either a pre-existing posterior retinal break or a break created with endodiathermy, usually just superior and nasal to the optic disc).
      D. Infuse air while draining subretinal fluid using the Charles fluted needle or using active suction.
    II. Indirect ophthalmoscope-guided technique.
      A. Introduce fluted needle through one of the superior sclerotomies under visualization with the indirect ophthalmoscope and a 20 D or 28 D lens.
      B. Turn on air infusion after having directed needle tip over the drainage retinotomy.
    III. Usually work with an infusion pressure of 35 mm Hg.
  ii. Perform endo- or indirect laser photocoagulation (3–4 rows) around the flattened retinal tear, bringing treatment up to the edge of the tear and not treating bare retinal pigment epithelium (RPE).
  iii. If peripheral retinal breaks are present and vitreoretinal traction is present on the breaks, consider placing scleral buckle (usually a 2.5 mm wide (e.g., #240, Dutch Ophthalmic) or 4 mm wide (e.g., #42, Dutch Ophthalmic) silicone band) to support the vitreous base.

Perform scleral buckling procedure as necessary (see Chapter 64). When necessary, the buckle is placed around the eye, and sutures holding the buckle in place (particularly in inferior quadrants) are tied before fluid-air exchange is performed. This approach may facilitate retinal reattachment if there is unrelieved retinal traction (e.g., in severe PVR).

22. Close each sclerotomy site with a 7–0 Vicryl suture (**Fig. 63.15**).
23. Perform air–gas exchange or silicone oil infusion if needed. Gas provides temporary retinal tamponade but has greater surface tension than silicone oil. Thus, gas is better at functionally closing retinal breaks and reattaching retina and tamponades inferior retinal breaks effectively. Silicone oil (usually 1000 or 5000 centistoke sterile oil (we prefer 5000 cst) provides long lasting tamponade, can be associated with complications (e.g., corneal decompensation, cataract, and glaucoma), and

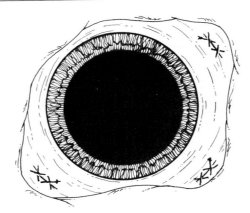

Figure 63.15

does not tamponade inferior retinal breaks as well as it has a lower specific gravity than water and will float above a meniscus of inferior intravitreal fluid in eyes with an incomplete fill.

a. Air–gas exchange.
  i. Infuse nonexpansile concentration of SF_6 (20%) or C_3F_8 (12–15%). SF_6 dissipates in ~2 weeks, and C_3F_8 dissipates to < 30% gas fill of the vitreous cavity in ~6 weeks (if aqueous humor is produced normally).
  ii. Many surgeons use SF_6 for phakic eyes and C_3F_8 for aphakic/pseudophakic eyes or eyes in which a long-lasting bubble is needed.
  iii. Insert tuberculin syringe (without a plunger) attached to 5/8 inch 30 gauge needle 3 mm (aphakic/pseudophakic eye) or 4 mm (phakic eye) posterior to limbus with one hand and introduce 20–50 ml syringe attached to a 5/8 inch 30 gauge needle containing a nonexpansile concentration of gas 3 or 4 mm posterior to the limbus with other hand.
  iv. Assistant gently depresses plunger of gas-containing syringe, thus forcing intraocular gas out of the tuberculin syringe.

b. Silicone oil infusion.
  i. Close superonasal sclerotomy with 7–0 Vicryl.
  ii. Place 7–0 Vicryl suture in superotemporal sclerotomy but do not tie suture.
  iii. Introduce silicone oil via inferotemporal sclerotomy.
    I. A 20 gauge angiocatheter is trimmed to 4 mm length and attached to a 10 ml syringe containing silicone oil.
    II. The silicone oil-containing syringe is connected to the vitrectomy machine. Using machine-pressurized mechanism, the oil is forced into the vitreous cavity. Infusion is stopped when silicone meniscus reaches the posterior lens capsule or the posterior surface of the iris diaphragm.
    III. If a machine-pressurized mechanism is not available, one can infuse the oil using a manually pressured device (silicone oil delivery device) (**Fig. 63.16**).

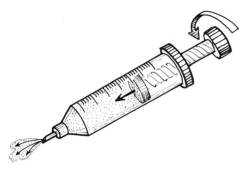

Figure 63.16

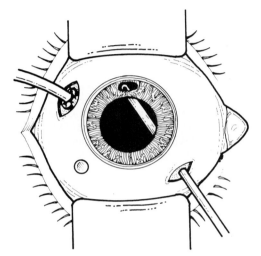

Figure 63.17

iv. In aphakic eyes, an inferior iridectomy should be created at 6 o'clock to prevent the development of pupil block secondary angle closure glaucoma (**Fig. 63.17**). Some surgeons also perform an inferior iridectomy in pseudophakic eyes.

v. Check intraocular pressure using Schiotz tonometer (underestimates correct intraocular pressure at very low and very high pressures). Generally, one attempts to leave intraocular pressure ≤ 21 mm Hg.

24. Remove rectus muscle sling sutures if placed previously.
25. Close conjunctiva (6–0 plain gut or 8–0 Vicryl).
26. Inject subconjunctival cefazolin (100 mg) and Decadron (4–8 mg).

 If patient is allergic to penicillin, consider substituting vancomycin (50 mg) for cefazolin.

27. Consider administering acetazolamide 500 mg intravenously if postoperative intraocular pressure elevation is anticipated and patient does not have a contraindication (e.g., sulfa allergy).

 Topical β-adrenergic antagonists (e.g., timolol), carbonic anhydrase inhibitors (e.g., dorzolamide), or α-adrenergic agonists (e.g., brimonidine tartrate 0.2%) can also be used if tolerated by patient.

28. Remove lid speculum, apply topical antibiotic ointment and atropine sulfate 1% (if not contraindicated) drops, apply patch, and place Fox shield.

Operative Procedure: Special Applications of Vitrectomy

Endophthalmitis

Vitreous biopsy is best performed via a pars plana one-, two-, or three-port vitrectomy. A single-port vitreous biopsy can be done in the office using a 23 gauge vitrectomy probe. If an automated vitrectomy probe is not available, the vitreous can be biopsied using a 1.5 inch 25 or 27 gauge needle attached to a tuberculin syringe. Use of a vitrectomy probe probably results in less vitreoretinal traction than aspiration with a syringe, and it does not increase the likelihood of obtaining false-positive culture results. Vitreous specimens (0.1–0.2 ml for aspirate, ~0.5 ml for vitrectomy probe-assisted vitreous biopsy, ~1 ml for two- or three-port vitrectomy) should be sent undiluted for culture and smear to increase the yield. If a two- or three-port vitrectomy is done, one should consider submitting the cassette fluid for culture. One study showed that when both vitreous biopsy and vitrectomy cassette specimens were cultured, the cassette specimens had a 76% positive culture rate; the vitreous biopsies had only a 43% positive rate.

If the view of the fundus is limited, preoperative echography should be done to detect the presence and amount of vitreous inflammation/debris, to detect choroidal detachment (particularly after trabeculectomy), and to rule out retinal detachment or intraocular foreign bodies (following trauma). Ultrasound also may indicate the presence of a posterior vitreous detachment, which can facilitate vitreous removal at surgery.

Vitreous Biopsy

1. Single-port vitreous biopsy: usually done in the office.
 a. Administer topical anesthetic (e.g., proparacaine).
 b. Place sterile lid speculum (wire-type preferred).
 c. Administer retrobulbar or subconjunctival anesthesia.
 d. Sterilize ocular surface with topical 5–10% Betadine.
 e. Biopsy can be done with patient sitting at slit lamp, as the stabilization of patient's head and the magnification of the biomicroscope facilitate placement of vitrectomy probe into the sclerotomy and visualization of the probe just posterior to the pseudophakos (IOL) or crystalline lens.
 f. To maintain visualization of sclerotomy, cauterize overlying conjunctiva at planned site of sclerotomy (3 mm posterior to limbus in aphakic/pseudophakic eyes or 4 mm posterior to limbus in phakic eyes).
 g. If vitrectomy probe is blunt-tipped, introduce 23 gauge sharp blade into anterior vitreous cavity to create sclerotomy.
 h. Introduce 23 gauge vitrectomy probe (Josephberg) into sclerotomy (facilitated by a slight twisting motion on entry). If using a vitrectomy probe with a sharp tip (which is preferred), neither previous incision with MVR blade nor twisting motion on entry is needed.

i. Have assistant very gently aspirate after probe is activated to maximum cutting rate and positioned in mid anterior vitreous cavity.

j. Stop suction before terminating automated cutting.

k. Remove vitrectomy probe from eye.

2. Vitrectomy in operating room: Patients with endophthalmitis and visual acuity of hand motions or better following cataract or secondary IOL surgery may be treated with vitreous biopsy and intravitreal antibiotics alone, but patients with severe inflammation appear to benefit from core vitrectomy plus intravitreal antibiotics. If a vitrectomy (versus vitreous biopsy) is indicated (e.g., a patient with light perception vision and acute postoperative endophthalmitis), a core vitrectomy should be performed, and, generally, one does not attempt to excise cortical or peripheral vitreous. In the setting of severe inflammation, the retina can be friable and more likely to tear.

a. It is best to avoid making sclerotomies near a filtering bleb so as not to disturb the bleb.

b. If media opacity or choroidal detachment precludes safe initial placement of infusion cannula, an infusion light pipe and a two-port pars plana vitrectomy can be a useful alternative to three-port vitrectomy.

c. Rarely, the crystalline lens or IOL has to be removed to aid in visualization of the probe or to completely remove all microorganisms (e.g., those adherent to IOL). This procedure is done using a three-port vitrectomy approach.

d. If inflammation prevents visualization of the pars plana infusion cannula and if infusing light pipe is not available, consider the following approach to cannula placement.

i. Using a 23 gauge butterfly needle, begin with limbal infusion into anterior chamber.

ii. With vitrectomy probe in the mid-vitreous, initiate the vitrectomy. Be sure limbal infusion is turned off initially, so an undiluted vitreous specimen can be obtained (see *e* below). Once specimen is obtained, turn on limbal infusion. (The vitrector should not be primed before taking the undiluted sample.)

iii. A pars plana infusion cannula (4–6 mm long) is introduced once sufficient anterior segment and vitreous opacities have been cleared to allow safe visualization of cannula in vitreous cavity.

e. Obtain undiluted vitreous biopsy.

i. Attach 10 ml syringe to vitrectomy aspiration line via "T" connector with line turned off to machine and on to syringe (**Fig. 63.18**).

ii. Assistant gently withdraws plunger of syringe with vitrectomy cutting mechanism activated to remove vitreous material.

iii. After ~0.5–1.0 ml of undiluted vitreous is obtained (or if globe collapses sooner), stop vitrectomy and turn on infusion again.

iv. Specimen is submitted for smear and culture immediately.

v. One can inoculate aerobic and anaerobic blood culture bottles in operating room for culture.

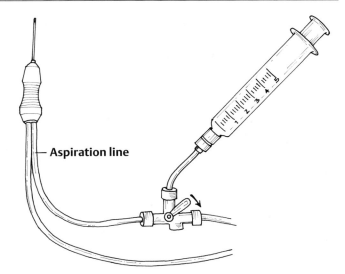

— **Aspiration line**

Figure 63.18

f. In aphakic or pseudophakic eyes, the probe can be directed into anterior chamber to remove debris that obscures visualization of posterior segment.

g. Attempt to continue to remove core vitreous until retina is visible or a bright red reflex is obtained, but not if visualization is inadequate.

h. Management of retinal breaks in this setting is difficult, and retinal detachment has a significant chance of developing PVR. (If a break is detected and one must treat the break and the endophthalmitis simultaneously, however, one can use full strength intravitreal antibiotics with a 50% gas bubble.)

i. At the time of one-, two-, or three-port vitrectomy, fibrin pupillary membranes can be removed with a sharp blade and/or a vitrectomy probe (via a limbal or pars plana incision) in aphakic/pseudophakic eyes to improve visualization of instruments in vitreous cavity. In phakic eyes, fibrin pupillary membranes sometimes can be engaged and retracted peripherally using flexible iris retractors.

j. Intravitreal antibiotic injections: Administration of intravitreal antibiotics is the mainstay of treatment of acute postoperative endophthalmitis. The infection is almost always seated in the vitreous cavity, and other routes of drug administration generally do not achieve satisfactory intravitreal drug levels. Because rapid initiation of therapy is important for successful treatment of endophthalmitis, antibiotics generally must be administered before culture results are available.

i. Currently, vancomycin is considered the drug of choice for the gram-positive organisms including methicillin-resistant *Staphylococcus* species and *Bacillus cereus* and is not toxic in the clinically recommended dose of 1 mg/0.1 ml.

ii. The best choice for antimicrobial treatment of gram-negative organisms is controversial. Aminoglycosides (gentamicin 0.1 mg/0.1 ml or amikacin 0.4 mg/0.1 ml) have been recommended traditionally for gram-negative coverage. Several clinical and laboratory reports have shown that aminoglycosides are toxic to the retina and RPE at doses close to therapeutic. Ceftazidime has been recommended as an alternative antibiotic to cover gram-negative organisms because of its broad therapeutic index, lower risk for retinal toxicity, and its in vitro antimicrobial activity, which is as effective as the aminoglycosides against gram-negative bacteria.

    I. Intravitreal ceftazidime is not associated with retinal-RPE toxicity in doses up to 10 mg/0.1 ml in primates.

    II. Ceftazidime has been reported to be physically incompatible with vancomycin causing the drugs to precipitate out of solution when combined. Precipitation can be avoided by injecting the two antibiotics from separate syringes.

iii. Currently, our recommendations for intravitreal therapy are: vancomycin (1 mg/0.1 ml) to cover gram-positive microorganisms and ceftazidime (2.25 mg/0.1 ml) to cover gram-negative microorganisms. In cases suspected of vancomycin-resistant Enterococci, ampicillin, an aminoglycoside, and systemic ciprofloxacin have been suggested as empiric therapy. In cases of suspected fungal endophthalmitis, amphotericin C 5 µg/0.1 ml is administered intravitreally. This dose can be repeated after 48 hours.

iv. Materials:

    I. Lid speculum.

    II. 5–10% povidone iodine.

    III. Tuberculin syringe attached to 5/8 inch 30 gauge needle.

    IV. Tuberculin syringe containing Vancomycin (2 mg/ 0.2 ml) attached to 5/8-inch 30 gauge needle.

    V. Tuberculin syringe containing ceftazidime (4.5 mg/0.2 ml) attached to 5/8-inch 30 gauge needle.

    VI. Topical anesthetic, or subconjunctival 2% lidocaine without epinephrine in a 1–3 ml syringe attached to a 5/8-inch 30 gauge needle, or 10 ml 2% lidocaine without epinephrine attached to 1.5-inch 25 gauge needle.

    VII. Castroviejo calipers (sterile).

v. Technique:

    I. Administer topical, subconjunctival, or retrobulbar anesthesia. Many patients can tolerate intravitreal antibiotic injection at the slit lamp under topical or subconjunctival anesthesia alone.

    II. Place lid speculum.

    III. Sterilize ocular surface with 5–10% povidone iodine.

    IV. If vitreous biopsy is to be done, do biopsy. (In this case, subconjunctival or retrobulbar anesthesia is done.) If vitreous biopsy is not to be done, perform anterior chamber paracentesis with tuberculin syringe entering at limbus (usually temporally).

    V. Insert tuberculin syringe 3 (aphakic/pseudophakic eye) or 4 mm (phakic eye) posterior to limbus as measured with calipers. Use separate syringes to prevent antibiotic precipitation.

    VI. Inject intravitreal antibiotic slowly (0.1 ml of each antibiotic) with the bevel of the needle facing anteriorly.

    VII. This technique permits adequate diffusion of antibiotic into the vitreous cavity, thus reducing the chance of retinal toxicity. The antibiotic solutions are rather viscous, and rapid injection with the bevel facing posteriorly favors delivery of the drug as a bolus over the macula.

    VIII. Repeat injection for second antibiotic-containing syringe.

vi. Repeat vitreous tap and injection of antibiotics (plus pars plana vitrectomy if not done originally) should be considered if no clinical improvement or if worsening is noted within 48 to 72 hours, since a single intravitreal injection is not adequate in some cases.

Removal of Intraocular Foreign Body

1. Magnetic foreign body ≤ 3 mm diameter located on the pars plana:

Even in this case some surgeons prefer a vitrectomy approach. One can use an external approach, however, as detailed below:

    a. Close entry site with suture.

    b. Isolate rectus muscles using 2–0 silk sutures.

    c. Localize IOFB externally using indirect ophthalmoscopy.

    d. Make sclerotomy over IOFB using #69 Beaver blade.

    e. Cauterize exposed choroid.

    f. Incise choroid.

    g. Place electromagnet over foreign body.

    h. Activate magnet and remove foreign body.

    i. Suture sclerotomy closed with 7–0 Vicryl suture.

    j. Consider laser- or cryoretinopexy in area just posterior to foreign body. In some cases, a segmental scleral buckle is needed also.

    k. If one cannot remove IOFB via an external approach, consider performing a pars plana vitrectomy ± lensectomy and IOFB removal via internal approach.

2. Nonmagnetic, posteriorly located (within 30 degrees of the optic nerve head or macula), or large (≥ 3 mm diameter) intraocular foreign bodies:

    a. Perform pars plana vitrectomy and excise vitreous attachments to IOFB.

    b. Introduce intraocular forceps and grasp IOFB firmly.

    c. Withdraw instrument and IOFB from eye.

    d. May need to enlarge sclerotomy to accommodate passage of IOFB out of eye.

        i. For large IOFB, a "T"-shaped sclerotomy may be helpful (**Fig. 63.19**)—"T" incision at pars plana).

        ii. Consider removal through original entrance site for very large IOFB.

            I. Culture IOFB.

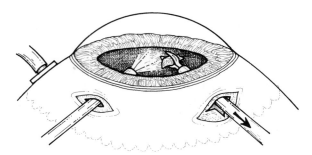

Figure 63.19

II. Suture sclerotomies closed and close conjunctiva as described above.

Repositioning of Posteriorly Dislocated IOL

1. Perform three-port vitrectomy.
2. Excise vitreous adherent to IOL.
3. Grasp IOL with intraocular forceps and deliver into anterior chamber.

May infuse perfluorocarbon to float IOL into retroiridal space. This maneuver prevents IOL from falling posteriorly and damaging retina during repositioning.

4. Use intraocular forceps to manipulate IOL haptics into ciliary sulcus (PCIOL, assuming adequate capsular support) or anterior chamber angle (ACIOL).
5. If PCIOL is dislocated and inadequate capsular support exists for sulcus fixation, consider replacing PCIOL with ACIOL via limbal incision or suturing PCIOL in position.
6. A technique for suturing PCIOL.
   a. Lens used is a Bausch & Lomb Model 6190B one-piece, PMMA with optic size 6.50 mm, biconvex, length 12.75 mm, displaying haptics with two midloop eyelets.
   b. Either 50%-thickness limbal-based triangular scleral flaps or circumferential 60%-thickness scleral incisions are created, centered at the 3 and 9 o'clock positions.
   c. Flexible iris retractors are placed at 2, 4, 8, and 10 o'clock via limbal incisions created with a sharp blade, and the pupil is dilated widely (**Fig. 63.20A**).
   d. If the eye has not previously undergone vitrectomy, a conventional three-port vitrectomy is done. Peripheral vitreous is dissected meticulously.
   e. A long 27 gauge bent needle is inserted ab externo 1 mm posterior to the limbus at 3 o'clock and exited at 9:15 o'clock in a ciliary sulcus location 1 mm posterior to the limbus (**Fig. 63.20A**).
   f. A straight, 16 mm long needle, carrying Ethicon 10–0 polypropylene (Prolene) suture, is swaged blunt end first into the barrel of the 27 gauge needle and maximally advanced.
   g. The entire assembly is withdrawn into the vitreous cavity (**Fig. 63.20B**).

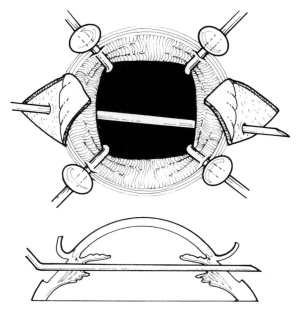

Figure 63.20A

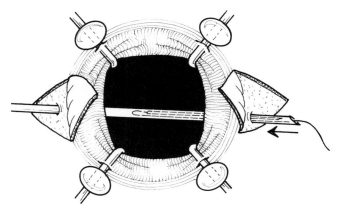

Figure 63.20B

h. The entire assembly is directed out of the eye through the ciliary sulcus at 8:45 o'clock 1 mm posterior to the limbus (**Fig. 63.20C**).
i. The 27 gauge needle is withdrawn from the eye. This maneuver creates an intraocular loop of 10–0 Prolene suture centered at the 9 o'clock position with two externalized sutures under the scleral flap (**Fig. 63.20D**).
j. A scleral tunnel or partial-thickness beveled limbal incision for PCIOL implantation is fashioned at 12 o'clock. If a limbal incision is made, the anterior chamber is entered with a sharp blade at 12 o'clock only (**Fig. 63.20E**).
k. The loop of 10–0 Prolene is externalized through the scleral tunnel using a hook (**Fig. 63.20F**).
l. A long 27 gauge bent needle is inserted ab externo 1 mm posterior to the limbus at 9 o'clock (between the Prolene sutures) and exited at 3:15 o'clock in a ciliary

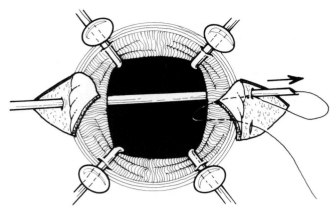

Figure 63.20C

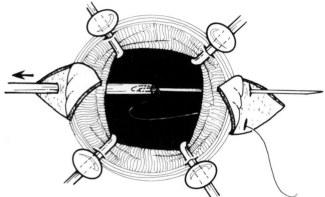

Figure 63.20D

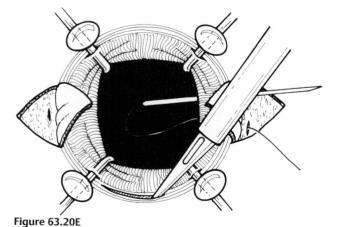

Figure 63.20E

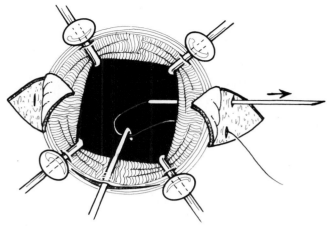

Figure 63.20F

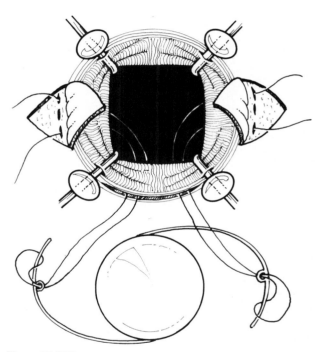

Figure 63.20G

n. The scleral tunnel is widened as needed, or the limbal incision is opened fully with a sharp blade to accommodate the IOL and visoelastic is injected into the anterior chamber.

o. The PCIOL is introduced into the eye; the haptics are seated in the ciliary sulcus, and the lens is centered in the sulcus by pulling up on the externalized sutures (**Fig. 63.20H**).

One can avoid intraocular suture tangles by pulling gently on the externalized sutures under the flaps so that the sutures are under mild tension. As the PCIOL is guided into the ciliary sulcus with one hand, the surgeon can use the other hand to pull up further on the free suture ends associated with the haptic that is entering the eye.

sulcus location. The same steps are followed in the 3 o'clock scleral bed to create the second externalized loop of 10–0 Prolene.

m. The loop is twisted and passed through the eyelet attached to the haptic. The Prolene suture is looped around the haptic without a knot (**Fig. 63.20G**).

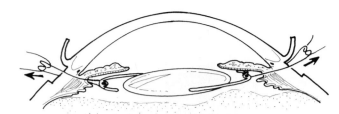

Figure 63.20H

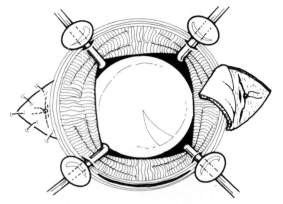

Figure 63.20I

p. The externalized sutures are tied and trimmed slightly long so that they lie flat against the sclera. The knots are buried under the scleral flaps, which are sewn shut with 10–0 nylon suture (**Fig. 63.20I**).

q. The scleral tunnel is closed with 10–0 nylon suture; the sclerotomies are closed with 7–0 Vicryl, and the conjunctival incisions are closed with 6–0 plain gut.

Macular Pucker

1. Perform three-port vitrectomy.
2. Place high magnification macula contact lens (34 degrees) on cornea.
3. Create cleavage plane between ERM and retina.
   a. First, try to use blunt pick to create cleavage plane between retina and ERM.
   b. The ERM edge at which dissection should be initiated may be present at the edge of retinal folds (**Fig. 63.21**).
   c. If one cannot develop an edge with blunt pick, one may use diamond-dusted cannula (Tano) or bent MVR blade to create cleavage plane.
      i. MVR: Indent MVR blade against lid speculum or other hard surface to create fine bend in tip. Be sure to scrape MVR blade gently on episclera to verify that bent tip is not fragile. If it is, it will break off in episclera. Once edge is created, peel ERM using intraocular forceps.
      ii. Tano cannula: Brush cannula against retinal surface gently in a sweeping motion. Start in area at ERM edge.
   d. If retina is detached, cleavage plane can also be extended using viscodissection.
4. Close eye as above.

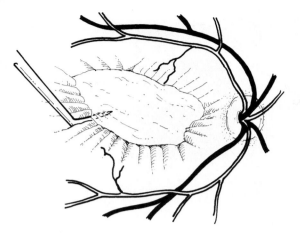

Figure 63.21

Macular Hole

1. Perform three-port vitrectomy with excision of PHF off of optic disc and macula.
2. Perform ILM dissection. Important for closure of macular holes in setting of reoperation. Two effective techniques are described below.
   a. Gently scrape retinal surface around macular hole with diamond-dusted cannula (Tano). Begin ~1.5 disc diameters away from margin of hole and scrape centripetally. When ILM is elevated, grasp edge with intraocular forceps and peel in a circumferential (i.e., capsulorrhexis) fashion away from edge of macular hole.
   b. Incise ILM ~1.5 disc diameters away from macular hole with MVR blade (**Fig. 63.22A**). Some surgeons use a Rice pick to elevate ILM at its cut edge (**Fig. 63.22B**). Some surgeons skip this step and proceed directly to grasp the edge of ILM with fine-tipped intraocular forceps and peel the ILM in a capsulorrhexis-like maneuver (**Fig. 63.22C**).
3. Perform air–fluid exchange as described above. Some surgeons use humidified air to reduce likelihood of developing postoperative visual field defects.
   a. Under visualization with a biconcave corneal contact lens (or 166 D wide angle lens), aspirate fluid over optic disc using a fluted needle.
   b. Aspirate fluid from center of macular hole using fluted needle (infusion pressure usually set to 25–35 mm Hg). Edges of hole should come into apposition if traction has been relieved adequately.
   c. Wait 5–10 minutes, reenter eye, and repeat fluid aspiration.

Submacular Surgery for Choroidal Neovascular Membrane Excision

1. Perform three-port vitrectomy.
2. Excise PHF.
3. Create localized retinal detachment over choroidal new vessel (CNV) by introducing bent 33 gauge cannula into subretinal space inferotemporal to edge of CNV.

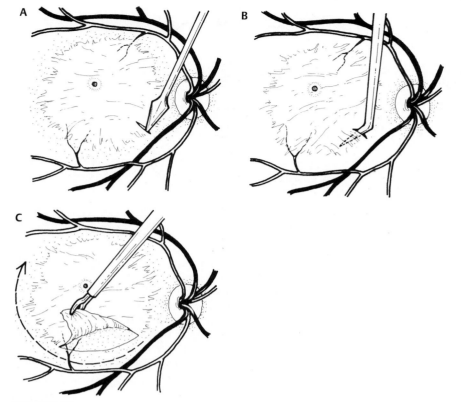

Figure 63.22

a. Observe retina carefully for presence of retina–CNV adhesions. These will be evident as areas in which the retina does not achieve a convex configuration as subretinal fluid is injected.
b. Stop infusion if retina–CNV adhesions are detected.
c. Use cannula to gently separate adhesions joining retina to subjacent CNV. Can also use subretinal pick.
d. If substantial subretinal fluid is present initially, this step can be omitted.
4. Elevate IOP sufficient to close central retinal artery.
5. Use cannula or subretinal pick to gently displace CNV until ~180 degrees of CNV perimeter near retinotomy is freely mobile in subretinal space.

One can project preoperative fluorescein angiogram in operating room to be certain of location of CNV perimeter.

6. Introduce subretinal forceps into subretinal space and gently grasp free edge of CNV.
7. Withdraw CNV from subretinal space in a single, slow, steady movement. Occasional side-to-side pulling will free up undissected CNV edges.
8. Either excise CNV from eye with intraocular forceps or remove CNV with vitrectomy probe.

Large CNVs can create retinal dialyses when removed from the eye, particularly if the sclerotomy has not enlarged and the peripheral vitreous has not been excised sufficiently.

9. Examine peripheral retina and identify any breaks.
10. Perform fluid–air exchange.

11. If peripheral retinal breaks are present, treat them and perform air-gas exchange.
12. Close sclerotomies.
13. Close incisions and dress eye as above.

Endophotocoagulation

1. Perform three-port vitrectomy as above.
2. After membrane peeling, retinal reattachment, etc., introduce endophotocoagulation probe into superior sclerotomy.
3. Instruct circulating nurse to provide protective goggles (appropriate to laser wavelength being used) to all operating room personnel not shielded by filter on operating microscope.
4. Instruct circulating nurse to turn laser on "Treat" with settings at continuous duration, and power setting of 150–300 milliwatts power (depending on degree of pigmentation of patient).
   a. Some surgeons prefer to set treatment duration to 0.1 seconds. If continuous duration is used, the foot pedal must be released as soon as moderate RPE-retinal whitening is observed.
   b. Some surgeons prefer to use the repeat mode where as some prefer to depress foot pedal to activate laser delivery for each laser burn application.
5. Aiming beam intensity is set to convenience of surgeon.

6. Apply laser treatment in pattern appropriate to purpose:
   a. Retinal break: surround retinal break with three rows of confluent white burns, each ~300–500 μm in diameter.
   b. Panretinal photocoagulation (PRP): Apply moderate burn intensity spacing burns 1–2 burn widths apart. Do not bring treatment closer than 500 μm to optic nerve head nasally or 2.5 disc diameters to fovea temporally.
7. Indirect laser ophthalmoscope permits application of burns in periphery.
8. Wide-angle viewing systems (e.g., AVI, Volk) using the wide-angle lens permit wide field of view for laser application even with endophotocoagulation probe. Biconcave contact lens (90 D) in fluid- or air-filled eye also permits wide field of view for PRP application.

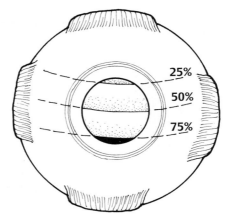

Figure 63.23

Postoperative Procedure

1. Keep patch and shield placed until patient is examined on postoperative day 1.
2. Generally, patients are discharged on day of surgery. Exceptions occur in patients who are medically unstable (e.g., poorly controlled diabetic patients) or patients with endophthalmitis receiving intravenous antibiotics.
3. Postoperative activity: Quiet, ambulatory activity unless head positioning is necessary.

Appropriately position head if intraocular gas has been used. (Generally, strict face-down position except for meals and bathroom privileges in phakic eyes.)

4. Topical antibiotics (e.g., gatifloxacin or moxifloxacin drops 4 times per day; avoid use of ointments, which obscure view of fundus).
5. Steroid drops (e.g., prednisolone acetate 1%) 4 times per day (or more frequently if indicated) for 3–6 weeks, tapered as inflammation permits.
6. Scopolamine 0.25% or atropine 1% drops twice per day for cycloplegia.
7. Control intraocular pressure with β-adrenergic antagonists (e.g., timolol), α-adrenergic agonists (e.g., brimonidine tartrate 0.2% twice per day), and/or carbonic anhydrase inhibitors (including topical dorzolamine 2% 3 times per day) as needed and as tolerated.
8. If patient has been admitted, discharge patient when stable (usually postoperative day 1 unless patient is receiving intravenous antibiotics for endophthalmitis).

Follow-up Schedule

1. Examination on daily basis while in hospital.
2. Check visual acuity.
3. Measure intraocular pressure.
4. Examine anterior chamber to rule out hypopyon, fibrinoid reaction.
5. Document clarity of crystalline lens (if present).
6. Document size of intravitreal gas bubble (**Fig. 63.23**).
   a. With patient sitting at slit lamp, looking straight ahead, and pupil dilated to 6 mm, if inferior meniscus of gas bubble is tangential to superior margin of pupil, then 25% gas fill is said to be present.
   b. If inferior meniscus of gas bubble bisects pupil, then 50% gas fill is said to be present.
   c. If inferior meniscus of gas bubble is tangential with inferior margin of pupil, then 75% gas fill is said to be.
7. Perform indirect ophthalmoscopy.
8. Examine at ~1, 3, and 6 weeks postoperatively and then as necessary.

Complications

1. Endophthalmitis (~0.05%)
2. Transient elevation in intraocular pressure
3. Central retinal artery occlusion
4. Choroidal infarction
5. Anterior chamber shallowing and secondary angle closure glaucoma
6. Persistent corneal epithelial defect (especially in diabetic patients)
7. Vitreous hemorrhage
8. Choroidal effusion
9. Choroidal hemorrhage
10. Iatrogenic retinal breaks and detachment (including PVR)
11. Cystoid macular edema
12. ERM
13. Rubeosis iridis and neovascular glaucoma (particularly in diabetic patients)
14. Cataract formation
15. Subretinal gas (if vitreoretinal traction inadequately relieved, intravitreal gas can enter subretinal space)
16. Bullous keratopathy
17. Sympathetic ophthalmia (e.g., ~0.1% after surgery in traumatized eyes)
18. Complications associated with scleral buckling (if buckle placed)
19. Complications associated with retrobulbar anesthesia (if administered)
20. Complications associated with general anesthesia (if administered)

64

Retinal Detachment Repair
Scleral Buckling and Pneumatic Retinopexy

■ Scleral Buckling

Principles

Several techniques are used in the repair of rhegmatogenous retinal detachments. These vary depending on the nature of the detachment and preference of the surgeon. The principles of the various techniques of retinal reattachment surgery, however, are the same. These include:

■ Localization of all retinal breaks.
■ Creation of chorioretinal adhesion at the margins of the breaks.
■ Relief of vitreoretinal traction either permanently (e.g., scleral explant or implant or direct relief via vitrectomy) or temporarily (e.g., episcleral balloon, intraocular gas bubble).
■ The following protocol outlines one general method of primary retinal reattachment surgery. Particular operations and the modalities employed therein should be tailored to the requirements of the specific case and the surgeon's preference.

Preoperative Procedure

See Chapter 3.
1. Schedule surgery expeditiously.
   a. If the macula is attached and threatened by progression of the detachment or if the macula has been detached for less than several days, then, in general, surgery should be performed within 24–72 hours if possible.
      i. Generally, in nonvitrectomized eyes, inferior extramacular detachments spread into the macula slowly.
      ii. Chronic detachments probably can be repaired on a nonemergent basis. Signs of a chronic detachment include: demarcation line (hyper- or hypo-pigmented) separating attached from detached retina; retinal cysts; subretinal fibrosis.
   b. If the macula has been detached for a lengthy period, surgery may be scheduled electively.
   c. Impose activity limitations as the nature of the detachment warrants. Strict bed rest with bilateral eye patching can promote substantial resolution of subretinal fluid in a minority of patients.
2. Complete retinal evaluation: Identify and diagram all retinal breaks.
3. Clip lashes 24 hours preoperatively, if possible.
4. Dilate pupil (e.g., cyclopentolate 1% plus phenylephrine 2.5% every 15 minutes starting 1 hour before surgery).

Instrumentation

■ Lid speculum (preferably self-retaining, e.g., Maumenee-Park)
■ Toothed tissue forceps (e.g., 0.3 or 0.5 mm forceps, Bishop-Harmon)
■ Westcott scissors
■ Stevens scissors
■ Cautery
■ Cotton-tipped applicators
■ Sutures (2–0 cotton, 4–0 white silk or Mersilene on spatula needle, 6–0 double-armed black silk on a spatula needle, 6–0 plain gut)
■ Muscle hooks (including fenestrated hook)
■ Needle holder
■ Utility tying forceps (e.g., Alabama)
■ Schepens retractor
■ Indirect ophthalmoscope
■ Retinal break localizer (modified thimble-type scleral depressor [Gass depressor])
■ Straight scleral depressor
■ Marking pen
■ Cryosurgical unit with retina cryoprobe
■ Silicone buckling elements
■ Hemostat (small)
■ Beaver #69 and #66 blades

■ Needle for drainage of subretinal fluid (e.g., small-gauge taper-point surgical needle, 2.5 mm diathermy pin)
■ Schiotz tonometer
■ Tuberculin syringe with $^{5}/_{8}$ inch 30 gauge needle
■ 20 ml syringe with 30 gauge needle, Millipore filter

Operative Procedure

1. Local anesthesia with sedation is preferred unless the patient is unlikely to be able to lie flat during surgery (e.g., kyphoscoliosis, congestive heart failure) or cannot communicate with the surgeon. Patients with severe myopia might undergo general anesthesia to avoid the risk of globe perforation associated with retrobulbar injection. One approach in the latter setting is to have the patient sedated, prepped and draped first. Then, after topical proparacaine and/or lidocaine gel is applied, make a conjunctival incision, separate the Tenon fascia from the globe, and provide retrobulbar anesthesia using a blunt-tipped cannula. Usually, surgery is done as an outpatient procedure.
2. Prep and drape. Adhesive-backed plastic drapes help to keep the eyelashes (if present) out of the surgical field.
3. Place lid speculum.
4. Perform a 360 degree conjunctival peritomy at the limbus. Two radial relaxing incisions can be made (Westcott scissors, tissue forceps).
5. Secure hemostasis with cautery.

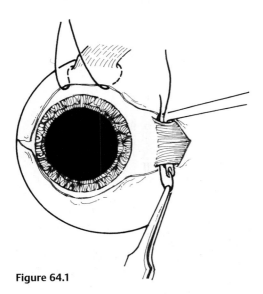

Figure 64.1

6. Isolate and sling rectus muscles (**Fig. 64.1**).
7. Buttonhole the Tenon capsule and intermuscular septum between muscles (Westcott or Stevens scissors; may use cotton-tipped applicator to bluntly dissect between and expose muscles).
8. Isolate muscle with muscle hook (see Chapter 37).
9. Sling each rectus muscle with a 2–0 silk suture (without a swaged-on needle).

10. The suture is placed through a fenestrated muscle hook, which is then passed under the muscle. The suture is pulled from the hook with forceps, slinging the muscle.
11. Alternatively (but less desirable due to risks associated with needle passage near the globe), one may use 4–0 silk with swaged-on needle (pass hub of needle under muscle).

Sling superior rectus muscle last, using the other traction sutures to achieve adequate exposure. The muscle hook should be passed in a temporal to nasal direction to avoid slinging the superior oblique tendon.

12. Tie knot at distal end of each suture.
13. Inspect sclera for abnormalities (e.g., thinning).
14. May rotate globe with traction sutures and retract conjunctiva with Schepens retractor.
15. Use cotton-tipped applicator to move tissue and inspect sclera in all four quadrants, respectively.
16. Examine retina completely with scleral depression (indirect ophthalmoscope, cotton-tipped applicator or straight depressor for scleral depression).
17. Localize and mark location of all retina holes and tears.
18. Indent sclera with retinal break localizer and mark depressed spot with marking pen, cautery, or diathermy.
19. For small holes and tears, mark directly over site.
20. For larger tears, mark posterior, anterior, and lateral margins of break.

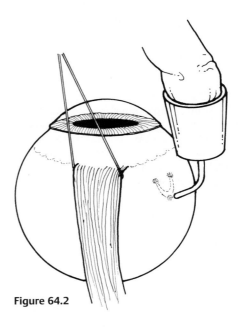

Figure 64.2

21. Apply cryotherapy to all retinal holes, tears, and areas of lattice degeneration (see Chapter 65). (**Fig. 64.2** illustrates marking of a large retinal break.)
22. Test cryoprobe (desired temperature should be –60 to –80°C).
23. Position eye with traction sutures.
24. Examine fundus with indirect ophthalmoscopy.

25. Position cryoprobe at edge of retinal break.
26. Treat breaks in undetached or shallowly detached areas first. (The eye softens as the sclera is depressed with treatment, subsequently allowing easier access to the more bullous areas surrounding a break.)
27. Indent sclera with probe tip (keep tip perpendicular to sclera), avoiding compression with instrument shaft.
28. Activate cryo-unit.
29. Terminate cryo-application when whitening of retinal pigment epithelium (RPE)-retina is observed through ophthalmoscope.
30. If no reaction is observed in several seconds after the cryo-unit achieves its lowest temperature, terminate the application and verify position of probe tip.

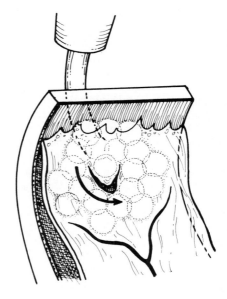

Figure 64.4

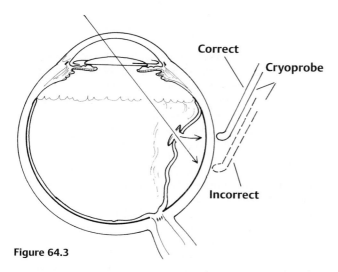

Figure 64.3

31. If retina is bullously detached, excessive freezing will be required to induce retinal whitening, and one should terminate the cryo-application once whitening of the underlying RPE is observed. Parallax can lead to incorrect identification of the location of RPE underlying the retinal break. (**Fig. 64.3** illustrates parallax effect.)
32. After cryoprobe thaws, move probe to adjacent area around break.
33. In this manner, make additional applications until the break is surrounded by treatment.

Note: Cryo spots must overlap each other slightly to completely seal the break.

34. A 1–2 mm treatment zone should surround the retinal break. The anterior-lateral margins of the retinal break should be treated precisely, as failure to do so is a common cause of recurrent retinal detachment (**Fig. 64.4**).
35. Treatment should extend to the posterior margin of the vitreous base for breaks in the anterior periphery.
36. Select style and size of buckling element to be used.
37. A wide variety of buckling elements is available. Among the most common are:
    a. Segmental silicone sponges (e.g., one half thickness 5 mm diameter sponge for radial buckle).
    b. Encircling, solid silicone bands with or without grooves (e.g., 7 mm wide, 3 mm thick, 2.5 mm grooved silicone #287 exoplant).
    c. Factors favoring placement of segmental element:
       i. Single break located anterior to the equator.
       ii. Multiple retinal breaks (one per quadrant) anterior to the equator in different quadrants.

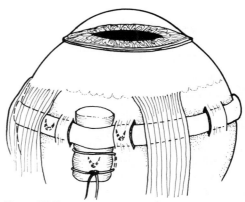

Figure 64.5

iii. Retinal break located just posterior to and unsupported by an encircling element. (**Fig. 64.5** illustrates combination encircling and radial element.)
iv. History of sickle cell disease or sickle trait.
v. Presence of advanced glaucomatous optic atrophy.
d. Factors favoring placement of encircling element:
   i. Multiple retinal breaks anterior to the equator in the same or different quadrants.
   ii. Presence of peripheral vitreoretinal pathology (e.g., lattice degeneration) in other quadrants that should be supported by the scleral buckle.
   iii. Presence of proliferative vitreoretinopathy (e.g., starfold formation).
   iv. No breaks found on exam.
   v. All breaks not definitively localized.
   vi. Aphakic/pseudophakic detachments.

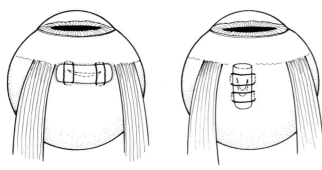

Figure 64.6

38. Determine element size by measuring dimensions of breaks using localization marks. (**Fig. 64.6** illustrates support of retinal break by scleral buckle.) Element should completely encompass break.
39. For radial buckles, the buckle should be centered on the meridian of the retinal break and extend ~2 mm posterior to the posterior margin of the retinal break.
40. For encircling buckles, all retinal breaks should be supported on the buckle, and the most posterior retinal break should be supported by at least the posterior slope of the scleral buckle.
41. Soak elements in bacitracin solution before use (if tolerated).

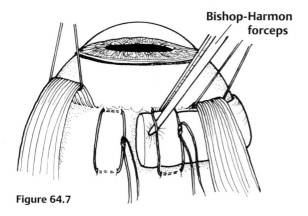

Bishop-Harmon forceps

Figure 64.7

Preplace mattress sutures to be used in securing buckle (4–0 white silk or Mersilene or 5–0 nylon) (**Fig. 64.7**).

42. Position globe with traction sutures.
43. Suture passes should be placed parallel to the buckling element (i.e., parallel to equator for encircling and circumferential segmental elements, perpendicular for radial elements).
44. Suture passes should be ~4 mm long through partial thickness sclera.
45. Visualize needle tip as it is placed through sclera to avoid perforating globe.
46. Thin sclera:
   a. Short suture passes at the corners of the mattress sutures can be taken if the sclera is thin or if there is another reason to avoid long intrascleral suture passes.
   b. For encircling elements, creation of partial thickness scleral tunnels can be safer than passing sutures (**Fig. 64.8**).
      i. Make two vertical incisions with #69 Beaver blade. Incision width depends on buckle width (e.g., 2.5 mm wide for #240 band).
         I. Anterior margin of incision should support posterior margin of vitreous base (i.e., be located ~2.5 mm posterior to ora serrata).
         II. Incisions should be separated by 3–4 mm.
      ii. Make tunnel using #66 Beaver blade.
47. For radial buckles, separate suture passes by 2–3 mm more than width of exoplant, depending on the buckle height desired.
48. For circumferential buckles, the anterior suture pass should be at the ora seratta. The distance between the anterior and posterior suture passes should be 2.5–3.0 mm more than the width of the buckling.
   a. The ora seratta is usually located externally by the line of rectus muscle insertions (spiral of Tillaux), but in high myopes, it is located further posteriorly and should be directly localized using indirect ophthalmoscopy and a marking pen or diathermy.
49. Place buckle (see **Fig. 64.7**).
50. Position encircling element under rectus muscles.
51. Hold element with utility tying forceps (e.g., Alabama).
52. Have assistant retract globe using stay sutures to expose a quadrant.
53. Guide element through the sutures and under the rectus muscles using the toothed (0.3–0.5 mm) and a tying forceps or a hemostat.
54. Temporarily tie the buckle into position using the preplaced mattress sutures.
55. First throw is the standard three-loop throw (**Fig. 64.9**).
56. Second throw: make one-loop and then grab other end of suture near knot to incarcerate loop (**Fig. 64.10**).
57. To untie knot, pull the short free end. (This will remove the second throw and leave only the first triple throw.)
58. Alternatively, to make knot permanent at its current tension, cut the loop and remove the short end of the suture. (This leaves two secured throws. An additional throw will produce a standard 3-1-1 knot.)
59. Verify proper positioning of buckle over retinal breaks by indirect ophthalmoscopy.

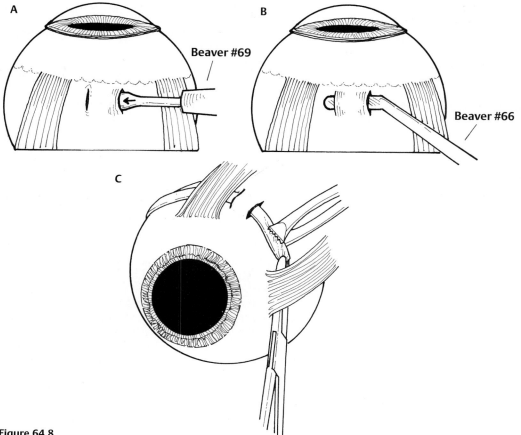

A

Beaver #69

B

Beaver #66

C

Figure 64.8

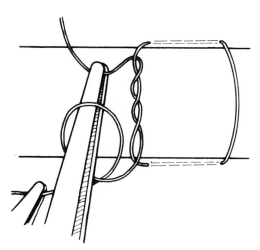

Figure 64.9

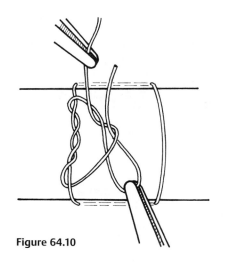

Figure 64.10

60. If drainage of subretinal fluid is anticipated, untie sutures to loosen buckle and expose drainage site, unless drainage site will not be supported by the buckle.
61. Drain subretinal fluid if indicated.
62. Drainage may not be necessary when detachment is low, and retina can be brought close to underlying retinal pigment epithelium through tightening of buckle sutures.
63. Drainage may be indicated in the following settings:
    a. Intraocular pressure must be lowered (as a result of elevating the scleral buckle, injecting a gas bubble, or due to preexisting conditions such as glaucoma, sickle cell trait, or sickle cell disease).
    b. High retinal detachment or giant retinal tear (i.e., lack of apposition of detached retina and subjacent RPE).
    c. Retinal breaks at or posterior to the equator (e.g., macular hole present).
    d. Multiple retinal breaks in three or more quadrants unless all are located near the ora serrata or unless there is little subretinal fluid.
    e. Significant vitreoretinal traction (e.g., proliferative vitreoretinopathy) is present.
    f. Longstanding retinal detachment (i.e., viscous subretinal fluid).
    g. No identifiable retinal breaks.
    h. Reoperations.

64. Drainage site selection. Usually just anterior to the equator.
    a. Choose area under bullous detachment or epiretinal membrane formation to avoid retinal perforation/incarceration.
    b. Place site under buckle if possible, especially for encircling buckles.
    c. Avoid areas overlying retinal breaks to avoid vitreous incarceration in drainage site, unless one wishes to drain liquid vitreous to create additional softening of the globe (e.g., insufficient subretinal fluid present).
    d. Avoid vortex veins. (Therefore, it is preferable to drain near horizontal rectus muscles where exposure is also better.)
65. For encircling elements, a drainage site 180 degrees away from the retinal break is preferred to permit tightening of sutures, elevation of the buckle, and closure of the break during drainage.
66. Drainage from a nasal quadrant reduces the chance for submacular hemorrhage if bleeding occurs during drainage.
67. Incise sclera down to suprachoroidal space (dark blue color) with a sharp blade (e.g., #69 Beaver blade). (**Fig. 64.11** illustrates drainage technique.)
68. Make incision radial and ~3 mm in length. Keep blade perpendicular to the sclera when creating the sclerotomy (**Fig. 64.11A**).

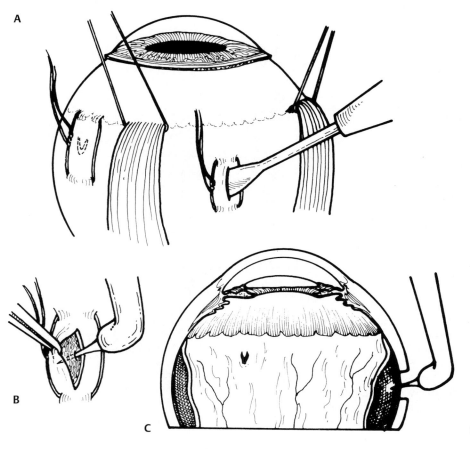

Figure 64.11

69. Examine exposed choroid for any large vessels, which should be avoided when performing drainage.
70. Preplace double-armed 6–0 black silk horizontal mattress suture, with suture passes tangential to the anterior and posterior margins of the sclerotomy.
71. Cauterize exposed choroid using electrocautery with a tapered point.
72. Enough current should be used to induce slight contraction of sclera and choroid when cautery is activated.
73. The cautery can be pretested on an exposed episcleral vessel.

Perform drainage. (**Fig. 64.11B** illustrates entry of needle into subretinal space with sclera grasped by forceps.)
   a. Use small-gauge taper-point surgical needle, 30 gauge needle, or tip of 2.5 mm diathermy pin.
   b. Release traction on eye.
   c. Some surgeons secure sclera at edge of drainage site with forceps.
   d. Carefully introduce needle ~1 mm through choroid into subretinal space just until a bead of subretinal fluid appears.
      i. Enter subretinal space tangentially to avoid retinal damage.
      ii. At this point instruct assistant to release all traction on eye.
   e. Use gentle pressure with a cotton-tipped applicator to help express subretinal fluid.
   f. Place cotton-tipped applicators in episcleral space as drainage proceeds to maintain more normal intraocular pressure. May also tighten buckle sutures to maintain intraocular pressure.
   g. If drainage site is not to be covered by buckle, close site with preplaced 6–0 silk suture. (If covered, it may be left unsutured.)

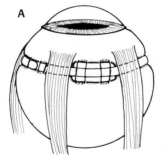 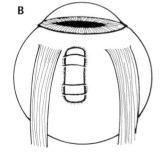

Figure 64.12

74. Secure element, applying enough suture tension to cause scleral edges to imbricate against the edges of the buckle. May choose to tie sutures temporarily (**Fig. 64.12**).
75. Examine retina by indirect ophthalmoscopy.
76. Verify buckle location and elevation over breaks.
77. Inspect drainage site. Rule out retinal incarceration, subretinal hemorrhage. If retinal incarceration is present, support site on buckle.

78. Ascertain patency of central retinal artery.
79. Observe disc color, presence of arterial pulsations.
80. If intraocular pressure (IOP) is too high, loosen sutures (if temporarily tied) and resecure buckle. If sutures permanently tied, see step 87 below.
81. Secure buckling elements permanently.
82. Make temporary sutures permanent.
83. Join ends of encircling element together either with tantalum clip (e.g., #240 band), Watzke sleeve (e.g., #42 band), or suture.
84. Trim buckling elements with scissors as necessary.
85. Irrigate operative field with bacitracin solution.
86. Check intraocular pressure (with Schiotz tonometer and again ascertain patency of central retinal artery by direct observation with ophthalmoscope).
87. If IOP is too high:
   a. Perform one or more anterior chamber paracenteses using a tuberculin syringe with $^5/_8$-inch 30 gauge needle (see Chapter 7) waiting ~5 minutes between attempts, and/or
   b. Perform vitreous tap using long 27 gauge needle positioned directly over optic nerve head using indirect ophthalmoscopic guidance and/or
   c. Perform limited vitrectomy and/or
   d. Administer osmotic agent (e.g., mannitol, 1–2 g/kg; may be contraindicated, e.g., in congestive heart failure) and/or
   e. Loosen encircling band.
   f. Again verify patency of central retinal artery.

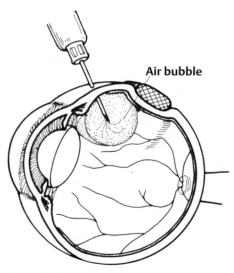

Air bubble

Figure 64.13

88. If globe is hypotonous, inject air or balanced salt solution (30 gauge needle on 5 ml syringe, Millipore filter) (**Fig. 64.13**).
89. Technique of air injection:
   a. Draw air into syringe through Millipore filter for sterilization.

b. Insert needle 3 mm (aphakic, pseudophakic) or 4 mm posterior to limbus (phakic). Ideally, the needle should penetrate only ~1 mm into vitreous cavity, and entry into the globe is at a superior location. If needle penetrates deeply into center of vitreous cavity or if entry is at an inferior location, then there is increased chance for creating many small bubbles ("fish eggs"), which sometimes can enter the subretinal space if the retina is detached and the retinal break is large.

c. Rapidly inject air, keeping needle tip within air bubble to create one bubble, rather than many small adherent bubbles.

d. Inject balanced salt solution or air until satisfactory intraocular pressure restored.

e. **Note:** Pars plana air injection is also useful for flattening horseshoe tears which "fishmouth" over the buckle.

90. Close peritomy.
    a. Secure the Tenon capsule directly to episclera with absorbable suture (e.g., 6–0 plain gut) to cover silicone sponge elements to prevent postoperative extrusion. May also choose to suture the Tenon capsule to the episclera at each side of muscle insertion in area of solid silicone buckling element.
    b. Remove rectus sling sutures as one proceeds with Tenon closure.
    c. Close conjunctiva with absorbable suture (e.g., 6–0 plain gut).

91. Inject subconjunctival cefazolin (100 mg) and Decadron (4–8 mg) or triamcinolone acetate (40 mg) unless there is a contraindication (e.g., penicillin allergy for cefazolin, history of glaucoma for triamcinolone).

92. Remove lid speculum, apply topical atropine 1% drops and antibiotic ointment, and patch and place Fox shield.

Postoperative Procedure

1. Keep patch and shield placed until patient is examined on postoperative day #1. This is usually an outpatient procedure.
2. Postoperative activity: Bed rest with bathroom privileges and head positioning as necessary.
   a. If gas bubble is in eye, position head so that bubble is apposed against retinal breaks.
   b. If one wishes to promote settling of retina on the buckle and gas has not been used, bed rest in supine position is appropriate.
3. Topical antibiotics (e.g., moxifloxacin drops 4 times per day; avoid ointments to avoid obscuring fundus view).
4. Scopolamine 0.25% or atropine 1% drops twice daily for cycloplegia.
5. Prednisolone acetate 1% drops 4 times daily.

Use drops more frequently or administer oral steroids (unless contraindicated) if inflammation is severe.

6. Percocet (5 mg oxycodone/325 mg acetaminophen or 7.5 mg/500 mg acetaminophen), one tablet by mouth every 6 hours for eye pain (unless contraindicated).

7. Examine on postoperative day #1:
   a. Rule out presence of hypopyon with slit lamp exam.
   b. Measure IOP (applanation or pneumatonometry).
   c. Note: Schiotz tension is falsely low secondary to decreased scleral rigidity.
   d. Treat elevated IOP with topical medications (e.g., β-adrenergic antagonists such as timolol 0.5% twice per day; carbonic anhydrase inhibitors such as Trusopt 1% 3 times per day) or oral agents (e.g., Diamox 250 mg every 6 hours or Neptazane 50 mg every 8 hours).

8. Funduscopy:
   a. Observe proper buckle location in relation to retinal breaks.
   b. Break should lie flat on buckle.
   c. Residual subretinal fluid should slowly resorb. Verify continued absorption of subretinal fluid during follow-up visits.
   d. Look for choroidal detachments (e.g., posterior to scleral buckle); can be a cause of persistent subretinal fluid despite closed retinal breaks.

Follow-up Schedule (in uncomplicated cases)

1. Postoperative day #1 and daily if hospitalized.
2. Approximately 1 week after discharge.
3. Three weeks, 6 weeks, and 3 months postoperatively, and then as case warrants.

Complications

1. Central retinal artery occlusion
2. Increased IOP
3. Anterior chamber shallowing and angle closure glaucoma
4. Incomplete cryotherapy of or relief of vitreoretinal traction on retinal breaks with consequent persistence of subretinal fluid
5. Chorioretinal/vitreous inflammation
6. Serous choroidal detachment
7. Hemorrhagic choroidal detachment
8. Exudative retinal detachment
9. Retinal and/or vitreous incarceration in drainage sites
10. Vitreous hemorrhage
11. Anterior segment ischemia
12. Infection and/or extrusion of buckling element
13. Endophthalmitis
14. Cystoid macular edema
15. Proliferative vitreoretinopathy
16. Cataract secondary to lens trauma during pars plana injections, due to gas bubble apposition against posterior capsule, or due to metabolic alterations following placement of an encircling element
17. Extraocular muscle imbalance
18. Change in refractive error secondary to distortion of globe by buckle
19. Globe perforation due to retrobulbar or subconjunctival (less likely) anesthesia

■ Pneumatic Retinopexy

Indications

■ Rhegmatogenous retinal detachment without proliferative vitreoretinopathy
■ Retinal breaks located in the superior 240 degrees, i.e., 8–4 o'clock (clockwise) all within 90 degrees of each other

Contraindications

■ Proliferative vitreoretinopathy
■ Inability to position head properly after surgery
■ Inappropriate location of retinal breaks

Relative Contraindications

■ Inability to tolerate elevated IOP (e.g., advanced glaucoma, sickle cell disease)
■ Extensive lattice degeneration
■ Properly selected cases of giant retinal tears 8–4 o'clock (clockwise) can be managed using the steamroller maneuver and a modification of the pneumatic retinopexy procedure described here (see below)

Instrumentation

■ Indirect ophthalmoscope
■ 20 and/or 28 diopter lens
■ Lid speculum (wire)
■ Cryosurgical unit
■ Millipore filter
■ Intraocular gas: either sulfur hexafluoride (SF_6), or perfluoropropane (C_3F_8)
■ Two tuberculin syringes, each with attached $^5/_8$-inch 30 gauge needle
■ 10% povidone iodine
■ 2% lidocaine without epinephrine for subconjunctival and retrobulbar injection
■ 10 cc syringe
■ 1.5-inch 25 gauge needle
■ 1.5-inch 27 gauge needle or 23 gauge vitrectomy probe
■ Sterile calipers (Castroviejo)
■ Two sterile cotton-tipped applicators
■ Cefazolin (100 mg/1 ml) for subconjunctival injection
■ Long-acting cycloplegic (e.g., atropine 1%)
■ Pneumatonometer

Operative Procedure

1. Place sterile lid speculum.
2. Inject 2% lidocaine subconjunctivally in quadrants of retinal breaks.
3. Localize and treat retinal breaks with cryotherapy as described above.
4. Some surgeons administer retrobulbar anesthesia using 5–10 ml 2% lidocaine via 1.5-inch 25 gauge needle after cryotherapy. In our experience, this step is unnecessary provided that subconjunctival anesthesia is administered in the quadrants in which intravitreal injections and cryotherapy will be done.
5. Sterilize ocular surface with instillation of topical povidone iodine × 2; let iodine dry after applications.
6. Draw up pure intraocular gas through Millipore filter into a tuberculin syringe. Cap syringe tightly to prevent dilution of gas by room air.
7. Perform anterior chamber paracentesis with tuberculin syringe attached to short 30 gauge needle. This maneuver softens eye, which enhances tolerance of the intraocular gas injection and reduces the risk of gas egress into the subconjunctival space (step 9 below).
8. Mark site of gas injection 3 mm (aphakia/pseudophakia) or 4 mm (phakic eye) posterior to limbus inferotemporally.
9. Inject 0.3 cc C_3F_8 or 0.5 cc SF_6 at site of caliper mark via tuberculin syringe attached to $^5/_8$-inch 30 gauge needle.
   a. Rapid smooth injection minimizes chance of multiple small bubble formation; small bubbles ("fish eggs") can enter the subretinal space through large retinal breaks.
   b. Insert needle, entering the globe at a superior location. Withdraw the needle so that it penetrates ~1 mm into the vitreous cavity. Deep penetration into vitreous cavity or entry at an inferior location increases the chance for fish egg formation. Excessive withdrawal of the needle will result in gas injection into the suprachoroidal space.
   c. Immediately tamponade injection site after gas injection with sterile cotton-tipped applicator to prevent egress of gas into subconjunctival space.
10. Instruct patient to position head so that gas bubble is direct away from meridian of retinal breaks.

If the detachment does not involve the macula, have the patient first position head face down. Patient then rotates head toward side of detachment to avoid forcing subretinal fluid into submacular space.

11. Check IOP with sterile pneumatonometer.
12. Visualize fundus with indirect ophthalmoscopy to verify patency of central retinal artery and to verify location of bubble in vitreous cavity.
   a. If small clusters of bubbles are seen (fish eggs), one may gently tap globe in quadrant of bubbles several times to break bubbles up into a single large bubble.
   b. If subretinal gas is present, rotation of head so that bubble rests against retinal break followed by gentle tapping of globe may dislodge bubble into vitreous cavity; otherwise, the patient will require vitrectomy to remove subretinal gas and reattach retina.

13. If central retinal artery remains closed for ≥ 5 minutes or if intraocular pressure is ≥ 40 mm Hg, perform repeat anterior chamber paracentesis or perform aspiration of vitreous using either long 27 gauge needle directed over optic nerve head under indirect ophthalmoscopic guidance or 23 gauge vitrectomy probe. For vitreous aspiration:

    a. Resterilize ocular surface with povidone-iodine.
    b. Introduce 27 gauge needle or vitrectomy probe 3 mm (aphakia/pseudophakia) or 4 mm (phakic eye) posterior to the limbus. If indirect ophthalmoscopy will be used to visualize the needle/probe tip, it is helpful to place the needle/probe in the quadrant on the side of the surgeon's nondominant hand.
    c. For 27 gauge needle, carefully guide needle tip just over optic nerve head and have assistant pull gently on syringe plunger to aspirate liquid vitreous. Several attempts may be necessary before identifying a pocket of liquid vitreous.
    d. For 23 gauge vitrectomy probe, have assistant gently pull on plunger attached to syringe that is coupled to the probe via plastic tubing. Cutting rate should be on maximum (use audible cues to assess cutting rate), and probe can be in mid-vitreous (phakic eye) or in anterior vitreous (aphakia/pseudophakia) cavity.

14. Inject subconjunctival cefazolin (unless contraindicated) in quadrant away from sclerotomy (to avoid diffusion of antibiotic into vitreous cavity).
15. Instill 1–2 drops of atropine 1% into eye.
16. Place light patch on eye.
17. Instruct patient to position head so that bubble is located in a quadrant away from retinal breaks for the first 6 hours after procedure. After this time the bubble will have enlarged to ~50% of its final size, and patient should position head so that bubble rests directly against retinal breaks.
18. If macula is attached, and there is bullous superior retinal detachment or temporal retinal detachment, steamroller maneuver should be employed.

    a. Patient first positions head face-down.
    b. If breaks are located between 10 and 2 o'clock (clockwise), patient then slowly (several degrees elevation every 5–10 minutes) sits upright, to force subretinal fluid out of retinal breaks while maintaining retina reattachment.
    c. If breaks are located in temporal quadrant, patient slowly rotates head away from the detachment while maintaining face-down posture.
    d. Head rotation maneuver can be repeated to force fluid from subretinal space into vitreous cavity while maintaining macular attachment.
    e. This maneuver can be performed in the surgeon's office the day after the procedure, which permits direct visualization of the process.

19. Unless contraindicated, administer 500 mg Diamox Sequel at bedtime to prophylax against IOP rise.
20. Tylenol 325–650 mg by mouth every 6 hours (unless contraindicated) is administered for pain.
21. Patient is instructed to call the surgeon for pain unrelieved by Tylenol, as this symptom may be due to sight-threatening, elevated IOP or endophthalmitis.
22. Giant retinal tears. Giant tears are usually managed with vitrectomy, installation of perfluorocarbon, photocoagulation of the reattached retina, removal of perfluorocarbon, and intravitreal gas tamponade. Cases with giant tears located 8–4 o'clock (clockwise), with no folding of the posterior margin of the retinal tear, and no evidence of epiretinal membrane formation or retinal stiffness can be managed with pneumatic retinopexy. Eyes with giant retinal tears often have a substantial amount of liquid vitreous present, which permits installation of a large volume of intravitreal gas.

    a. Administer retrobulbar anesthesia.
    b. Place lid speculum.
    c. Instill povidone iodine to sterilize ocular surface.
    d. Perform anterior chamber paracentesis using tuberculin syringe attached to 30 gauge needle. Usually, a substantial volume of fluid (~0.75 ml) can be removed before the anterior chamber collapses.
    e. Inject ~0.75 ml 20% SF_6 into the mid vitreous cavity as described above.
    f. Have the patient assume a face-down position for several minutes to force subretinal fluid into the vitreous cavity.
    g. Depending on size of giant tear (and corresponding size of gas bubble needed to reattach retina), repeat anterior chamber paracentesis and intravitreal gas injection, sterilizing the ocular surface again between each cycle.
    h. Inject subconjunctival cefazolin (unless contraindicated), instill cycloplegic drops, and patch eye as described above.
    i. Have patient lie face-down over night. If the tear is located between 8 and 11 or 1 and 4 o'clock (clockwise), the bubble may be positioned directly over the break ~6 hours after gas injection by having the patient lie on the side opposite that of the giant tear. If the tear is located between 10 and 2 o'clock (clockwise), the patient may sit upright ~6 hours after gas injection to tamponade the retinal tear.
    j. If the retina is folded down over itself superiorly (e.g., superior giant tear), the flap can be unfolded by having the patient start from a face down position and then perform backward somersaults.
    k. If the retina is folded down over itself temporally, the flap can be unfolded by having the patient rotate head nasally while maintaining face-down position; the patient rotates temporally to unfold a nasal tear.
    l. The day after gas injection, the retina should be completely reattached. Laser photocoagulation can now be applied to the retinal tear.
    m. If the retina is not reattached, either the gas bubble is too small, the patient has not positioned the head properly, or the retina is too stiff to be managed by this technique.

n. If the retina is attached, rotate the head so that the gas bubble is directed to the quadrant away from the tear and apply 3–5 rows of laser photocoagulation to the posterior margin of the tear taking care to treat for 1 clock on either side of the edges of the tear all the way up to the ora serrata. A 28 D lens may facilitate viewing through the gas bubble.

If poor visualization precludes application of laser photocoagulation, cryopexy can be administered as described above with care taken to treat attached retina along the posterior margin of the vitreous base for one clock hour on either side of the edges of the giant tear.

Postoperative Procedure

1. See patient on postoperative day #1.
2. Check visual acuity, IOP, slit lamp exam (to rule out hypopyon, cataract, and to assess gas bubble size).
3. Examine fundus. Normally all or most subretinal fluid will have resorbed. (Chronic detachments may take longer for subretinal fluid resorption.) In any case, there should be a definite decrease in the amount of subretinal fluid.
4. If the amount of subretinal fluid is not less or has increased, suspect that there is an additional (or new) retinal tear that is not tamponaded by the gas bubble. Such tears are often located in the inferior periphery.
5. Depending on the location of the additional (new) retinal tear, the break might be tamponaded by additional gas injection (and retinopexy) versus scleral buckling versus vitrectomy surgery.

6. Maintain proper head position with bubble apposed against retinal break(s) for 1 (laser photocoagulation) to 2 (cryotherapy) weeks after surgery.
7. See patient in follow-up at 1, 3, 6, 12, and 24 weeks after surgery and annually thereafter in uncomplicated cases, more often as the need arises.

Complications

Similar to those of scleral buckling with the following observations.

1. Retinal and vitreous incarceration in drainage sites will not occur, as this is a nondrainage procedure.
2. Anterior segment ischemia is unlikely to occur, as there is no manipulation of the rectus muscles or encircling of the globe.
3. Infection and/or extrusion of buckling element cannot occur.
4. Extraocular muscle imbalance is highly unlikely to occur, as there is no manipulation of the rectus muscles. It can occur, however, as a result of anesthetic-induced damage to the muscle.
5. Change in refractive error will not occur secondary to distortion of globe by buckle. It could arise as a result of changes in the crystalline lens.

65

Retinal Cryotherapy

Indications

1. Prophylaxis of selected retinal tears and areas of abnormal vitreoretinal adhesion (e.g., lattice degeneration).
2. Rare cases of progressive retinoschisis.
3. Treatment of selected retinal tumors and vascular malformations (e.g., Coats disease).
4. Peripheral panretinal cryotherapy to induce regression of neovascularization in:
   a. Selected cases of neovascular glaucoma.
   b. Proliferative retinopathies refractory to panretinal photocoagulation (PRP) or in eyes in which PRP is not possible (e.g., media opacities).

Preoperative Procedure

1. Complete retinal evaluation: Identify and draw all retinal breaks or other areas of pathology (e.g., lattice degeneration, retinal telangiectasia).
2. Dilate pupil (e.g., cyclopentolate 1% + phenylephrine 2.5%).

Instrumentation

- Indirect ophthalmoscope
- Scleral depressor
- Cryosurgical unit with retinal cryoprobe
- Tuberculin syringe and 5/8-inch 30 gauge needle
- 2% lidocaine without epinephrine
- Lid speculum (preferably wire type)

Operative Procedure

1. Treatment of retinal breaks
   a. Localize and draw all retinal breaks (indirect ophthalmoscope, scleral depressor).

b. Open gas valve and test cryoprobe (desired temperature should be −60 to −80°C; usually requires nitrogen gas tank pressure > 600 psi).
c. Apply anesthesia.
   i. Subconjunctival lidocaine 2% without epinephrine to quadrants that will be treated.
   ii. Retrobulbar anesthesia (± lid block) may be used in patients receiving extensive treatment (e.g., panretinal cryopexy) but usually is not necessary if extensive subconjunctival anesthesia is used.

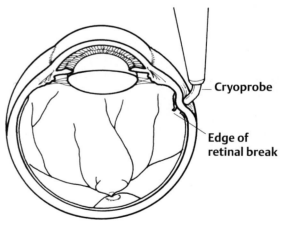

Figure 65.1

d. Apply cryoprobe directly over conjunctiva at edge of retinal break (**Fig. 65.1**).

Ensure that probe tip is perpendicular to globe. A common mistake is to indent the sclera with the shaft, not the tip of the cryoprobe. This error can lead to treatment of areas posterior to the retinal break.

e. Use indirect ophthalmoscope to visualize fundus, indent sclera with cryoprobe tip, and indent retina up to edge of retinal break.

f. While indenting sclera with probe tip, activate cryounit (usually foot pedal mechanism).

g. Terminate cryoapplication as soon as RPE-retina whitening is observed through the ophthalmoscope. If no reaction is observed in several seconds after the cryounit achieves its lowest temperature, terminate the application and verify position of probe tip. Also check to be sure that the operative field is dry, that the sleeve connecting the gas tank to the cryoprobe is intact, and that the gas pressure is adequate.

h. After the whitening dissipates, move probe to contiguous area around break.

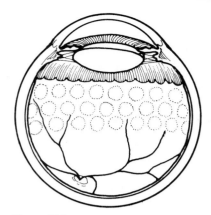

Figure 65.3

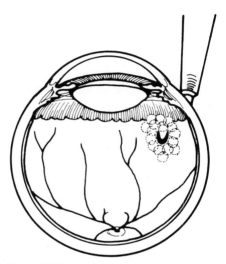

Figure 65.2

i. Apply additional applications to surround the break with treatment (**Fig. 65.2**).
   i. Cryo spots should overlap slightly to completely seal the break.
   ii. Breaks should be surrounded by a 1–2 mm zone of treatment.
   iii. For breaks anterior to the equator, we recommend extending treatment to the ora serrata.

2. Peripheral panretinal cryotherapy
   a. Location of cryoapplications (**Fig. 65.3**):
      i. Apply directly through conjunctiva.
      ii. Place treatment between ora serrata and equator.
      iii. Apply ~3–4 applications per clock hour (i.e., 9–16 applications per quadrant).
      iv. May apply for entire 360 degrees.
      v. Sometimes, one can treat posterior to the equator with this approach, although treatment extending as far posterior as the temporal arcades usually requires conjunctival peritomy to permit posterior probe application.
   b. Apply treatment under direct observation with indirect ophthalmoscope as described previously.
   c. If unable to view retina, may apply treatment in "blind" fashion.
      i. First determine the time required for an application, using ophthalmoscopy to observe a freeze in an area in which visualization is possible, as described in "Treatment of retinal breaks" on page 348.
      ii. For subsequent applications, apply probe to desired location, activate unit, and terminate treatment after the predetermined time interval.

3. Treatment of Coats Disease: Generally the retinal vascular lesions are treated with laser photocoagulation. If significant subretinal fluid is present, however, laser uptake is impaired, and cryoretinopexy is more likely to be effective.
   a. Place lid speculum, apply local anesthesia as above.
   b. Apply cryoprobe to area of peripheral retinal telangiectasia.
   c. Activate cryounit with foot pedal under visualization with indirect ophthalmoscope.
   d. Terminate freeze after intraocular ice ball envelops retinal vascular abnormalities.

Postoperative Procedure

1. Cycloplegia (e.g., scopolamine 0.25% or atropine sulfate 1% twice per day).
2. Analgesics for pain control (e.g., usually acetaminophen 650 mg q 6 hours suffices, but occasionally Percocet (e.g., oxycodone 5 mg/acetaminophen 350 mg) is needed).
3. For horseshoe tears, restrict activity until there is pigmentation at the cryosite, suggesting formation of chorioretinal adhesion (usually, ~2 weeks).
4. Follow-up at ~1, 2, and 3–6 weeks after treatment and thereafter as required. In the case of retinal breaks, scleral depression of the treatment site is not recommended for 1–2 weeks after treatment.

Complications

1. Incomplete treatment of retinal break. Most common error is to treat inadequately the anterior margins of the retinal break.
2. Development of new retinal breaks. New retinal breaks occur in ~10% undergoing pneumatic retinopexy. Thus, development of a new break need not indicate a complication of treatment. However, new breaks can develop in association with cryoretinopexy (usually at the posterior margin of previous treatment), presumably due to vitreoretinal traction on iatrogenically thinned retina.
3. Inflammation with breakdown of blood–retinal barrier (controversial).
4. Cystoid macular edema.
5. Formation of epiretinal membranes.
6. Vitreous hemorrhage.
7. Scleral perforation during scleral depression.
8. Conjunctival laceration during scleral depression.

66

Pars Plana Lensectomy

Indications

- Select cases of traumatic, subluxed, and/or dislocated cataractous lenses. A pars plana approach is particularly useful in cases where zonular rupture with vitreous prolapse into the anterior chamber precludes a safe phacoemulsification, extracapsular, or intracapsular cataract extraction approach.
- Select congenital cataracts.
- Other cases in which lens removal combined with posterior vitrectomy is indicated.

Preoperative Procedure

See Chapter 3.
1. Complete retinal evaluation.
2. Ultrasound examination of retina and vitreous if cataract precludes direct visualization.
3. Dilate pupil.
   a. Cyclopentolate 1% and phenylephrine 2.5% every 10 minutes × 3, starting 1 hour before surgery.
   b. Can use flexible iris retractors intraoperatively if iris dilates poorly (e.g., posterior synechiae).
4. *Optional:* Topical nonsteroidal anti-inflammatory agent (e.g., flurbiprofen) every 30 minutes starting 2 hours before surgery (to minimize intraoperative miosis).

Instrumentation

- Lid speculum
- Fine-toothed tissue forceps (e.g., 0.12 mm straight Castroviejo and/or Colibri)
- Westcott scissors
- Cautery, bipolar or disposable (optional)
- Castroviejo calipers
- Marking pen (optional)
- 20-gauge microvitreoretinal (MVR) blade
- Needle holder
- 4 mm infusion cannula (6 mm cannula in cases with choroidal detachment, 2.5 mm cannula in pediatric cases)
- Sutures (4–0 silk or 6–0 Vicryl, 7–0 Vicryl, and 8–0 Vicryl or 6–0 plain gut)
- Cotton-tipped applicators
- 23 gauge butterfly needle
- Ultrasonic phacofragmentation unit with 20 gauge tip

Note: In this chapter, the Alcon Accurus vitrectomy machine's phacofragmentation unit is used for illustrative purposes. The authors recognize that other excellent machines are available and settings may differ based on machine. The authors have no financial interest in the Accurus system.

- Vitrectomy suction/cutting instrument
- Intraocular forceps
- Fiber optic illuminator
- Corneal ring
- Contact lenses
  - Traditional lens system (TLS): 20 degrees and 30 degrees prism, wide angle (48 degrees), macula (34 degrees), and biconcave (90 D) lenses.
  - Wide angle lens system (WAS): wide-angle lens (Ocular 155D or Volk's Mini Quad/Quad XL), equator lens (Ocular 91 D lens or Volk's Central Retinal lens), macula lens (Ocular 66D or Volk's Super Macula).
- Scleral plugs
- Indirect ophthalmoscope
- 20 D and/or 28 D lens
- Fluted needle (Charles) with or without silicone tip
- Retinal cryopexy unit and/or indirect laser ophthalmoscope
- Heavier than water liquid (e.g., perfluoro-octane), optional

Operative Procedure

1. Anesthesia: General or retrobulbar ± lid block.
2. Prep and drape eye.
3. Place lid speculum.

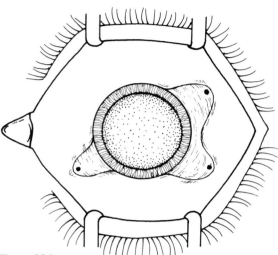

Figure 66.1

4. Perform conjunctival peritomy at limbus 4 clock hours temporally and superonasally in area of planned entry sites (Westcott scissors, toothed forceps) (**Fig. 66.1**).
5. Secure hemostasis with cautery (optional).
6. Place infusion inferotemporally (unless contraindicated, e.g., due to choroidal detachment) and two sites for bimanual manipulation superotemporally and superonasally at 10 and 2 o'clock, respectively.
   a. Sclerotomies should be 3.0 mm from limbus (measure with calipers).
   b. Sclerotomy sites should be parallel to the limbus.
   c. Mark location of sites with cautery (optional).
   d. Prepare infusion site.

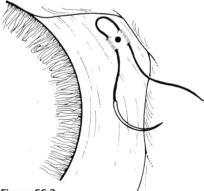

Figure 66.2

i. Preplace 4–0 white silk (or 6–0 Vicryl) mattress suture through partial-thickness sclera spanning the sclerotomy site (**Fig. 66.2**).

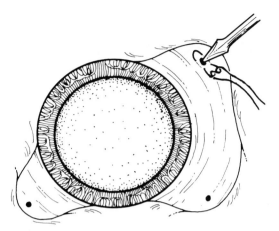

Figure 66.3

   ii. Enter eye with MVR blade (**Fig. 66.3**).
      I. Hold blade perpendicular to eye, aiming toward anatomical center of globe.
      II. Enter eye with enter eye with controlled firm pressure, and penetrate pars plana completely.
      III. Visualize knife tip through pupil to verify penetration.
   iii. Place infusion cannula through sclerotomy (a twisting motion facilitates entry of cannula).
   iv. View cannula directly through pupil or with indirect ophthalmoscope to ascertain its proper position and penetration through pars plana.
      I. Use of the endoilluminator probe can facilitate visualization of the cannula tip through the pupil. Direct the light source toward the infusion cannula through the pupil.
      II. Do not start infusion if cannula cannot be visualized.
      III. If view is obscured by cataract, use the butterfly needle (to be placed in Step 11 below) for infusion until enough lens is removed to allow direct visualization of the cannula or use a 6 mm infusion cannula.

Note: if preoperative ultrasound indicates a large choroidal detachment, then it is best to infuse via limbus until enough lens material has been removed to permit direct visualization of cannula tip in vitreous cavity.

   v. Secure infusion cannula to sclera with the preplaced suture.
7. At one premarked site (side of dominant hand), perform sclerotomy with MVR blade.
8. Through the superior sclerotomy of the dominant hand, incise the lens capsule at or just anterior to the equator with the MVR blade.

9. Insert ultrasonic phacofragmentation probe through the sclerotomy and into the lens through the lens capsule incision.
10. Remove lens nucleus with ultrasound probe.
    a. Ensure that fragmenter is properly tuned.
    b. Use ultrasound to fragment nucleus.
        i. Settings: proportional vacuum (vacuum ranges from 0–200 mm Hg), ultrasound typically power ranges from 15–50% of maximum, depending on the degree of nuclear sclerosis.
        ii. Some surgeons also set the fragmatome on pulse mode, usually 4–8 pulses/second.
    c. Start at mid-depth of the nucleus near incision site and carefully fragment the nucleus while proceeding across the lens.
    d. Avoid disruption of lens capsule.
    e. If vitreous presents at the ultrasound tip, replace the fragmatome with a vitrector and remove the vitreous before proceeding. Do not sonicate or aspirate vitreous with the ultrasound unit.
11. If the crystalline lens is unstably fixated, consider maneuvers to stabilize the lens.
    a. Infuse perfluoron into the vitreous cavity to float the lens into the posterior chamber, or

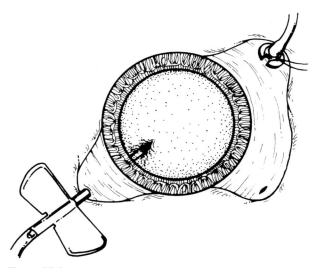

Figure 66.4

    b. Through the other sclerotomy site, insert a 23 gauge butterfly needle and spear the lens at the equator (**Fig. 66.4**).
        i. Bend needle ~30 degrees before insertion to facilitate manipulation.
        ii. Avoid pushing needle forcibly into a hard nucleus to prevent exacerbation of lens subluxation.
        iii. Needle is connected to irrigation and initially can be used for infusion if the cannula placed in Step 6 above cannot be visualized because of cataract.

        iv. May use butterfly needle both to manipulate nuclear material into the fragmatome port and to irrigate into and inflate the capsular bag (**Figs. 66.5 and 66.6**).
12. Remove ultrasonic probe.

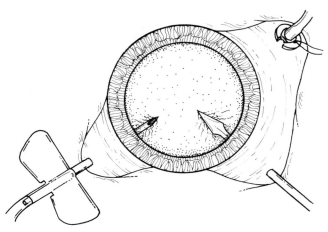

Figure 66.5

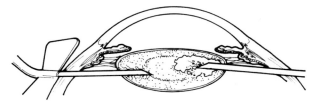

Figure 66.6

13. Insert vitrectomy instrument into capsular bag via previously made equatorial incision in lens capsule.
14. Set vitrectomy instrument parameters for cortex removal.
    a. Cutting rate: Accurus 800 probe: ~800 cpm; InnoVit: 1000–1200 cpm; Accurus 2500: 1000–1500 cpm.
    b. Vacuum: ~150–180 mm Hg.
    c. Infusion pressure: 25–35 mm Hg, depending on vacuum setting.
    d. For excision of firmer material (e.g., fibrous pupillary membranes), decrease cutting rate and increase suction.
    e. Some probes also permit control of the port size. For such instruments, open the port size maximally to optimize incarceration of material into the probe, thus permitting better cutting.

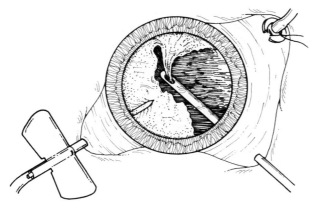

Figure 66.7

15. Remove residual cortex with vitrectomy probe (**Fig. 66.7**).
    a. May strip and aspirate cortex using *only* suction mode if cortical material aspirates easily.
    b. If necessary, cut and aspirate residual cortex using parameters as outlined above.

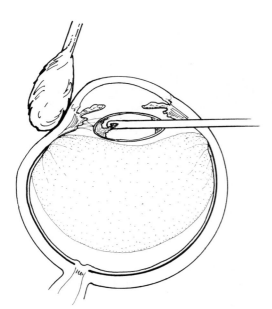

Figure 66.8

c. Peripheral cortex can be visualized for removal using scleral indentation and the coaxial illumination of the operating microscope (**Fig. 66.8**).

Alternatively, flexible iris retractors can be placed via limbal incisions (2, 4, 8, and 10 o'clock) to dilate the pupil widely and improve visualization of peripheral lens cortex.

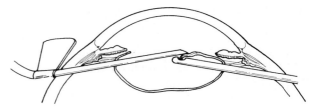

Figure 66.9

16. *Optional:* Remove central portion of anterior capsule (**Fig. 66.9**).

    Set initial vitrectomy parameters and vary as needed.

    a. Cutting rate: Accurus 800 probe: ~300 cpm; InnoVit and Accurus 2500 probes: ~1000 cpm.
    b. Vacuum: ~150–200 mm Hg.
    c. Infusion pressure: 25–35 mm Hg, depending on vacuum.
    d. May use butterfly needle to feed material into vitrector port.
    e. When removing peripheral capsule, turn vitrector port downward or toward pupillary space to avoid iris; otherwise keep vitrector port in view.
17. If posterior capsule is ruptured and vitreous is presenting:
    a. Try to preserve posterior capsule for support of a posterior chamber intraocular lens. Even if central posterior capsule is disrupted, often one can place a sulcus-fixated posterior chamber intraocular lens if the anterior capsule is intact in this setting. Direct vitrectomy port so that vitreous in the posterior chamber and anterior $1/3$ of the vitreous cavity is removed without disturbing the residual capsule.
    b. In cases with proliferative vitreoretinopathy (PVR), it may be best to remove the lens capsule in its entirety as it may serve as a scaffold for future scar tissue proliferation with formation of anterior PVR and secondary hypotony. In such cases, one can remove residual lens capsule using intraocular forceps, grasping the lens capsule and drawing it centrally. Occasionally, one must sever zonular fibers with the MVR blade or with intraocular scissors.

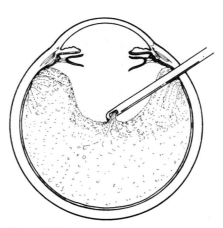

Figure 66.10

18. Perform subtotal vitrectomy as necessary (see Chapter 63) (**Fig. 66.10**).
    a. Vitrectomy parameters:
        i. Accurus 800 probe: cutting rate 800 cpm, vacuum 150 mm Hg, infusion pressure 25–35 mm Hg.
        ii. InnoVit probe: cutting rate 1200 cpm, vacuum 150–200 mm Hg, infusion pressure 35 mm Hg.
        iii. Accurus 2500 probe: cutting rate 2500 cpm, vacuum 150, infusion pressure 35 mm Hg.
    b. May perform an anterior vitrectomy without a contact lens.
    c. If a deeper vitrectomy is needed (i.e., posterior two thirds of the vitreous cavity),
        i. Suture the lens ring using a 4–0 white silk or 6–0 Vicryl suture at either 3 and 9 o'clock meridian or at 6 and 12 o' clock meridian ~3 mm from the limbus.
        ii. Use a corneal contact lens and fiber optic illuminator for visualization (see Chapter 63).
    d. Goals:
        i. Remove vitreous from anterior and posterior chambers to prevent iridovitreal adhesions.
        ii. Remove vitreous opacities.
        iii. Using the wide-angle corneal contact lens (e.g., 48 degree high refractive index lens, Ocular 155D, or Volk's Mini Quad/Quad XL), examine fundus for any lens fragments that may have fallen into the vitreous. If large (e.g., ≥ ¼ size of nucleus) nuclear or cortical fragments are found, a vitrectomy should be performed with aspiration or sonication of the residual lens fragments (see Chapter 64).

19. If large lens fragments fall posteriorly, heavier than water liquids, such as perfluorocarbons, can be used to float the fragments into the midvitreous cavity to avoid retinal damage during phacoemulsification.
20. Place intraocular lens, if appropriate, via limbal or clear corneal incision.
21. Remove instruments. If vitreous prolapses through sclerotomy sites, cut it flush with sclera using Westcott scissors or activate vitrectomy probe at high cutting rate (e.g., 800–2500 cpm) and low suction (e.g., 25–50 mm Hg) just internal to sclerotomy. When infusion fluid egresses from the sclerotomy readily, the sclerotomy can be closed.
22. Place scleral plugs in sclerotomics to prevent globe decompression.
23. Examine fundus with indirect ophthalmoscopy and scleral depression. If retinal tears are present, treat them with retinopexy (either laser photocoagulation or cryotherapy) and perform a fluid–air exchange using the indirect ophthalmoscope to visualize the fluted needle positioned over the optic nerve head.

If retinal breaks are treated, an air-gas exchange using nonexpansile SF_6 (20%) or C_3F_8 (12–15%) should be done once the sclerotomies are closed.

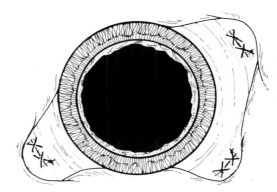

Figure 66.12

24. Close each sclerotomy site with a 6–0 or 7–0 Vicryl suture (**Fig. 66.12**).
25. Close conjunctiva (e.g., 6–0 plain gut or 8–0 Vicryl).
26. Inject subconjunctival cefazolin (100 mg) (unless allergic) and Decadron (4–8 mg) or triamcinolone acetate (40 mg) (unless contraindicated).

If the patient is allergic to penicillin, consider using vancomycin (50 mg) instead of cefazolin.

27. Remove lid speculum.
28. Apply topical antibiotic, steroid ointment, and atropine sulfate 1% drops.
29. Apply patch and place Fox shield.

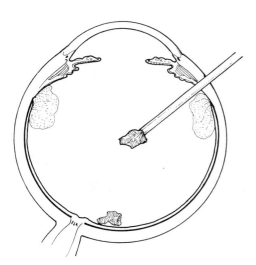

Figure 66.11

Small lens fragments can be removed with a fluted needle (**Fig. 66.11**).

Postoperative Procedure

1. Keep patch and shield placed until patient is examined on postoperative day #1.
2. Topical antibiotics (e.g., gatifloxacin [Zymar, Allergan, Inc.]) 4 times per day for 3 weeks.
3. Steroid drops (e.g., prednisolone acetate 1% 4 times per day) tapered over 3–6 weeks as inflammation warrants.
4. Control intraocular pressure with β-adrenergic antagonist (e.g., timolol), α-adrenergic agonist (e.g., brimonidine tartrate 0.2%), and/or carbonic anhydrase inhibitors (e.g., dorzolamide 2% topically t.i.d. or Diamox 250 mg by mouth every 6 hours) as necessary and as tolerated.
5. Scopolamine ¼% or atropine 1% drops b.i.d. for cycloplegia.

Follow-up Schedule

1. Postoperative day #1.
2. Approximately 1, 3, and 6 weeks postoperatively and then as necessary.

Complications

1. Retinal tears and detachment.
2. Hemorrhagic choroidal detachment.
3. Incomplete removal of lens material with subsequent inflammation caused by lens/vitreous admixture.
4. Vitreous hemorrhage.
5. Cystoid macular edema.
6. Preretinal membrane.
7. Retained intraocular perfluorocarbon.
8. Central retinal artery occlusion (due to postoperative increase in intraocular pressure).
9. Outer retinal ischemia secondary to choroidal infarct (due to intraoperative increase in intraocular pressure, usually the result of excessive elevation of infusion pressure but occasionally due to reduced ocular perfusion pressure).
10. Endophthalmitis.
11. Corneal decompensation.
12. Nonarteritic anterior ischemic optic neuropathy.

67

Retina Laser Procedures

■ Panretinal Photocoagulation

Indications

1. Diabetic retinopathy.
   a. The Early Treatment Diabetic Retinopathy Study (ETDRS) has shown that panretinal photocoagulation (PRP) decreases the incidence of severe visual loss in patients with "high risk" proliferative diabetic retinopathy (i.e., risk of severe visual loss was ~50% over 5 years among untreated patients versus ~25% among treated patients). "Severe visual loss" is defined as visual acuity < 5/200 on two consecutive visits separated by 3 months. The following clinical features define high risk proliferative diabetic retinopathy (HRPDR):
      i. Neovascularization at or within 1 disc diameter of the optic disc (NVD) that is larger than NVD in a standard photograph (~$1/4$–$1/3$ disc area in size).
      ii. Any NVD in the presence of vitreous or preretinal hemorrhage.
      iii. Moderate to severe neovascularization elsewhere (NVE) (i.e., neovascularization ≥$1/2$ disc diameter in size), in the presence of vitreous or preretinal hemorrhage.
   b. PRP should probably be offered to most type II diabetic patients with PDR even in the absence of "high risk" characteristics.
   c. PRP is somewhat beneficial for patients who have severe nonproliferative diabetic retinopathy (NPDR). One should consider offering PRP to such patients if they cannot be followed properly or if the fellow eye has been lost due to complications of PDR. It may be offered to patients with bilateral severe NPDR. PRP should probably be deferred in patients with clinically significant macular edema (CSME) and severe NPDR until either high risk features develop or the macular edema resolves (e.g., in response to focal macular laser photocoagulation). Severe NPDR can be defined using the "4-2-1" rule:
      i. 4 quadrants of "severe" intraretinal hemorrhage, or
      ii. 2 quadrants of "severe" venous beading, or
      iii. 1 quadrant of "severe" intraretinal microvascular abnormalities (IRMAs).
      iv. "Severe" is defined as a degree of abnormality greater than or equal to that present in standard photographs used during the ETDRS.
   d. Rubeosis iridis even in the absence of neovascularization of the posterior pole. This occurs uncommonly but can be seen particularly after pars plana vitrectomy or in the setting of complete posterior vitreous detachment.
2. Retinal branch vein occlusion.
   a. The Branch Vein Occlusion Study showed peripheral scatter photocoagulation is effective in:
      i. Decreasing the incidence of neovascularization following retinal branch vein occlusion and
      ii. Decreasing the incidence of vitreous hemorrhage (VH) in patients who have developed retinal neovascularization (30% incidence among treated patients versus 60% among controls).
   b. The study investigators recommended that patients without NV should be followed until new blood vessels develop, at which point they should be treated.

Approximately 40% of patients with areas of retinal capillary nonperfusion ≥ 5 disc diameters in size develop NV. Among patients with NV, ~60% develop VH. Among patients with VH, ~12% develop a loss of 5 Snellen lines of vision. Thus, scatter photocoagulation is not recommended until NV develops.

   c. **Note:** Laser treatment of retinal branch vein occlusion is placed only in the area drained by the occluded vein. This does not involve four-quadrant scatter photocoagulation such as is applied in the treatment of PDR. Generally, treatment is applied no closer than 2 disc diameters away from the edge of the foveal avascular zone.

3. Central retinal vein occlusion (CRVO) with rubeosis iridis or with retinal NV and VH.
4. Sickle cell retinopathy: Scatter photocoagulation applied in the quadrant around areas of peripheral retinal NV is the preferred method to treatment patients with recurrent vitreous hemorrhage and/or retinal neovascularization secondary to proliferative sickle cell retinopathy (most common in patients with SC disease). One should avoid direct treatment over the long posterior ciliary arteries to reduce the chance for anterior segment ischemia.
5. Radiation retinopathy: Radiation can damage retinal vascular cells and produce a retinal microangiopathy that resembles diabetic retinopathy clinically. Usually, patients must be exposed to radiation doses of 35 Gy or more for retinopathy to develop. Concurrent administration of chemotherapy or coexisting disease such as diabetes mellitus lowers the threshold for the development of radiation retinopathy. To treat proliferative radiation retinopathy, scatter photocoagulation is applied as described for PDR.

Preoperative Procedure

1. Complete retinal examination to evaluate presence of NV and retinal ischemia.
2. Fluorescein angiogram to evaluate capillary dropout (in cases of retinal vein occlusion or rubeosis iridis secondary to PDR without posterior pole retinal neovascularization) and to distinguish venous collaterals (BRVO) and IRMA (diabetic retinopathy) from NV.

Instrumentation

- Argon green (514–527 nm), krypton red (647 nm), tunable dye (577–630 nm), or diode (790–830 nm) laser. The longer wavelengths (e.g., krypton red and diode modalities) are especially useful for eyes with nuclear sclerotic cataracts or vitreous/preretinal hemorrhage.
- Fundus contact lens.
- Goldmann 3-mirror lens:
  - Image is oriented with same spatial relationships as retina undergoing treatment.
  - May use mirrors to treat peripheral fundus.
  - Burn size = spot size set on laser.
- Rodenstock, quadraspheric, or transequator lenses:
  - Image is inverted and backward (similar to image obtained with indirect ophthalmoscope).
  - A much larger area in a given field may be treated than with the Goldmann lens.
  - Burn size ≅ approximately twice the spot size set on laser (e.g., 250 μm setting gives approximately a 500 μm spot size).

Operative Procedure

1. Anesthesia: Topical (e.g., proparacaine) is preferred. Retrobulbar anesthesia may be necessary in a patient who has experienced excessive pain on previous treatment or who is unable to maintain steady fixation. If retrobulbar anesthesia is administered, the surgeon should be prepared to manage infrequent systemic complications such as respiratory depression and seizures.
2. Place contact lens with methylcellulose solution.
3. Establish clear view of fundus and identify landmarks.
4. Focus aiming beam, tilting the contact lens as necessary to produce a round, not elliptical, spot.

Laser Parameters

1. Spot size:
   a. 500 μm (set laser at 200–300 μm if using Rodenstock, quadraspheric, or equator plus lens).
   b. 200 μm if treating within vascular arcades.
2. Duration: 0.05–0.2 seconds.

   Short durations (e.g., 0.05 second) tend to be associated with less discomfort.

3. Power: Start at ~150 mW (100 mW for krypton) and adjust as necessary to produce desired effect.
4. Typical treatment schema:
   a. Number of laser applications:
      i. PRP for PDR: Apply ~1500 spots over two sessions. It is probably best not to focus on the number of treatment spots but to focus on the total surface area treated. The usual goal is to treat the retina outside the temporal arcades as far peripherally as the equator for 360 degrees.
      ii. PRP for CRVO: Apply treatment as above. Patients with rubeosis iridis may require treatment extending to the ora serrata.
      iii. Scatter photocoagulation for BRVO: Treatment is confined to the quadrant involved by the vein occlusion.
      iv. Scatter photocoagulation for sickle cell retinopathy: Treatment is applied surrounding areas of peripheral retinal NV out to the ora serrata and for 1 clock hour on either side of the NV. For patients in whom follow-up is uncertain, one may elect to treat the periphery for 360 degrees. One should avoid direct treatment to long posterior ciliary arteries to reduce the chance of anterior segment ischemia.
      v. Total number of spots and density of burns varies with clinical response to treatment.
         I. Clinical response to treatment typically requires ~3 weeks.
         II. Clinical response is evident as a loss of the capillary brush border of the NV, the development of fibrosis of the NV, and/or as regression of the NV.
      vi. Separate treatment sessions by ~1–2 weeks.

b. Space spots ¹/₂ –1 burn width from each other.
c. Some surgeons apply test burns in peripheral area of relatively normal retina to obtain baseline power for treatment.
d. Adjust laser power to produce a gray-white (not intense white) burn.
e. Session 1:

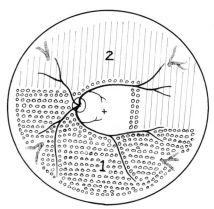

Figure 67.2

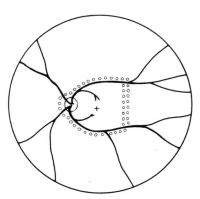

Figure 67.1

i. Circumscribe area not to be treated with 1–2 rows of spots (**Fig. 67.1**).
   I. Do not treat papillomacular bundle.
   II. Do not treat closer than one third disc diameter to optic nerve head nasally.
   III. Usually avoid treatment within vascular arcades temporally (may place a few spots just inside arcades if they are greater than 2 disc diameters from the edge of the foveal avascular zone).
   IV. Temporally: place 1–2 rows of burns, no closer than 2 disc diameters from the edge of the foveal avascular zone (assuming a relatively normal sized foveal avascular zone of 300–500 μm is present). Do not treat nasal to this demarcation.
ii. Select a section of retina for treatment (i.e., inferior fundus at first session [especially if vitreous hemorrhage is present]; superior half of fundus at second treatment session).
   I. Apply enough evenly scattered spots to cover the target area.
   II. Vary power as needed to obtain uniform burn intensity.
   III. If Rodenstock or transequator lens is used, may switch to Goldmann or quadraspheric lens to reach far periphery if necessary.
   IV. To facilitate treatment of peripheral retina, have patient look away from the mirror of a Goldmann lens or in the direction of the quadrant to be treated with a Rodenstock and quadraspheric lens.
f. Subsequent sessions:
   i. Treat previously untreated regions.
   ii. May treat more peripherally in previously treated quadrants.

iii. An example of one possible multiple-session treatment sequence is illustrated (**Fig. 67.2**).
g. Treatment tips:
   i. May directly treat small areas of flat NVE with confluent application of laser burns if they do not regress in response to scatter (i.e., indirect) treatment.
   ii. Do not treat NVD directly.
   iii. Do not treat areas of fibrovascular traction or elevated retina (to avoid inducing retinal breaks).
   iv. Do not treat directly over retinal vessels (to avoid inducing vascular occlusion).
   v. If patient is uncomfortable (e.g., when treating horizontal meridian near ciliary nerves), decrease laser duration and power.
   vi. Repeatedly verify landmarks and aiming beam position to avoid inadvertently treating the macula.

Postoperative Procedure

1. Usually prescribe oral analgesic (e.g., Tylenol, 650 mg p.o.) for headache. Some surgeons treat with topical atropine 1% b.i.d. and prednisolone acetate 1% q.i.d. after extensive treatment (e.g., entire fundus in cases of rubeotic glaucoma) to prevent development of secondary angle closure due to laser-induced choroidal detachment. For treatments involving fewer spots, it may be reasonable to prescribe oral analgesic only.
2. Follow-up in ~1 week.

Complications

1. Inadvertent foveal burn
2. Vitreous hemorrhage
3. Choroidal effusion with possibility of secondary angle closure glaucoma
4. Macular edema with possible permanent decrease in visual acuity
5. Epiretinal membrane formation
6. Retinal tear formation

7. Break in the Bruch membrane with choroidal hemorrhage, choroidal and/or choroidovitreal neovascularization
8. Constriction of visual field (usually with extensive scatter photocoagulation)
9. Decreased dark adaptation
10. Decreased accommodative amplitude

■ Laser Photocoagulation for Macular Edema

Indications

Macular Edema in Diabetic Retinopathy

Treat eyes with retinal thickening involving or threatening the center of the macula (clinically significant macular edema [CSME] as defined by the ETDRS). CSME is defined as:

1. Thickening of the retina at or within 500 µm of the center of the macula, or
2. Hard exudates at or within 500 µm of the center of the macula associated with adjacent areas of retinal thickening, or
3. Areas of retinal thickening one disc diameter or larger any part of which is within one disc diameter of the center of the macula.
4. Macular edema is defined by the presence of retinal thickening on clinical exam. Dye leakage seen on fluorescein angiography may or may not indicate retinal thickening, depending on how well the RPE and retina clear the fluid delivered to the retina via incompetent retinal vessels. Also, areas of nonperfused retina may be thickened. Optical coherence tomography (OCT) detects macular edema more sensitively than clinical exam. One study showed that clinicians cannot reliably detect thickened retina with contact lens biomicroscopy unless the thickness is > 300 µm. OCT-3 can detect thickness of 200–300 µm reliably. Use of OCT measurements to guide treatment recommendations for CSME is not standardized at this time.
5. Given a patient with CSME the ETDRS defines treatable lesions as:
   a. Discrete points of hyperfluorescence or leakage on the fluorescein angiogram (e.g., microaneurysms [MAs], IRMAs, capillaries).
   b. Diffuse sites of leakage within the retina (e.g., leaking capillary bed).
   c. Thickened avascular areas of retina.
6. Among untreated patients, moderate visual loss (doubling of visual angle or a 3-line loss of vision on the ETDRS vision chart) occurred in ~24% during 3 years of follow-up versus ~12% who underwent macular photocoagulation.
   a. The treatment benefit was most marked for patients with thickening involving the macular center.
   b. Only ~3% of patients experienced moderately improved visual acuity after treatment, so the major goal of treatment is to *stabilize* vision, not to improve it.

Macular Edema in Branch Retinal Vein Occlusion

The Branch Vein Occlusion Study concluded that eyes with visual acuity of 20/40 or less secondary to macular edema benefit from photocoagulation to the involved area.

1. Patients are eligible for treatment if:
   a. Visual acuity is 20/40 or worse and not spontaneously improving, and
   b. BRVO is at least 3 months old, and
   c. Decreased vision is not due to blood in the fovea and/or macular capillary nonperfusion, and
   d. Fluorescein angiography documents fluorescein leakage in the macula.
2. Among untreated patients, after 3 years of follow-up, 34% had visual acuity ≥ 20/40 versus 60% of treated patients.

Preoperative Procedure

1. Perform stereoscopic contact lens fundus exam to evaluate location and extent of retinal thickening from macular edema.
2. Perform fluorescein angiogram and color fundus photos to precisely identify areas of focal and diffuse leakage as well as areas of macular capillary nonperfusion.
3. Perform baseline OCT exam to document severity of macular thickening and to serve as comparison for future measurements after treatment (optional).

Instrumentation

- Argon green (514–527 nm), krypton red (647 nm), tunable dye (577–630 nm), or diode laser (790–830 nm):
  - Some surgeons prefer argon green or dye yellow for discrete areas of vascular leakage (e.g., MAs and IRMA) since these wavelengths are absorbed well by hemoglobin.
  - Krypton red, dye red, and diode laser may be preferred for macular grid treatments since these wavelengths are not absorbed well by retinal blood vessels or macular xanthophyll pigment, thus sparing (relatively) the overlying retina. Although these wavelengths may also be advantageous in situations where blood partially obscures the planned treatment area, one should not treat over blood in this setting, as it may stimulate epiretinal membrane formation or produce undesirably intense retinal burns.
- Fundus contact lens:
  - Goldmann three-mirror lens or macular contact lens:
  - Image is oriented with same spatial relationships as eye undergoing treatment.
  - Burn size = spot size set on laser.
- Rodenstock lens: probably should be avoided for macular treatments due to image inversion and relative minification of view.

Operative Procedure

Treatment of Diabetic Macular Edema

1. Project recent representative fluorescein angiogram for reference during treatment.

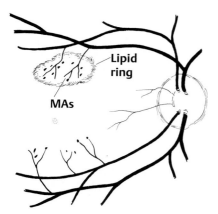

Figure 67.3

a. In some cases (e.g., pregnancy, allergy to fluorescein dye), a fluorescein angiogram cannot be done. In this situation, if there is a circinate lipid ring, the leaking lesions are almost always located in the center of the lipid ring, and treatment can be directed to this area (**Fig. 67.3**).

If there is no lipid ring, grid treatment can be considered, but the patient must be cautioned that the treatment may be placed too close to the edge of or even within the foveal avascular zone (FAZ) inadvertently with resultant symptomatic scotomata or loss of central visual acuity. This situation is perhaps more likely to arise if there is pathological enlargement of the FAZ.

2. Anesthesia: Topical (e.g., proparacaine) is preferred. Retrobulbar anesthesia may be necessary in a patient who has experienced excessive pain on previous treatment (rare in this setting) or who is unable to maintain steady fixation.
   a. If retrobulbar anesthesia is administered, the surgeon should be prepared to manage infrequent systemic complications such as respiratory depression and seizures.
   b. Also, after a perfect retrobulbar injection, some torsional eye movement is possible because the superior oblique muscle will not be paralyzed by the injection.
3. Place fundus contact lens with methylcellulose solution.
4. Establish clear view of fundus and identify landmarks.
5. Focus aiming beam, tilting the contact lens as necessary to produce a round, not elliptical, spot.
6. Treat focal areas of leakage.
   a. Use argon green or dye yellow laser.
   b. Treat all discrete points of hyperfluorescence or leakage that lie within 2500 μm of the center of the macula as determined with the angiogram. One may

also treat thickened retina that is nonperfused. Treatment of nonleaking lesions (e.g., MAs versus intraretinal hemorrhage) less than 125 μm in diameter is optional.
   c. Do not treat lesions closer than 500 μm to center of the macula during the initial treatment.
   d. Do not treat the edge of the FAZ.
   e. If retinal thickening involves the center of the macula and visual acuity is 20/40 or better, treat leaks no closer than 500 μm to the macular center at the initial treatment.

After ~3 months follow-up, if CSME persists and if vision is 20/40 or better, consider treatment of leaking lesions located 300–500 μm from the center of the macula provided that the treatment spares the edge of the FAZ and patient understands and accepts the risk of developing paracentral scotomata or central visual loss.

   f. One may treat intraretinal hemorrhages ≤ 125 μm in diameter that lie 1500 μm or more from the macular center and outside the papillomacular bundle.
   g. Do not treat flame-shaped hemorrhages.
7. Laser parameters:
   a. Spot size: 50–100 μm.
      i. Recommend 50 μm spot when treating 300–500 μm from center of FAZ.
      ii. Recommend 100 μm spot when treating > 500 μm from center of FAZ.
   b. Duration: 0.05–0.1 seconds. Consider using 0.05s when treating close to the edge of FAZ to avoid inadvertent treatment of foveola due to saccade.
   c. Power: Start at ~100 mW and increase as necessary to produce mild whitening of the RPE.
8. Patterns of focal treatment: Direct versus grid laser photocoagulation.

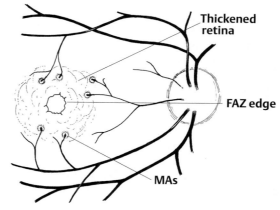

Figure 67.4

   a. Direct treatment: Laser spot is targeted only to leaking lesions in thickened retina (**Fig. 67.4**).
      i. Size: 50–100 μm spot.
      ii. Duration: 0.05–0.1 second
      iii. Power: enough to create mild whitening of RPE under treated lesion. When treating MAs ≥ 40

μm in size, may consider increasing the power enough to whiten the MA, although it is not clear that this intensity of treatment is required to elicit a clinical response.

iv. When treating with the goal of whitening MAs, consider first treating the subjacent RPE with a 100 μm spot to produce mild RPE whitening. This may reduce the power needed to create whitening of the MA.

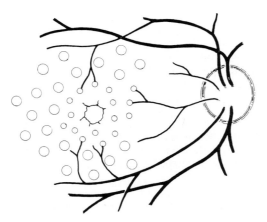

Figure 67.5

b. Grid treatment: Laser spots are applied in a "grid" pattern in areas of retinal thickening without any specific attempt to treat leaking lesions (**Fig. 67.5**).
   i. Size: 50–200 μm (usually, 100 μm).
   ii. Spacing: 1–2 burn widths apart depending on the degree of retinal thickening (close spacing for marked thickening).
   iii. Duration: 0.05–0.1 sec (usually 0.1 sec).
   iv. Power: enough to create mild whitening of RPE.
   v. Distribution: above, below, and temporal to fovea. Extend treatment to PRP burns, if present.
   vi. Treat conservatively in the papillomacular bundle and use 50 μm spots.
   vii. Stay at least 500 μm from macular center and from margin of optic nerve head.

9. Treatment tips:
   a. Sometimes, resolution of retinal thickening can be brought about through medical management (e.g., control of hypertension, elimination of fluid overload, especially in dialysis patients).
   b. Avoid treating near the edge of FAZ to prevent the development of symptomatic paracentral scotomata.
   c. Avoid placing numerous, closely spaced laser spots in papillomacular bundle.
   d. Areas of markedly thickened retina usually require more power per spot size to produce RPE whitening than do areas of less thickened retina. Therefore, try to treat the less thickened retina first and increase laser power if necessary as more thickened retina is treated. When switching from treating more thickened retina to treating less thickened retina, be sure to reduce the laser power before treating.

e. When switching from 100 to 50 μm spot sizes, be sure to reduce laser power to avoid excessive energy delivery with associated risk of Bruch membrane perforation (associated with risk of subretinal hemorrhage and choroidal neovascularization) and retinal hole formation. Short duration of treatment (e.g., 0.05 second) also increases the likelihood of Bruch membrane perforation (at a given power).

f. When treating within 300–500 μm of the center of the macula, consider using a 50 μm spot size and 0.05 second duration to avoid creating symptomatic scotomata and avoid creating a foveolar burn inadvertently due to an unanticipated saccadic eye movement.

g. Apply grid photocoagulation to areas of thickened retina with diffuse leakage or capillary nonperfusion.

h. May use argon green, krypton red, dye red, or diode laser.

i. Treat thickened areas of diffuse leakage or capillary nonperfusion within two disc diameters of, but not closer than 500 μm to, the center of the macula.

10. Re-treatment
   a. Often three to four treatments are required to produce resolution of retinal thickening.
   b. Space treatment sessions by ~3 months to judge the effects of treatment.
   c. Consider obtaining repeat fluorescein angiogram to determine site of persistently leaking lesions and to reassess location of FAZ.
   d. If clinical exam unclear, consider obtaining repeat OCT to assess response to previous laser treatment.
   e. Apply additional laser treatment to leaking lesions or in grid pattern as above.
   f. Additional grid photocoagulation may be applied to sites of diffuse leakage not treated originally.

Treatment of Macular Edema in Retinal Branch Vein Occlusion

1. Prepare patient and instrumentation as in Steps 1–7 above.

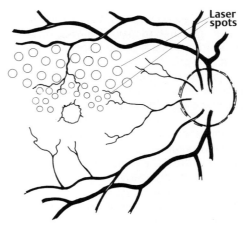

Figure 67.6

2. Apply Grid photocoagulation to ischemic foci and areas of leakage as detailed above (**Fig. 67.6**).
   a. Either argon green, dye red, krypton red, or diode laser may be used.
   b. Treatment may be extended up to the edge of FAZ and peripherally to the major vascular arcade (i.e., 2 disc diameters from the edge of FAZ).
   c. Avoid direct treatment of shunt vessels, the perifoveal capillary network, and areas of intraretinal hemorrhage.

Postoperative Procedure

1. No medications necessary.
2. Consider repeating stereoscopic examination of macula, fluorescein angiogram, and OCT ~3 months after laser treatment. Follow-up sooner if decreased vision is noted.
3. Consider retreating any focal areas of leakage if CSME persists. Additional grid photocoagulation may be applied to sites of diffuse leakage not originally treated.

Complications

1. Symptomatic scotomata or decreased central visual acuity.
2. Breaks in the Bruch membrane.
3. Subretinal hemorrhage.
4. Choroidal neovascularization: May occur with or without clinically evident breaks in the Bruch membrane. Can be difficult to detect on the basis of clinical findings alone as these patients may already have intraretinal blood and lipid (e.g., diabetic maculopathy) and decreased visual acuity. Fluorescein angiography is very helpful in confirming the diagnosis, and OCT can sometimes reveal the choroidal new vessel more clearly than angiography.

■ Focal Photocoagulation of Choroidal Neovascularization

Indications

1. The Macular Photocoagulation Study (MPS) demonstrated the efficacy of argon and krypton laser photocoagulation in decreasing the incidence of severe visual loss secondary to choroidal neovascularization in: (1) age-related macular degeneration; (2) the presumed ocular histoplasmosis syndrome; and (3) idiopathic choroidal neovascularization (ICNV).
2. The effectiveness of laser photocoagulation in treating choroidal new vessels (CNVs) has been proved only in the case of well-defined CNVs.
3. Despite the fact that the MPS demonstrated that laser photocoagulation of subfoveal CNVs is better than observation, in most cases, subfoveal CNVs are not treated with laser photocoagulation due to the availability of superior treatment alternatives (e.g., intravitreal injection of vascular endothelial growth factor [VEGF]-A inhibitors

and photodynamic therapy [PDT]). With this caveat in mind, we describe the use of laser photocoagulation to treat subfoveal CNVs for completeness.

Preoperative Procedure

1. Complete retinal examination including stereoscopic contact lens examination of the macula.
2. Perform fluorescein angiogram and color fundus photography to precisely localize CNV. A recent fluorescein angiogram (less than 72–96 hours old) is necessary to guide treatment.

Instrumentation

- Argon green or krypton red laser.
  - Argon blue-green laser treatment was the modality shown to be effective in the MPS treatment of extrafoveal CNVs. When treating within the FAZ, argon green is preferable, since the green wavelength light is not absorbed by macular xanthophyll pigment.
  - Krypton red is absorbed by melanin in the retinal pigment epithelium and inner choroid. It is not well absorbed by blood vessels, free blood, and xanthophyll pigment. Thus, the krypton laser may be preferable in treating near the fovea, particularly at sites where blood obscures the CNV. Krypton red laser may be more likely to induce RPE tears, however, particularly if a CNV is associated with an RPE detachment.
  - While laser photocoagulation can be used to treat juxtafoveal CNVs, many retinal surgeons prefer to treat such lesions with PDT (e.g., Verteporfin) or with intravitreal injection of VEGF-A inhibitors (e.g., Lucentis).
- Fundus contact lens:
  - Magnification ~1.05–1.1, depending on the lens used (e.g., Goldmann lens).

Operative Procedure

1. Project recent (≤ 72 hours old for extra- and juxtafoveal CNV; ≤ 96 hours old for subfoveal CNV) representative fluorescein angiogram ± color fundus photograph for reference during treatment.
2. Anesthesia: Retrobulbar or topical (e.g., proparacaine). Generally, the treatment is not painful, and topical anesthesia is preferred unless the patient has difficulty maintaining steady fixation. Even a "perfect" retrobulbar block is associated with some torsional eye movement due to sparing of the superior oblique innervation.
3. Place fundus contact lens with methylcellulose solution.
4. Establish clear view of fundus and identify landmarks.
5. Laser parameters:
   a. Spot size: 200–500 μm. Outline CNV border with 200 μm spots (start on foveal side first) and fill in center with 500 μm spots.

b. Duration: 0.2–0.5 sec. (For krypton red, consider using longer duration to minimize risk of choroidal hemorrhage.)

c. Power: Start at ~150 mW and adjust as necessary to create uniform, intensely white burns.

6. Focus aiming beam tilting the contact lens as necessary to produce a round, not elliptical, spot.

7. Apply treatment.

a. Estimate necessary power.

i. Place test spots away from foveal edge of CNV.

ii. When using argon green, start at ~150 mW and adjust as necessary to produce a hot white burn.

iii. When using krypton red, adjust as necessary to produce a gray-white or yellow-white burn. (An intense white burn suggests unwanted power that may cause rupture of the Bruch membrane and choroidal hemorrhage.)

iv. If hemorrhage obscures the CNV, consider reducing power to produce a slightly less intense reaction in retina.

b. *Optional:* Delineate the CNV with noncontiguous 100 μm spots before treating perimeter continuously with 200 μm spots.

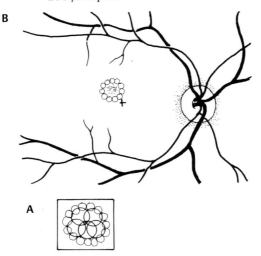

Figure 67.7

c. Treat foveal side of the CNV first to avoid iatrogenic bleeding into fovea from subsequent laser spots (**Figs. 67.7A and 67.7B**).

i. Place a row of overlapping 200 μm, 0.2 sec burns at the foveal edge of the CNV.

ii. Extend burns ~100 μm past the edge of the CNV or contiguous pigment and hemorrhage unless, in the case of extra- or juxtafoveal CNVs, such treatment would involve treating foveal center.

d. Complete treatment of the perimeter of the CNV.

i. Place burns in overlapping fashion.

ii. Extend burns ~100 μm past the nonfoveal edge of the CNV complex.

iii. If nonfoveal edge of CNV is obscured by blood, extend the treatment ~125 μm beyond the edge of the hemorrhage.

e. Treat the remainder of the CNV with overlapping 200–500 μm burns of 0.5 sec duration.

i. Burns should be intensely white. (Laser application should be stopped before full 0.5 sec period if developing spot appears excessively hot, however.)

ii. Ensure complete coverage of the CNV.

Extra- versus Juxta- versus Subfoveal Treatment

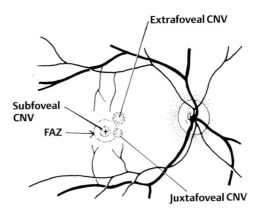

Figure 67.8

1. Extrafoveal CNVs: (**Fig. 67.8** illustrates extra-, juxta-, and subfoveal location).

a. MPS definition and eligibility: Foveal edge of CNV 200–2500 μm from FAZ center; best-corrected visual acuity ≥ 20/100; peripapillary CNV treatment must spare 1.5 clock hours of temporal nerve fiber layer.

b. Treatment: Argon green laser, retrobulbar (optional) versus topical anesthesia, fluorescein angiogram 72 hours old or less, intense uniform whitening, treatment extends 100 μm beyond edge of the CNV, if the CNV is 300 μm or more from the center of the FAZ; if not, then simply cover the CNV. Repeat treatment if fluorescein angiogram shows leakage at the edge of the treatment scar, and this edge is 200 μm or more from the center of the FAZ.

c. Results: (5-year follow-up in MPS studies) (**Table 67.1**).

d. Recurrence following treatment of extrafoveal CNV:

i. Risk factors: Cigarette smoking (age-related macular degeneration [AMD], ICNV); confluent drusen or disciform scarring in fellow eye (AMD).

ii. Definition: Leakage of fluorescein dye noted at the perimeter of the treatment scar later than 6 weeks after treatment (new leakage within 6 weeks after treatment is defined as persistence); subretinal blood, fluid, or lipid is usually present.

iii. Retreat the recurrence if it is well-defined (see below).

iv. Recurrences are infrequent after 2 years in AMD, POHS, and ICNV; 73% occur within the first year, overall.

Table 67.1 Results (with 5-Year Follow-up in MPS Studies)

	AMD*	POHS*	ICNV*
Mean visual acuity without treatment	20/200	20/80	20/80
Mean visual acuity with treatment	20/125	20/40	20/64
≥ 6 line loss of vision: without treatment	64%	41%	45%
With treatment	46%	10%	23%
Relative risk	1.5	3.6	2.3
Recurrence	54% (8% independent)	26% (7% independent)	34%

*AMD, age-related macular degeneration; POHS, presumed ocular histoplasmosis syndrome; ICNV, idiopathic choroidal neovascularization.

    v. Visual outcome is worse with recurrence.

2. Juxtafoveal CNVs:

  a. MPS definition and eligibility: CNV with posterior edge between 1–199 μm from the FAZ center or 200–2500 μm from the FAZ center if blood extends within 200 μm of the FAZ center; blood or blocked fluorescence can extend through the entire FAZ; visual acuity ≥ 20/400; peripapillary CNV are treatable if treatment can spare 1.5 hours of temporal retina.

  b. Treatment: Krypton red laser, fluorescein angiogram 72 hours old or less, retrobulbar anesthesia, treatment extends 100 μm beyond the hyperfluorescence border away from the fovea and extends 100 μm into the blood on the foveal side if hyperfluorescence is 100 μm or farther from the FAZ center; follow-up at 2, 4, 6 weeks, then 3, 6 months, then every 6 months.

  c. Results (AMD):

    i. Persistence 32%, recurrence 47% of CNV at 5-year follow-up.

    ii. Mean visual acuity without persistence or recurrence is 20/80–20/100; with persistence is 20/200; with recurrence is 20/250.

    iii. Risk factors for persistence: small CNV, failure to cover 10% or more of the foveal half of the CNV, nongeographic atrophy in the fellow eye.

    iv. Risk factors for recurrence: extensive drusen, nongeographic atrophy, or disciform scarring in the fellow eye. Without risk factors, recurrence is 40%.

  d. Juxtafoveal persistent or recurrent lesions are treated as described above.

  e. At 3-years follow-up, 49% with treatment versus 58% without treatment lost 6 lines or more vision. The mean visual acuity was 20/200 with treatment versus 20/250 without treatment.

    i. There was no statistically significant treatment benefit if definite hypertension was present (defined as diastolic blood pressure > 94 mm Hg, or systolic blood pressure > 159 mm of Hg, or using antihypertensive medications).

    ii. Without hypertension, 65% without treatment versus 31% with treatment lost 6 lines or more vision.

3. Subfoveal CNVs (AMD):

  a. Definition and eligibility: Note that at this time, most patients with subfoveal CNVs are treated with intravitreal injection of anti-VEGF-A agents or, in some cases, with PDT. Some retinal surgeons also employ combination therapy (e.g., combined intravitreal Lucentis and Verteporfin-PDT).

    i. Fluorescein angiogram < 96 hours old.

    ii. CNV with well-demarcated boundaries.

    iii. CNV ≤ 3.5 disc areas (DA) in size (1 disc area = 1.77 mm²) with new vessels under the geometric center of the FAZ.

    iv. Visual acuity 20/40 to 20/320.

    v. The lesion must have classic CNV; classic or occult CNV has to comprise most of the lesion.

  b. Treatment:

    i. Confluent intense white burns covering all areas of classic and occult CNV and other components (e.g., thick blood, elevated blocked fluorescence, serous pigment epithelial detachment [PED]) and extending 100 μm beyond the border of the lesion (except blood).

    ii. In the MPS study, retrobulbar anesthesia was recommended, but it is not required. Most patients are treated with topical anesthesia.

    iii. 200–500 μm spot size with 0.2–0.5 sec duration applied to boundaries and 200–500 μm spot size with 0.5–1.0 sec duration applied within boundaries.

    iv. Fluorescein angiography at 3 and 6 weeks, 3 and 6 months, and every 6 months thereafter; in the MPS, there was random assignment to Krypton red versus Argon green laser.

  c. Results:

    i. Failure to be eligible: Most often due to poorly demarcated CNV, CNV less than one half the entire lesion, lesion component other than CNV under the FAZ center, lesion > 3.5 disc areas.

    ii. Visual outcome (MPS) (**Table 67.2**).

    iii. Reading speed: Three months after treatment, reading speed was better in the no treatment group than in the treatment group; by 24 months, reading speed was greater in the treatment group. After 4-year follow-up, 30% treated versus 48% untreated were not able to read any words (20/1500) using study eye.

    iv. Contrast threshold (with better contrast threshold, one is better able to perform functional tasks at a given Snellen acuity) (MPS) (**Table 67.3**):

Table 67.2 Visual Outcome (MPS) after Laser Treatment of Subfoveal CNVs (AMD)

	3 Months Follow-Up	24 Months Follow-Up	48 Months Follow-Up
Mean visual acuity without treatment	20/200	20/400	20/500
Mean visual acuity with treatment	20/320	20/320	20/320

Table 67.3 Contrast Threshold (MPS) after Laser Treatment of Subfoveal CNVs (AMD)

	Initial Visit	3 Months Follow-Up	24 Months Follow-Up	48 Months Follow-Up
With treatment	14%	14%	14%	14%
Without Treatment	14%	20%	28%	28%

v. Initial lesion size, initial visual acuity, and conformity with eligibility criteria affected pattern of visual loss.
  I. Small lesion (≤ 1 MPS DA):
    A. VA ≤ 20/125, then the treatment group had better vision than the no treatment group throughout follow-up (0% versus 14% with ≥ 6 line decrease at 3 months and 13% versus 35% with ≥ 6 line decrease at 48 months).
    B. VA ≥ 20/100, then the treatment group had worse vision than the no treatment group at 6 months (32% versus 19% with ≥ 6 line decrease); by 12 months, the treatment group did better (27% versus 38% with ≥ 6 line decrease).
  II. Medium lesion (>1 to ≤ 2 MPS DA):
    A. VA ≤ 20/200, then treated eyes better throughout follow-up (see above).
    B. VA ≥ 20/160, then treated eyes worse at 6 months; substantially better 12 months after treatment (see above).
  III. Large lesion (> 2 MPS DA):
    A. VA ≤ 20/200, then treated eyes slightly better throughout follow-up (treated and untreated have ~3% with ≥ 6 line decrease at 3 months.)
    B. VA ≥ 20/160, then treated eyes substantially worse for 18 months (46% versus 13% with ≥ 6 line decrease at 3 months), little difference thereafter (50% versus 55% with ≥ 6 line decrease at 48 months).
4. Recurrent subfoveal CNVs.
  a. Definition and eligibility (AMD): Note that at this time, most patients with subfoveal CNVs are treated with intravitreal injection of anti-VEGF-A agents or, in some cases, with PDT. Some retinal specialists also employ combination therapy (e.g., combined intravitreal Lucentis and Verteporfin-PDT).
    i. Fluorescein angiogram < 96 hours old.
    ii. CNV under FAZ center continuous with scar from prior treatment, or CNV within 150 μm of the FAZ center contiguous to the scar from earlier laser treatment that has developed atrophy extending under the fovea.

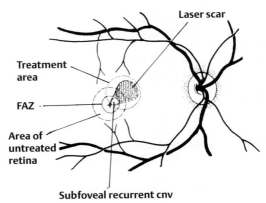

Figure 67.9

    iii. CNV plus scar ≤ 6 MPS disc areas; some portion of the retina within 1 disc diameter of the FAZ center (four disc areas centered on the fovea) not to be treated (**Fig. 67.9** illustrates eligibility).
    iv. Visual acuity between 20/40 and 20/320.
    v. Age ≥ 50 years.
  b. Treatment
    i. Cover classic and occult CNV and other components of recurrence 100 μm beyond the perimeter of lesion components (except blood) and 300 μm into the scar along the perimeter bordered by the CNV.
    ii. If a feeder vessel is present, it should be covered 100 μm either side of feeder vessel and 300 μm radially beyond base of feeder into the scar (**Fig. 67.10**).
    iii. Retrobulbar anesthesia optional.
    iv. In the MPS, krypton red versus argon green laser was randomly assigned.
    v. Follow-up was at 3 and 6 weeks, 3 and 6 months, and every 12 months thereafter.
  c. Visual outcome (MPS) (**Table 67.4**):
  d. Reading speed was worse with treatment at 3 months, but better with treatment by 24 months follow-up.

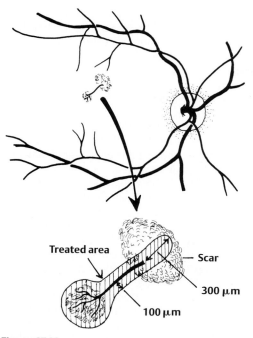

Figure 67.10

e. Contrast sensitivity (MPS) (**Table 67.5**).
f. Probability of recurrence and persistence was 26% and 22%, respectively, at 24 months follow-up (equally likely with krypton red versus argon green laser). Although visual acuity was worse with recurrence at 3-months follow-up, by 24 months it was not associated with worse visual outcome.
g. Expect an immediate 2.5-line decrease in vision after treatment with stable vision thereafter (a bigger decline should be anticipated if patients have relatively good visual acuity). There was no significant visual benefit noted with treatment until 12 months after enrollment.

Postoperative Procedure

1. No medications necessary.
2. Follow-up in 2–4 weeks with a repeat fluorescein angiogram to verify efficacy of vessel obliteration and retreat as necessary.
3. Follow patients for recurrence with daily Amsler grid self-examination, and in office at ~3, 6, 12, 24, 36, and 48 weeks, and every 6–12 months thereafter with fundus biomicroscopy and fluorescein angiography.

Complications

1. Inadvertent foveal burn (in setting of extra- or juxta-foveal CNV)
2. Rupture of the Bruch membrane
3. Choroidal hemorrhage
4. Pigment epithelial tear through fovea
5. Visual loss
6. Scotomata
7. Incomplete treatment (results in persistence of CNV)
8. Recurrence of neovascularization (i.e., CNV detected > 6 weeks after photocoagulation)
9. Epiretinal membrane formation
10. Retinal neovascularization at treatment site. Usually self-limited, but may be confused with persistent/recurrent CNV.

◼ Laser Photocoagulation for Retinal Breaks

Indications

▨ Acute symptomatic retinal break
▨ Retinal break with progressive subclinical retinal detachment
▨ Prophylaxis against retinal detachment in fellow eye

Table 67.4 Visual Outcome (MPS) after Laser Treatment of Recurrent Subfoveal CNVs

	3 Months Follow-Up	24 Months Follow-Up	36 Months Follow-Up
With treatment	20/250	20/250	20/250
Without treatment	20/200	20/320	20/320

Table 67.5 Contrast Sensitivity (MPS) after Laser Treatment of Recurrent Subfoveal CNVs

	Initial Visit	3 Months Follow-Up	24 Months Follow-Up	36 Months Follow-Up
Without treatment	10%	14%	20%	20%
With treatment	14%	14%	14%	14%

Instrumentation

- Lid speculum
- Topical anesthetic (may need subconjunctival or retrobulbar 2% lidocaine)
- 20 D or 28 D lens
- Scleral depressor
- Wide-angle viewing fundus contact lens (e.g., Rodenstock, quadraspheric, transequator, or Goldmann three-mirror lens)
- Argon, diode, or tunable dye laser with capacity for direct and/or indirect ophthalmoscope laser treatment (e.g., Novus Omni Laser by Lumenis)

Operative Procedure

1. Make careful retinal drawing of location of retinal break using indirect ophthalmoscopy.
2. Use indirect laser ophthalmoscope or contact lens laser delivery system.
   a. Indirect system may be easier to use for peripherally located retinal tears.
   b. Choice of wavelength:
      i. Argon green is usually adequate.
      ii. In the setting of nuclear sclerotic cataract or mild vitreous hemorrhage, longer wavelength light (e.g., krypton or dye red laser or diode laser) may penetrate better and give better uptake at level of RPE-choroid.
   c. Topical anesthesia is usually adequate. Subconjunctival anesthesia can be administered if needed and usually suffices if topical anesthesia is inadequate.

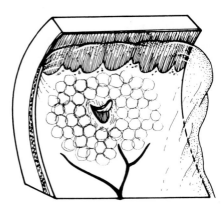

Figure 67.11

   d. Surround retinal break with three to four rows of confluent laser applications using 20 D or 28 D lens (**Fig. 67.11** illustrates laser around retinal break).
   e. Extend treatment to ora serrata for retinal breaks anterior to equator. Treating this area is particularly important for flap tears to prevent extension of the tear (due to ongoing vitreoretinal traction) and development of subretinal fluid around the lateral horns of the tear. If this area cannot be treated satisfactorily with laser photocoagulation, consider switching to cryotherapy (see Chapter 65) to complete this part of the treatment.
   f. Use sufficient power to achieve a moderately white burn.
   g. If have difficulty getting laser uptake:
      i. Be sure you are treating in attached retina. A white burn will not be achieved if there is significant subretinal fluid in treatment area.
      ii. Be sure laser spot is focused properly. Use of 20 D lens gives a higher magnification view than a 28 D lens, thus facilitating more precise focusing. On the other hand, a 28 D lens gives a larger spot size on the retina and a wider field of view.
      iii. Use adequate power and treatment duration to achieve energy delivery. If exceptionally high power/duration is needed (e.g., significant nuclear sclerotic cataract), the patient may require subconjunctival (occasionally, retrobulbar) anesthesia. With indirect delivery system, typically start with 0.05 or 0.1 sec duration and 250 mW power and increase duration and power as needed.
      iv. Contact lens delivery sometimes permits greater power delivery.
         I. Spot size: 500 µm (set laser at 200 µm if using Rodenstock, quadraspheric, or transequator lens).
         II. Duration: 0.05–0.2 sec.
         III. Power: Start at ~150 mW (100 mW for krypton) and adjust as necessary to produce desired effect.
      v. Consider switching to cryopexy if media opacity precludes adequate uptake.

Postoperative Procedure

1. Some surgeons suggest that patients restrict activity to bed rest with no reading.
   a. Approximately 7 days are required for a firm chorioretinal adhesion to form after laser photocoagulation (10–14 days are required following cryotherapy). During this time, eye movements can cause a detachment to develop or to progress through the laser treatment zone.
   b. Rapid eye movements (REMs) during sleep can promote development/extension of subretinal fluid. Some surgeons prescribe sedatives that are thought to reduce the period of REM sleep for this reason.
2. Follow-up approximately 1 week after treatment to assess stability of result.
3. Inform patient to follow-up immediately if new symptoms of photopsia, floaters, or decreased peripheral or central vision are noted.

Instruct patient to check vision monocularly at least once a day.

4. Follow-up at ~3, 6, 12, and 24 weeks and as needed thereafter.

Complications

1. Failure to surround retinal break
2. Choroidal rupture with complications such as choroidal neovascularization, vitreous hemorrhage, and/or retinal detachment
3. Failure of chorioretinal adhesion to stop accumulation of subretinal fluid
4. Cystoid macular edema (controversial, unlikely)
5. Epiretinal membrane (controversial, unlikely)

■ Photodynamic Therapy of Choroidal Neovascularization

Introduction

Visudyne is the commercial name for verteporfin for injection. Photodynamic therapy with Visudyne requires intravenous drug injection followed by properly timed exposure to nonthermal red light. Verteporfin, when activated by light in the presence of oxygen, generates singlet oxygen and other free radicals and initiates damage to vascular endothelium.

Indications

1. Lesion secondary to AMD in which classic CNVs comprise ≥ 50% of the lesion that involves geometric center of the FAZ as determined by fluorescein angiography. Among AMD patients with predominantly classic CNV lesions (defined as those in which the classic component of the CNV comprises 50% or more of the area of the entire lesion): 59% verteporfin-treated patients versus 31% of placebo patients lost less than 3 lines vision on the EDTRS chart at 24 months follow-up. Among AMD patients with predominantly classic CNVs that had *no* occult CNVs: 77% verteporfin-treated patients versus 27% of placebo patients lost less than 3 lines of vision on the EDTRS chart at 12 months follow-up. Because of the greater chance for moderate visual improvement using anti-VEGF-A agents, most retina specialists recommend intravitreal injection of an anti-VEGF-A agent (e.g., Lucentis) as a first-line approach when treating with monotherapy. Lucentis has been proved to be more effective than PDT for AMD patients with predominantly classic subfoveal CNVs.
2. Feeder vessels to recurrent CNVs that extend through the geometric center of the FAZ.

3. Pure occult subfoveal CNVs. Consider treating lesions ≤ 4 MPS disc areas in eyes or with visual acuity ≤ 20/50–1. Such eyes have a 49% chance of ≥ 3-line visual loss (on ETDRS chart) if treated with verteporfin versus 75% chance of ≥ 3-line loss in placebo-treated eyes at 2 years follow-up. As noted above, because of the greater chance for moderate visual improvement using anti-VEGF-A agents, most retina specialists recommend intravitreal injection of an anti-VEGF-A agent (e.g., Lucentis) as a first-line approach when treating with monotherapy.
4. Small studies indicate that PDT with Visudyne may be effective in patients with idiopathic CNV and CNV associated with high myopia, angioid streaks, or the ocular histoplasmosis syndrome. Some aspects of treatment described in this chapter (e.g., frequency of re-treatment after reappearance of dye leakage from CNV with fluorescein angiography) are not established through randomized clinical trials for all of these subgroups of patients. Management of these patients should be individualized and based on the judgment of the treating physician and desires of the patient.

Eligibility Criteria

- Women of childbearing potential should have a negative pregnancy test (blood or urine) at initiation of treatment and should not become pregnant during treatment. Negative pregnancy test is required before each treatment in such patients. Other eligibility criteria outlined above should be documented before treatment.
- Women who are nursing children should be warned that verteporfin may be secreted in breast milk.
- Patients with active hepatitis or clinically significant moderate to severe liver disease should be excluded.
- Patients with known porphyria or other porphyrin sensitivity or hypersensitivity to sunlight or bright artificial light should be excluded.

Preoperative Procedure

1. Complete retinal examination including stereoscopic contact lens examination of the macula. Perform fluorescein angiogram and color fundus photography to precisely localize CNV. A recent fluorescein angiogram (up to 2 weeks old) is necessary to guide treatment.
2. Prepare the patient.
   a. Dilate pupil (Cyclogyl 1% plus phenylephrine 2.5%).
   b. Place documentation of medical systems review, including specific questioning regarding liver disease and documentation of negative pregnancy test, in chart.
   c. Verify that patient has appropriate sun protection.
   d. Place treatment wrist band.

Table 67.6 Magnification of Various Fundus Cameras

Camera Model	Angle of View						
	20°	30°	35°	40°	45°	50°	60°
Topcon 50F/X/EX/IA	3.7X		2.5X			1.8X	
Zeiss FF 450/FF 450plus	4.33X	2.91X				1.87X	
Zeiss FF 4/3/2		2.5X					
Canon 60U				2.5X			1.7X
Nikon NFC 50/505	3.66X	2.41X				1.45X	
Kowa Pro 1/2/3	4.3X		7.5X			1.7X	
Kowa RC-XV	3.7X	2.5X			1.7X		
Kowa fx 500			2.6X			2.0X	

Used with permission from Carl Zeiss Meditec Inc.

3. Calculate spot size:
   a. The greatest linear dimension (GLD) of the lesion complex is measured with fluorescein angiography. All classic and occult CNV, blood and elevated blocked fluorescence, and associated serous pigment epithelial detachments constitute the lesion complex. The GLD as measured directly from the angiogram must be corrected for the magnification of the fundus camera (**Table 67.6**).
      i. For digital angiography, lesion can be measured with Topcon software; Camera: Topcon TRC 50 IA Imagenet digital image.
         I. Using software, draw circle around perimeter of CNV.

      II. Click and program indicates treatment spot size.
      ii. For angiography done with photographic film, the lesion is measured with a reticle: Topcon 50 IA: 2.5 magnification, Zeiss FF 450 30 degree: 2.6 magnification.
   b. Select an appropriate frame of the pretreatment fluorescein angiogram and record lesion GLD in millimeters as measured with reticle.
      i. Record camera magnification.
      ii. (GLD/mag) × 1000 + 1000 = treatment spot size in micrometers. Addition of 1000 ensures that treatment will extend at least 500 μm beyond the border of the lesion complex (if the treatment spot is centered properly).
   c. In the TAP and VIP studies, the greatest linear dimension of the entire CNV lesion was ≤ 5400 μm (approximately equivalent to the diameter of a 9 Macular Photocoagulation Study [MPS] disc area), and best-corrected distance visual acuity was 20/40–20/200 on an EDTRS chart. In practice, larger lesions are treated using a "painting" technique (see below for details).
4. Calculate dose of Visudyne needed:
   a. Patient will receive 6 mg/m² body surface area (BSA) and a total infusion volume of 30 ml.
   b. Calculate BSA using BSA nomogram (**Fig. 67.12**):
      i. Measure and mark patient's height.
      ii. Measure and mark patient's weight.
      iii. Draw line between height and weight marks.
      iv. Use BSA nomogram to identify patient's BSA (i.e., where line crosses central rule).
   c. Calculate Visudyne dose from BSA:
      i. BSA × 6 mg/m² = Total Visudyne dose.
      ii. Divide total Visudyne dose by 2 = total volume of reconstituted Visudyne solution needed.
      iii. Subtract total volume reconstituted Visudyne from the standard 30 ml to obtain volume dextrose 5% in water (D5W) required. Saline causes Visudyne to precipitate.

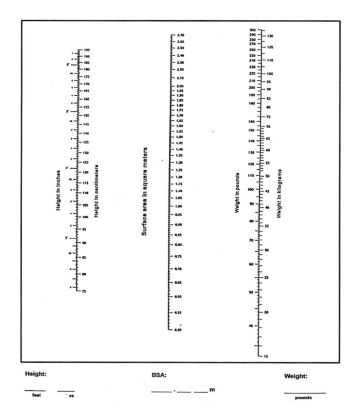

Height:

____ ____
feet   es

BSA:

____.__ __ m

Weight:

pounds

Figure 67.12

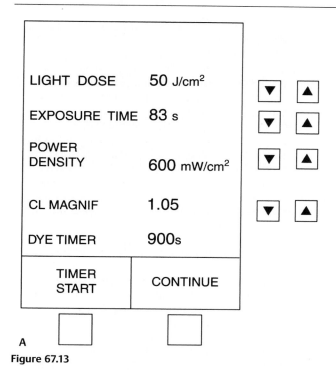

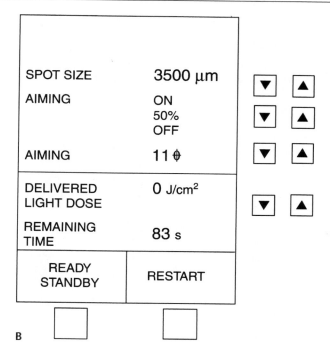

Figure 67.13

Instrumentation

- PDT laser
  - Laser system must deliver a stable power output at a wavelength 689 ± 3 nm. The following laser systems have been tested for compatibility with Visudyne and are approved for delivery of a stable power output at a wavelength of 689 ± 3 nm:
    - Coherent Opal Photoactivator Laser Console and LaserLink Adapter, Coherent, Inc., Santa Clara, CA, US.
    - Zeiss VISULAS 690s laser and VISULINK PDT adapter, Carl Zeiss, Inc., Thornwood, NY, US (**Figs. 67.13A and 67.13B**).
- Adjustable chairs for surgeon and patient
- Viewer projector for selected frame of angiogram
- Visudyne-related supplies:
  - One biohazard container
  - Three syringes (10 ml each)
  - One Y-shaped tubing extension set
  - One filter (1.2 μm)
  - One syringe (30 ml)
  - One D_5W bag (50 ml)
  - Five needles (18–20 gauge)
  - Alcohol wipes
  - One multidose vial of sterile H_2O
  - IV catheters/angiocatheters (18–22 gauge) with Y adapter
  - Extension tubing
  - Gloves
  - One-inch paper or silk tape
  - Visudyne vial
  - IV pump
  - Macula lens (e.g., Volk centralis lens, Mainster macula lens)

Operative Procedure

Visudyne

1. Prepare Visudyne solution
   a. Attach 18-gauge needle to a 10 ml syringe.
   b. Open Visudyne and sterile H_2O vials.
   c. Swab vial tops with alcohol wipe.
   d. Withdraw 7 ml sterile H_2O into the 10 ml syringe.
   e. Empty 7 ml sterile H_2O into the Visudyne vial and agitate solution until it is dissolved.
   f. Leave Visudyne vial attached to the needle and syringe and set aside.
   g. Reconstituted Visudyne (i.e., 7 ml plus caked powder in vial) yields a final volume of 7.5 ml and a concentration of 2 mg/ml.
      i. If stored, reconstituted Visudyne should be protected from light and used within 4 hours.

   Do not store Visudyne vial at temperatures > 77°F.

2. Attach 18-gauge needle to 30 ml syringe and withdraw volume of D_5W from 50 ml bag as determined by previous calculation.
   a. Aspirate air into D_5W-containing syringe to 30 ml mark to accommodate reconstituted Visudyne.
   b. Aspirate needed volume of reconstituted Visudyne solution needed according to previous calculation.

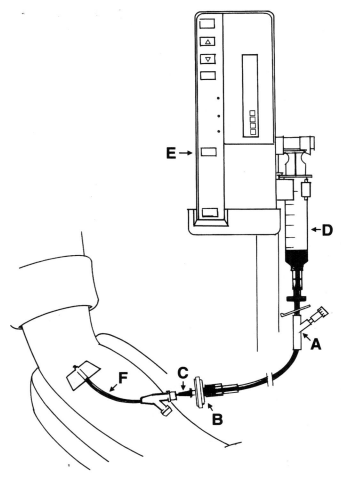

Figure 67.14

Assemble Infusion Apparatus (**Fig. 67.14**).

1. Attach Y-shaped extension set (A) to 30 ml syringe containing Visudyne solution.
2. Attach the 1.2 μm filter (B) to the extension set.
3. Attach an 18 gauge needle (C) to the other end of the 1.2 μm filter.
4. Depress plunger of the 30 ml Visudyne-containing syringe and prime the apparatus.
5. Clamp apparatus after it is primed.
6. Using two 18 gauge needles, fill two 10 ml syringes with 5 ml of D$_5$W solution and label them; these will be used to check that the infusion line is patent (before infusion) and to check that the remaining infusion in the IV tubing is flushed at the end of the infusion.

Infuse Visudyne (**Figs. 67.13A and 67.13B**)

1. Attach 30 ml syringe (D) containing reconstituted Visudyne to infusion pump (E).
2. Set infusion pump to an infusion time of 10 minutes at a rate of 3 ml/minute.
3. Insert 18–22 gauge IV catheter with Y adapter (F) into an arm vein (preferably antecubital; small veins are fragile and increase the likelihood of extravasation).
4. Withdraw needle from angiocath and dispose of it in biohazard sharps container.
5. Swab IV catheter nipple with an alcohol wipe.
6. Insert 18 gauge needle attached to a syringe containing 5 ml D$_5$W into nipple, pull back on plunger, and verify blood return; if there is blood return, flush the line with the D$_5$W solution; discard syringe in the biohazard sharps container.
7. Swab IV catheter nipple with an alcohol wipe and insert 18 gauge needle attached to primed infusion set apparatus.
8. Secure catheter firmly to patient's arm with tape.
9. Unclamp tubing.
10. Switch infusion pump on to start infusion.
11. Immediately activate stopwatch or timer that is set to count down from 15 minutes (preferably, use the internal timer on the laser).
12. At end of infusion, use dextrose flush to inject remaining volume of Visudyne into antecubital vein (A).
13. Remove filter extension set from IV extension set by withdrawing the 18 gauge needle.
14. Leave the IV line in place for 5 minutes after the termination of the infusion.
15. Cautions:
    a. Maintain sterility throughout this entire procedure (from Visudyne reconstitution through Visudyne injection).
    b. Measure volumes precisely (to within 0.1 ml).
    c. Exclude all air from the infusion line.
    d. Take every step possible to prevent extravasation.
    e. Timing should be precise; treatment should start exactly 15 minutes after the start of the IV infusion.
    f. If verteporfin extravasation occurs, stop infusion immediately and apply cold compresses; thoroughly protect area from direct light until swelling and discoloration have faded to prevent a local burn, which can be severe.
    g. If back pain occurs during infusion (reported in 2.2%), have patient stand up to help relieve the pain.
    h. Please read Visudyne package insert for information regarding carcinogenesis, mutagenesis, infertility, possible drug interactions, and reported adverse reactions.

Apply Laser Irradiation to CNV

1. 30 minutes-2 hours before treatment, dilate pupil of eye to be treated.
2. Adjust laser spot to size determined by pretreatment angiogram.
3. Adjust laser for magnification factor of the contact lens used (**Table 67.7**).
    a. Mainster standard lens: 1.05 magnification.
    b. Mainster wide field lens: 1.50 magnification.

Table 67.7 Magnification Factor Associated with Contact Lenses

Description	Lens Type	Lens Manufacturer	Magnification*
V.EQUATOR+	Equator Plus	Volk	2.27×
V.SUPERQUAD	SuperQuad 160	Volk	2.00×
V.QUADRASPH	QuadrAspheric	Volk	2.00×
O.PRP–165	PRP 165	Ocular Instruments	1.96×
O.MAINST-UF	Ultra Field PRP	Ocular Instruments	1.89×
O.MAINST-WF	Mainster Wide Field Laser Lens	Ocular Instruments	1.47×
V.TRANSEQUAT	Trans Equator	Volk	1.44×
O.FUNDUS	Fundus Laser Lens	Ocular Instruments	1.08×
O.YANNUZZI	Yannuzzi Fundus Laser Lens	Ocular Instruments	1.08×
O.3-MIRROR	Three Mirror Universal Laser Lens	Ocular Instruments	1.08×
O.MAINST-STD	Mainster Standard Laser Lens	Ocular Instruments	1.05×
V.AREACENTR	Area Centralis	Volk	0.94×
V.FUNDUS	Fundus	Volk	0.82×
O.MAINST-HM	Mainster High Mag	Ocular Instruments	0.80×

Used with permission from Carl Zeiss Meditec Inc.
* The magnification factor specified refers to the magnification of the laser spot by the contact lens.

4. Test laser function by selecting patient parameters and briefly releasing laser emission on a dummy target; if the laser is malfunctioning, an error code will appear; when test is complete, reset parameters.
5. Approximately 2–5 minutes before laser treatment, insert topical anesthetic drops into eye to be treated.
6. After installation of anesthetic drops, place lens on eye.
7. Bring area to be treated into proper focus.
8. Adjust intensity of illumination beam and aiming beam:
   a. Somewhat less than maximal intensity illumination will facilitate visualization of aiming beam.
   b. Aiming beam can be set to pulse on 50% of the time or constantly remain activated.
9. Memorize landmarks defining boundary of area to be treated by comparing projected angiogram to clinical exam findings.
10. Instruct personnel working in treatment room during laser application to put on laser goggles.
11. Begin laser irradiation of CNV 15 minutes after the start of the infusion; treatment is initiated by activating foot pedal with two rapid depressions and maintaining depressed position after second depression.
12. Laser is preset to deliver light dose of exactly 50 J/cm^2 at an intensity of 600 mW/cm^2 over 83 seconds. Some surgeons feel that a dose of 25 J/cm^2 provides adequate CNV treatment and reduces the chance for PDT-induced severe visual loss and adjust the machine settings accordingly.
13. It may be reassuring to patients to report to them how the treatment is proceeding during the 83-second irradiation.
14. Bilateral treatment:
   a. If neither eye has been treated before, consider treating just one eye at the first treatment (recall that 1–4% of treated patients experience vision loss of 4 lines or more within 7 days of treatment); the second eye can be treated a week later.
   b. If one of the two eyes has been treated previously with no untoward event, then consider treating both eyes at the same visit.
   c. If bilateral treatment is done, consider treating the more severely involved eye first at the 15-minute time point after infusion.
   d. Recalibrate the laser settings, then treat the second eye such that treatment of this eye is completed within 20 minutes of the start of the infusion.
15. After treatment, remove contact lens from the eye and rinse the eye with sterile saline to remove coupling medium.
16. Remove IV line from patient and inspect infusion site.
17. Cover infusion site.

Postoperative Procedure

Avoid exposure of skin or eyes to direct sunlight, bright indoor light, tanning salons, lighting in dentist's office or operating room, or exposure to halogen lighting for 5 days after Visudyne. Draw curtains or shades to block direct sunlight. Watching TV or going to the movies is fine as long as skin and eye protection is maintained appropriately.

1. The patient that goes outdoors during first 5 days after Visudyne treatment, should wear long-sleeved shirt and slacks (preferably tight-knit light colored fabrics), gloves, socks and shoes, sunglasses, wide-brimmed hat.
2. Sun block will not prevent burns, as visible light can photoactivate residual drug in the skin. Visudyne patients should wear sunglasses after treatment (upon leaving the doctor's office), and patients should wear the glasses whenever in direct sunlight or bright light for 5 days after Visudyne treatment.

3. Advise patient not to stay in dark after treatment; exposure to ambient indoor light will help inactivate the drug (photobleaching).
4. Some physicians instruct office staff to call the patient 2–4 days after Visudyne treatment to monitor the patient.
5. Schedule next follow-up appointment in 3 months, but immediately if the patient notices decreased vision or a problem at the infusion site.
6. AMD patients should be evaluated approximately every 3 months. If fluorescein leakage from the CNV is documented, then one should consider repeating the therapy provided that there has been no untoward reaction to treatment previously.
   a. The spot size for re-treatment includes the GLD of any area of leakage from CNV and contiguous hypofluorescence due to blood or hyperfluorescence due to a serous PED plus 1000 µm. Contiguous hypofluorescence not from blood (even if elevated) or hyperfluorescent staining of fibrous tissue is not included in the area to re-treat.
7. Instruct patient to contact you if there are any questions or problems.
8. Instruct patient to bring sunglasses and long-sleeved shirt for all follow-up visits.
9. Place wrist band which indicates that patient has just been treated with verteporfin.
10. Give patient wallet card.
11. If emergency surgery is necessary within 48 hours after treatment, as much of the internal tissue as possible should be protected from intense light.

68

Intravitreal Injection of Antivascular Endothelial Growth Factor Agents for Choroidal Neovascularization

Indications

Currently, intravitreal ranibizumab (Lucentis) injection (with or without associated verteporfin photodynamic therapy (PDT)) has provided the best visual results reported for treatment of subfoveal choroidal new vessels (CNVs) in patients with age-related macular degeneration (AMD). (Nonrandomized case series also indicate a benefit for treatment of myopia-associated CNVs and AMD using bevacizumab [Avastin].) Intravitreal ranibizumab has been proved to be effective in randomized clinical trials (including active controls with randomization to verteporfin PDT for patients with predominantly classic CNVs) regardless of lesion type (classic, occult, mixed), and presenting visual acuity. Overall, 90–95% patients experience less than 15 letters visual loss on the Bailey-Lovie visual acuity chart and 25–40% of patients experience moderate visual improvement when patients receive monthly intravitreal injections during the course of 1 year.

Preoperative Procedure

Complete retinal examination including stereoscopic contact lens examination of the macula. Fluorescein angiography and optical coherence tomography are done to document (or diagnose) presence of subfoveal CNV as well as amount of subretinal fluid present.

Instrumentation

- Sterile gloves
- Sterile lid speculum
- 2 Betadine swabs
- Topical proparacaine (fresh bottle)
- Lidocaine 1% without epinephrine (optional)
- Proparacaine-soaked pledget (optional)
- Lidocaine gel (optional)

- Topical antibiotic (e.g., moxifloxacin hydrochloride; be sure to inquire regarding drug allergies)
- Tuberculin syringe
- Sterile 30 gauge needle (½ inch)
- Becton Dickinson filter needle with 5 μm filter; 19 gauge, 11/2 inches (BD #305200); included in the vial box of Lucentis
- 1 bottle of Lucentis
- 1 package sterile cotton-tipped swabs
- 1 sterile alcohol wipe

Operative Procedure

1. Put on sterile gloves.
2. Place drop of sterile proparacaine in eye.
3. Place lid speculum.
4. Inject 0.3 ml of subconjunctival lidocaine at the clock hour of anticipated injection (optional) or apply proparacaine-soaked pledget against anticipated location of intravitreal injection (optional) or apply lidocaine HCl jelly 2% USP (optional).
5. Express Betadine onto ocular surface; use swab to wipe eyelid margins and, especially, eyelashes with Betadine; let Betadine dry, then repeat.
6. Withdraw Lucentis into tuberculin syringe using 19 gauge filter needle provided by Genentech.
7. Remove 19 gauge filter needle and attach sterile ⅝-inch 30 gauge needle to Lucentis-containing syringe.
8. Express all but 0.05 ml (0.5 mg) of Lucentis from tuberculin syringe.
9. *Optional:* Position patient at slit lamp.
10. Inject Lucentis entering 4 mm (phakic eye) or 3 mm (aphakic or pseudophakic eye) posterior to the limbus near 8:30 o'clock (right eye) or 3:30 o'clock (left eye). Withdraw needle from eye after ~10 seconds.
11. Tamponade injection site with sterile cotton-tipped swab.
12. Dress eye with topical antibiotic drops.

13. Remove lid speculum.
14. Wipe lid margin and lashes with sterile alcohol wipe to remove Betadine from skin.

Postoperative Procedure

1. Use topical antibiotic drop in injected eye every hour while awake. Some retina specialists recommend a regimen of 1 drop 4 times per day for 3 days after the injection. (Instruct patient to wash hands before placing drop in eye.) If patient uses eye drops for another indication (e.g., anti-glaucoma drops), instruct patient to use a fresh bottle in operative eye.
2. Follow-up exam within 1 week to identify complications (e.g., endophthalmitis, retinal tear, retinal detachment, vitreous hemorrhage), but follow up sooner if there is worsening vision, increasing floaters, or increasing pain in the eye.

Note: Some retina specialists have a technician do the follow-up exam or conduct follow-up assessment by phone interview or do not follow-up until the next scheduled time for injection unless there is a change in symptoms.

Complications

1. Traumatic cataract.
2. Retinal tear.
3. Retinal detachment.
4. Endophthalmitis.
5. Systemic: In three completed randomized studies, there was no statistically significant increased risk of stroke or heart attack associated with Lucentis injection.

Index